PRACTICAL ATLAS OF NUTRITION

AND FEEDING IN CATS AND DOGS

VOLUME II

Roberto Elices Mínguez

PhD in Veterinary Medicine by the Universidad Complutense de Madrid (UCM).

Professor of Production and Companion Animal Nutrition.

Veterinarian in the Small Animal Medicine Department (Endocrinology and Obesity) of the Veterinary Teaching Hospital of the School of Veterinary Medicine of Madrid (UCM).

Small animal veterinarian—medicine and surgery—in private clinics.

For this English edition:

Practical atlas of nutrition and feeding in cats and dogs. Volume II

Plaza Antonio Beltrán Martínez nº 1, planta 8 - letra I
(Centro empresarial El Trovador)
50002 Zaragoza - Spain

First printing: March 2017

This book has been published originally in Spanish under the title:
Atlas de nutrición y alimentación práctica en perros y gatos. Volumen II
© 2011 Grupo Asís Biomedia, S.L.
ISBN Spanish edition: 978-84-92569-57-1

Translation:
Anna Frandsen

ISBN: 978-84-16818-51-8
D.L.: Z 400-2017

Design, layout and printing:
Servet editorial - Grupo Asís Biomedia, S.L.
www.grupoasis.com
info@grupoasis.com

Servet is the publishing house of Grupo Asís

To my parents, family, and pets

Acknowledgments

To my right hand, Mercedes Morán Cuesta, for sharing her time. Thank you Mer, without your help and efforts, this would not have been possible.

To Silvia Miguélez for her collaboration in reviewing this publication.

To my colleague at the HCV, Dr. Lola Pérez Alenza, for her advice.

To my dear friends, Cristina Ortiz Díez de Tortosa, Mar Sanz Luengo, and Carmen Muñoz Serrano from the Library of the School of Veterinary Medicine of Madrid (UCM). Without your work and affection, collecting the bibliography would have been impossible.

To the editing and design team at Servet Publishing House, especially to Tatiana Blasco, for all of the hours shared sending emails back and forth, and to Javier Nuviala. I send my congratulations to the graphic designers for their magnificent work.

To all my friends, but especially to Carlos Recio, Raúl González Burguillo and Pablo Mantilla.

Wherever you are resting, to my best *four-legged friend*, Ramón, for your nearly fourteen years of selfless affection.

Prologue

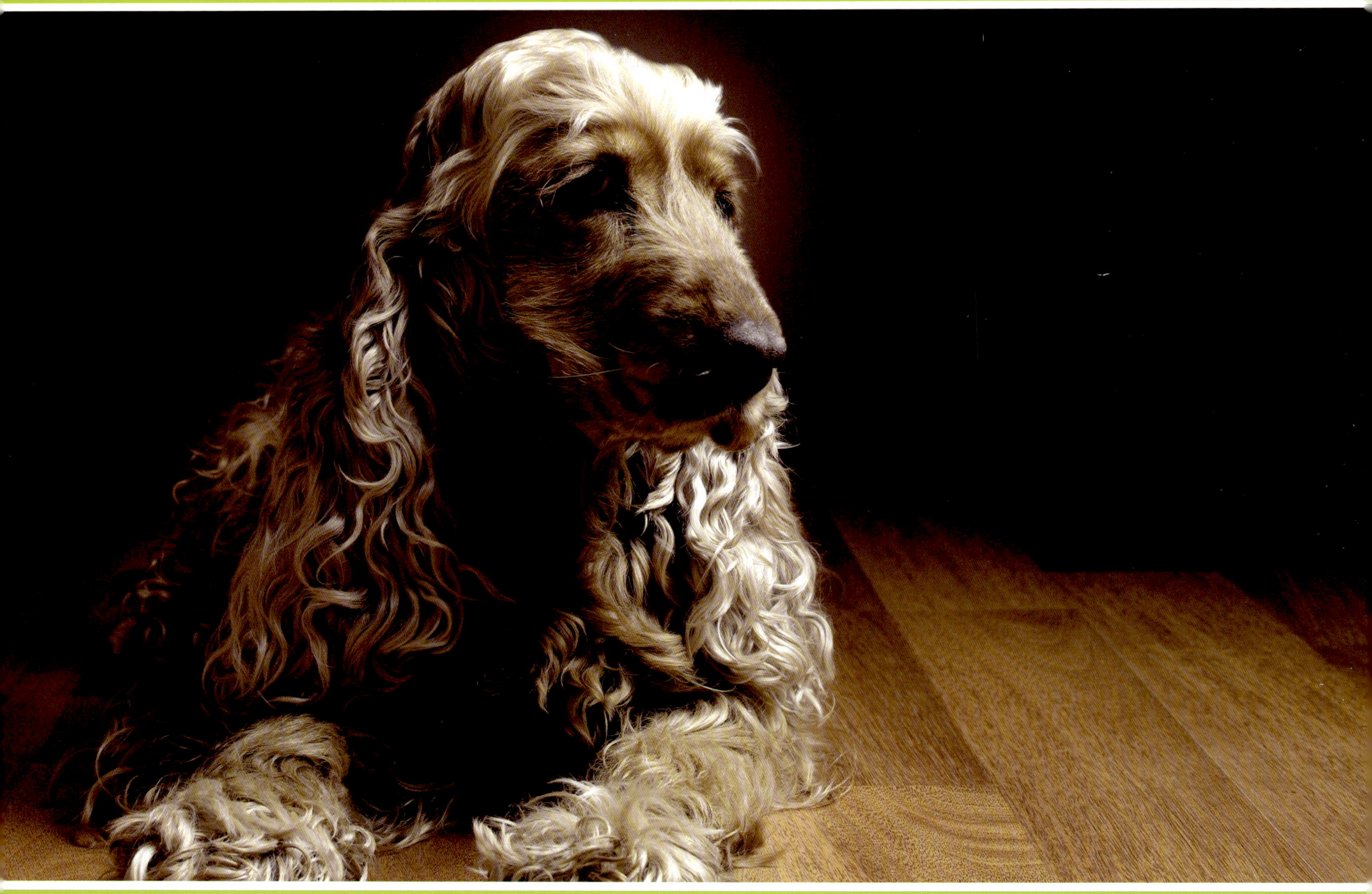

Once again we have taken on the demanding task of transforming dog and cat nutrition into images, and, although we now have the experience of creating the first volume, this was still a great challenge.

This time, the different graphic layouts in which the theoretical and practical content has been expressed are structured by sections in the index and according to the physiological states described, making them easier to find. In other respects, the spirit of this publication is the same that we poured into the first volume; that is, to accompany the text with images, drawings, diagrams, and other graphic elements to make reading and learning pet nutrition easier. Once again, our greatest wish is that the reader feels that we have met these objectives.

We would like to thank the author, Roberto Elices, who has embraced this project and allowed us to transform his experience and knowledge into this atlas, and we would also like to thank the members of the creative department who once again knew how to use their ingenuity and knowledge to visually express the content.

We hope that you enjoy your reading.

EDITORIAL SERVET
[SERVET PUBLISHING HOUSE]

Preface

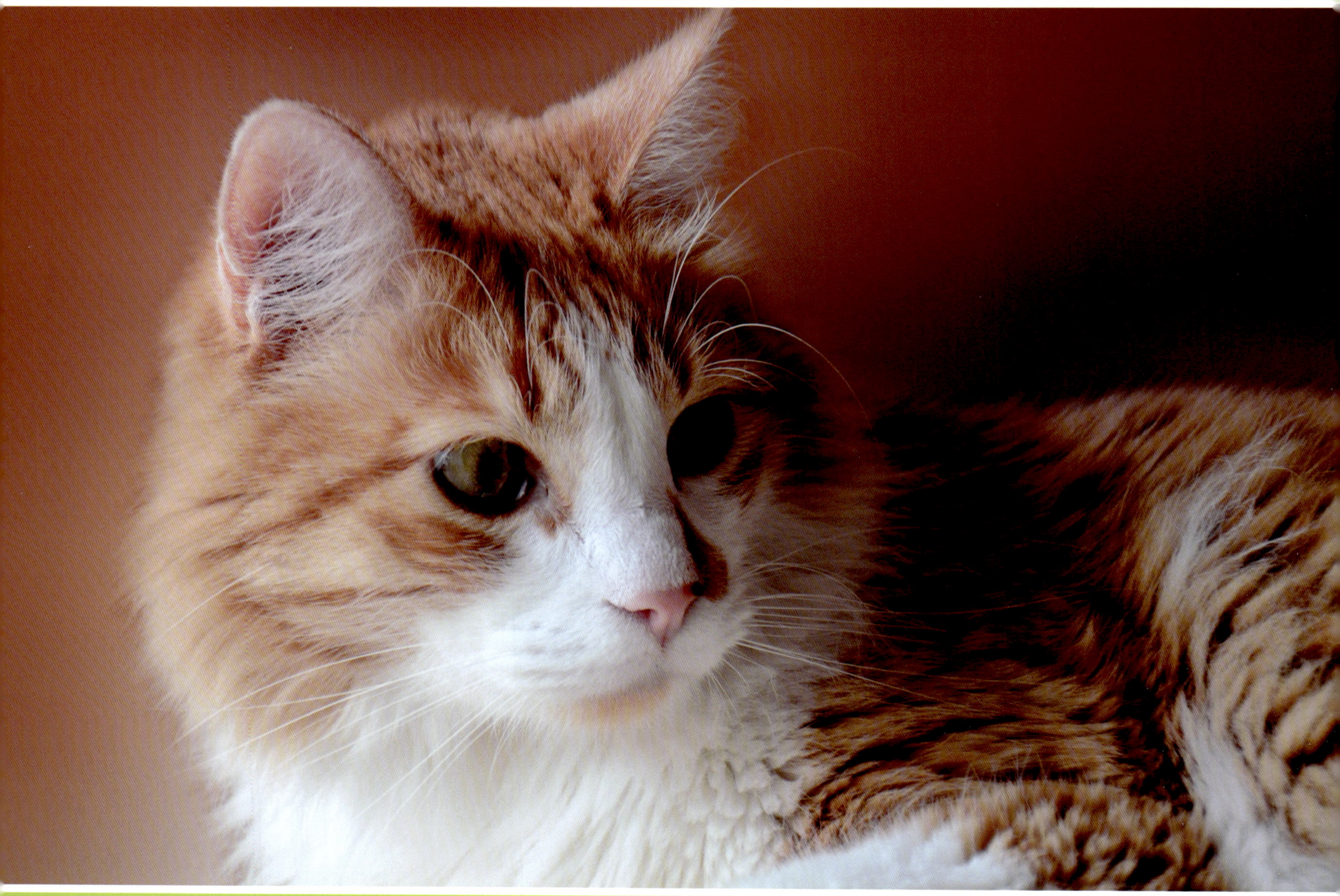

The first references on pet nutrition are from the 1920s. Specific publications started to appear around the mid 1990s. In spite of this, its presence in veterinary medicine publications was really scarce.

Just over a year ago, Servet publishing company contacted us and offered us the possibility of creating a publication on nutrition that would be different from any existing publication. The first volume of this project was created during that period. We had to start somewhere and decided that the contents provided in Volume I should cover the recommendations on the nutrition and feeding of adult dogs and cats in maintenance. That is exactly what we did. The different physiological states were left for future publications. With this volume that we hereby present to you, we hope to once again meet the goals with which this project was created.

We would like to thank our colleagues from the library of the Veterinary School of the UCM and the entire team from Servet Publishing House for the great efforts they made to create this new book.

Our wish is that reading this book offers a new perception on how we can help to achieve the greatest well-being in our pets.

Roberto Elices Mínguez
Madrid, May 2011

Index

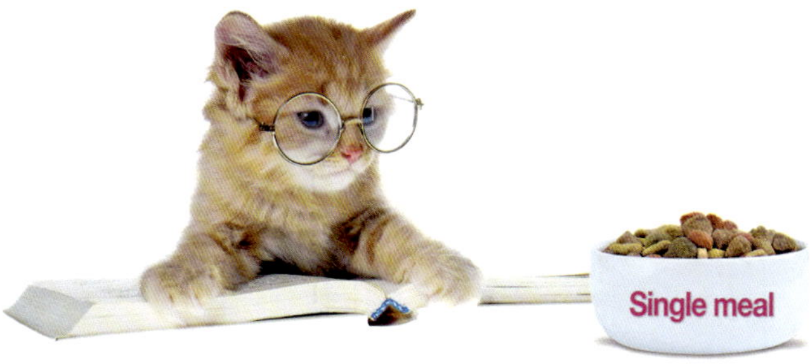

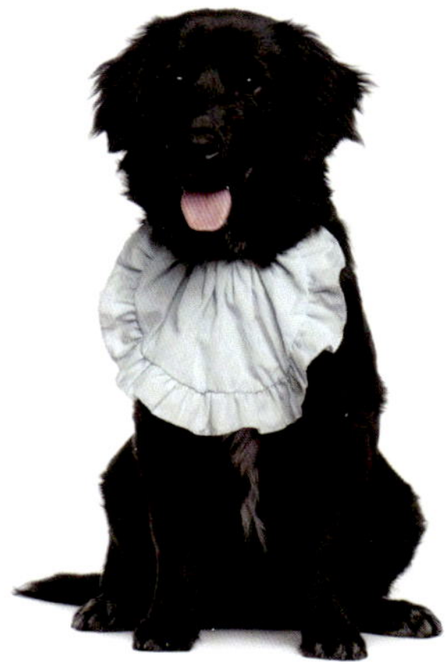

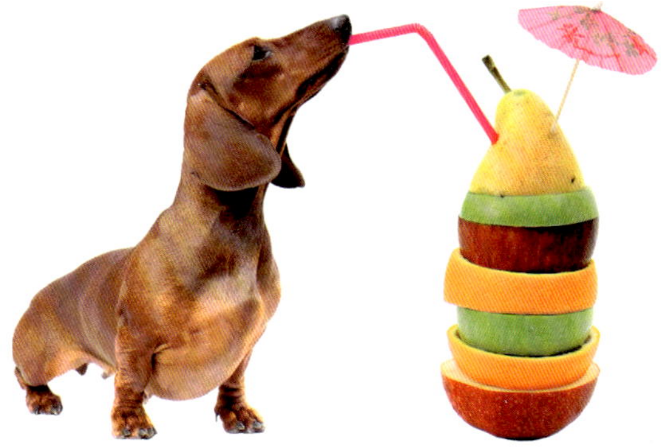

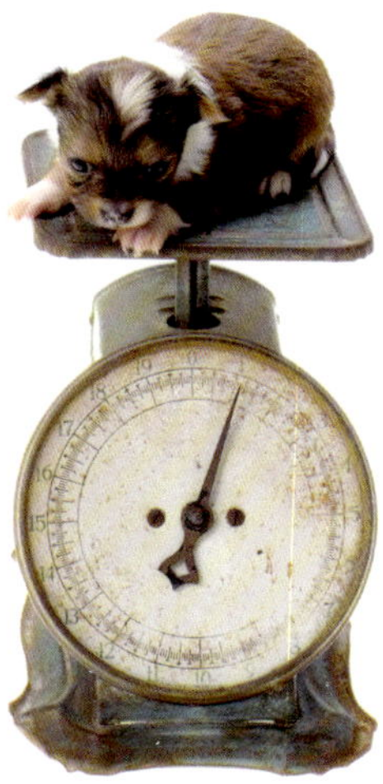
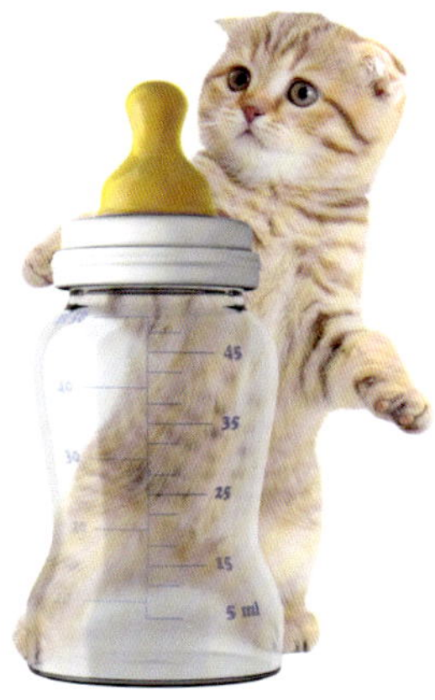
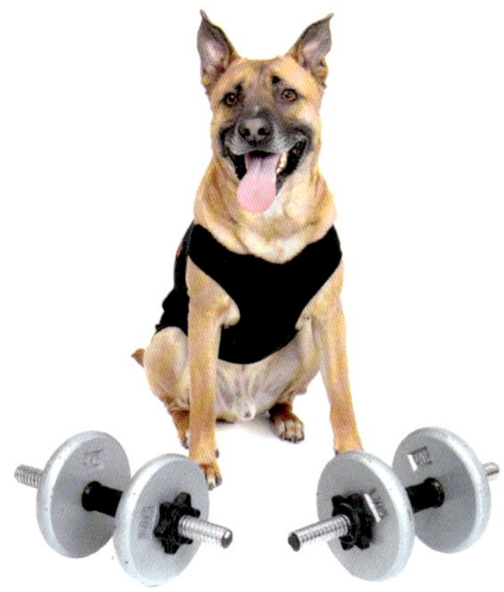
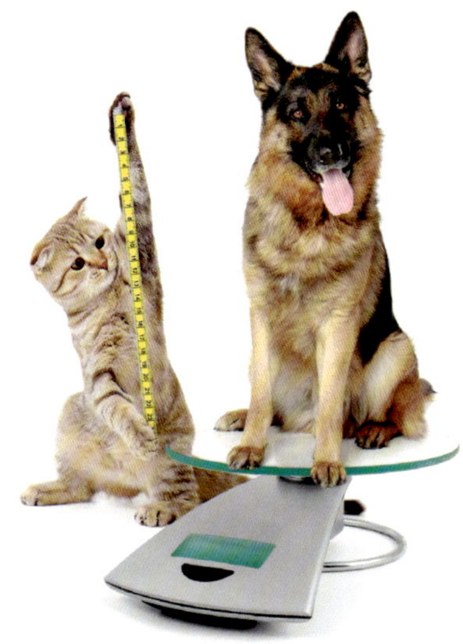

Feeding geriatric animals

Feeding sporting and working dogs

How should we

Are they being fed correctly?

✔ We often wonder in our clinical practice if pet owners are feeding their pets correctly. The causes of extreme thinness or obesity may be due to poor adjustment between the energy requirements (ER) and the food ration (R) or to incorrectly providing it.

✔ The pet's feeding regime, any possible changes to said regime, and the pet's environment (vacation periods in open areas, presence of other pets, elderly people, or children, the owner's health, etc.), should be reflected in the animal's medical records. Various factors can affect the frequency and quantity of food offered.

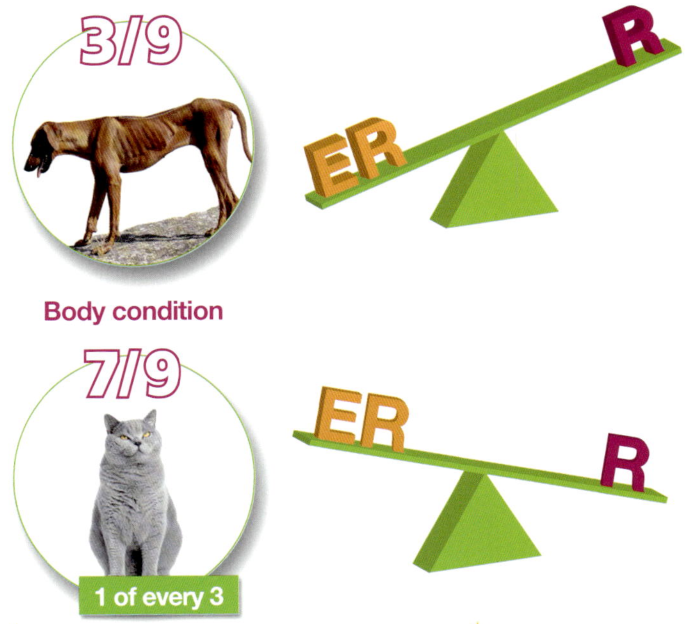

Feeding methods

✔ Studies show that most dog owners feed their dogs once daily (25-75 %), and the proportion that feeds them twice daily (<50 %) or three times per day is less, with the last option only present in the first year of the animal's life.

✔ We can distinguish three alternatives for feeding healthy animals. Each feeding regimen has its advantages and disadvantages.

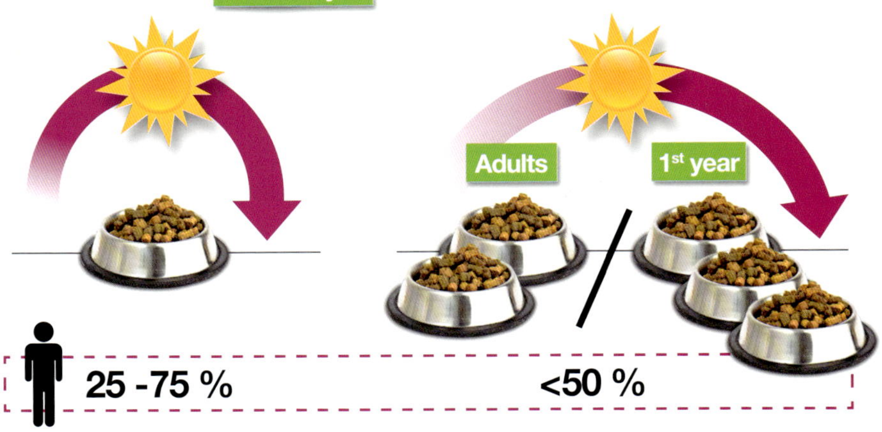

1 Free feeding (ad libitum)

✔ This consists of leaving a large amount of food permanently available to the pet. Special feeders of different sizes are generally used from 1.5 to 40 kg.

✔ There is one variation that is used especially with cats: food is released into the dish as it is consumed.

✔ Dry food is usually used in these cases. Using this feeding technique with wet foods has three main problems:

- Poor acceptance due to loss of freshness.
- Difficulty cleaning the dish.
- Microbial contamination of the food due its high water content.

✔ This type of feeding is frequent in animals that live in rural environments (working or hunting animals), shelters or adoption centers, and in homes with yards.

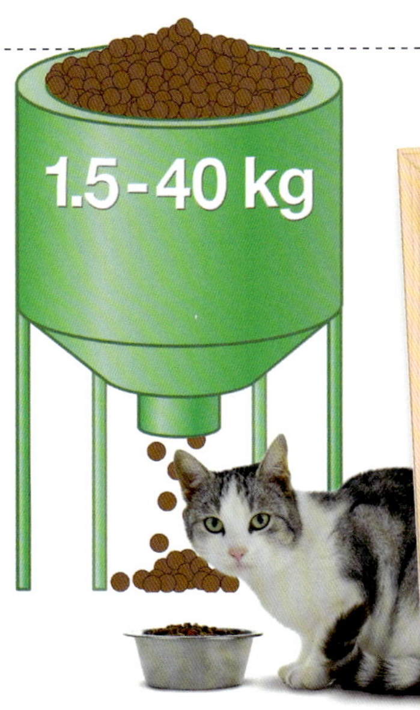

ADVANTAGES

✔ No continuous work is required nor special skills from the feeder.

✔ Problems of under-feeding and aggressiveness from dominance are avoided in large dog pounds, keeping the animals calmer.

DISADVANTAGES

✘ Less control over the animals' state of health.

✘ Less control over the ingestion of the food and its acceptance.

✘ Predisposition to obesity and vomiting due to excessive volume of food in the stomach.

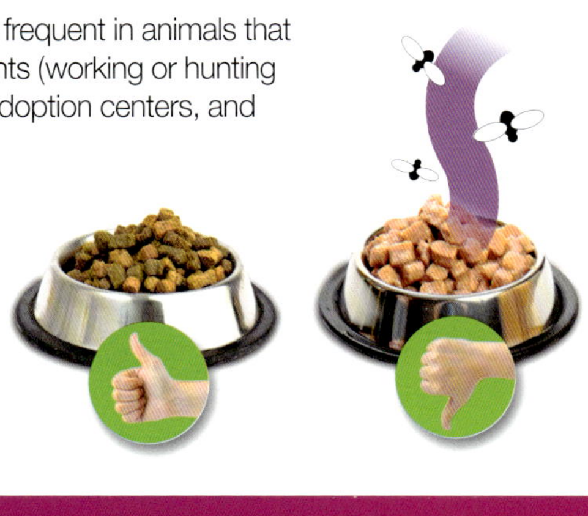

feed our pets?

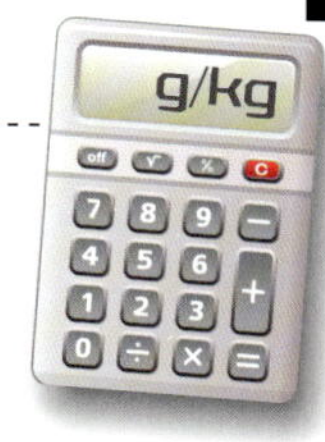

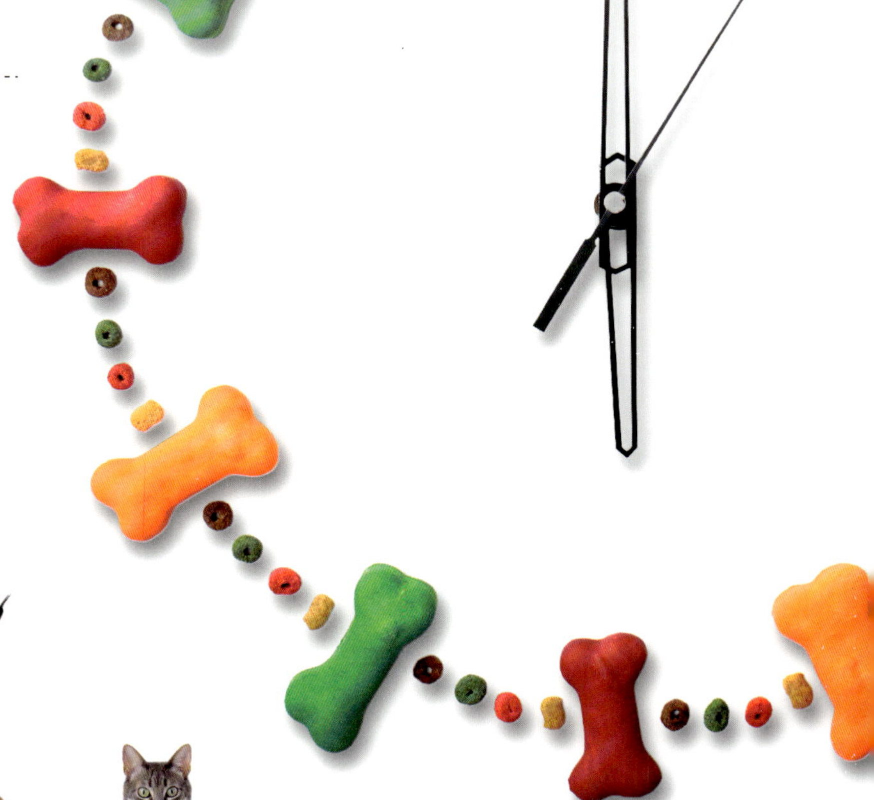

2 Restricted free feeding

- ✔ The daily ration is calculated for the pet's requirements and provided in a continuous manner in the feeder until it is completely consumed. This is likely the most widely used method for dogs and cats.
- ✔ It is the first choice system for cats as it is similar to their natural feeding patterns: several times per day in small amounts regardless of circadian rhythms.

ADVANTAGES AND DISADVANTAGES

- ✔ This ensures stricter control over the dose of food, the animals' appetite and their variations in weight and body condition.
- ✘ It requires a certain amount of attention and precision when preparing the food ration.
- ✘ The owner must dedicate time to this task.

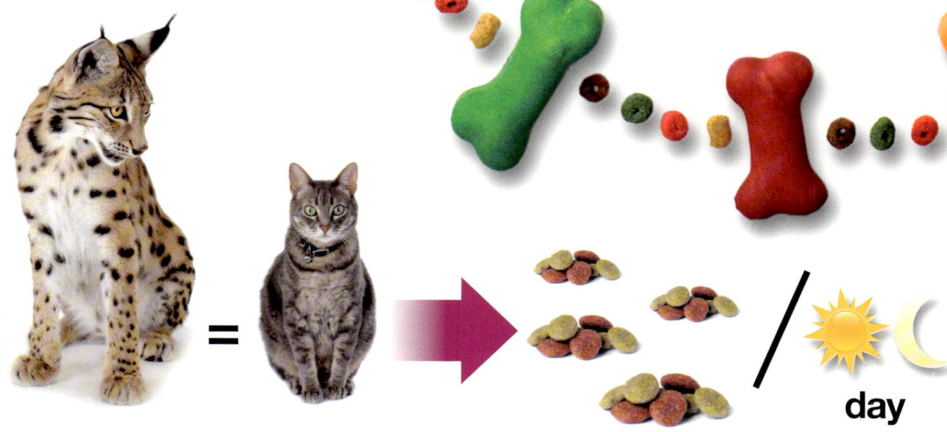

3 Fixed-schedule controlled feeding

- ✔ This is the most complex system of all. It requires the greatest responsibility, but it also achieves a greater bond between the owner and the pet.
- ✔ This is the ideal system. It is recommended for all pets on a treatment involving the use of dietary foods.
- ✔ Putting this method into practice from early ages is the best option, as if it were ever necessary in the future, the dog or cat would already be used to this regime (for example, diabetic patients or those predisposed to gastric dilation).
- ✔ This method is based on dividing the animal's total daily ration into two, or preferably three feedings with a limited time access of 10-20 minutes, and up to 1 or 2 hours in the case of some cats. The pet is called beforehand and the same location is always used for feeding (patio, kitchen, washroom...). After the aforementioned time, the food dish is removed and no more food is given until the next feeding.

ADVANTAGES AND DISADVANTAGES

- ✔ Correct management of the daily dose.
- ✔ Control of the appetite and the state of health.
- ✔ Prevention of weight gain.
- ✘ It requires a little more time, dedication, and habit changes from the owners.

- ✔ Any remaining food will not be given in the next feedings, with a few exceptions: some dogs and cats do not eat the same amount at each feeding and in this case, we can reduce the amount of food for the morning feeding and increase it equally in the other two feedings (for example, 40:40:20).

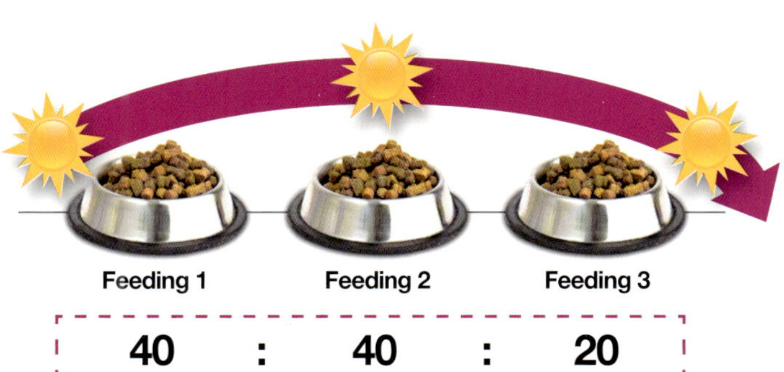

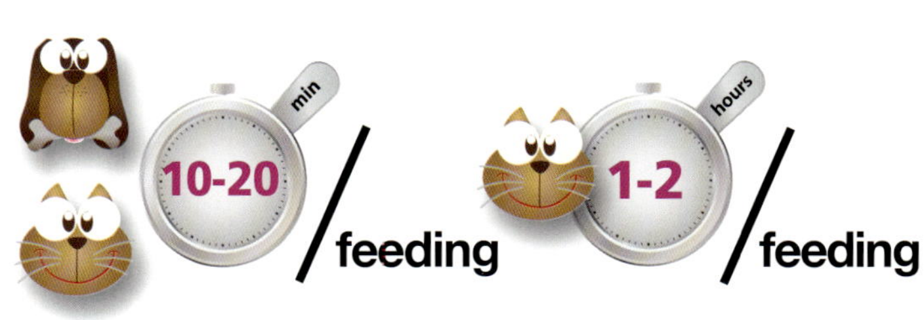

- ✔ For this type of feeding, we can combine dry and wet foods to find the greatest acceptance by the patient.

Learning

1 Guidelines for correct feeding

Except with free-choice feeding, a series of guidelines should be followed with all feeding systems:

- **Pets should be taught to eat:** from a very early age, cats and dogs develop a preference or aversion for certain types of food. In the same way, they will also prefer certain tastes and smells. Knowing and making the most of these preferences will thus allow us to correctly manage their diet.
- **Always in the same place:** pets should have a set place to eat.
- **In a quiet environment:** in order to avoid aggressive behavior or competition, every pet should be given a quiet area where to eat.
- **No pressure from the owners:** owners should not watch their pets eat or encourage them to eat.

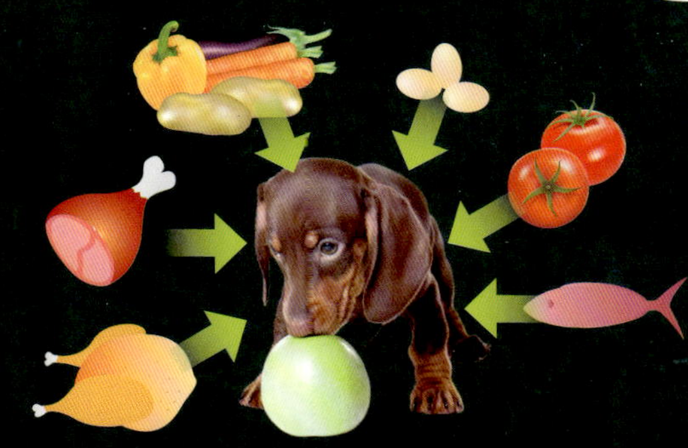

- **All pets should have their own bowl.**

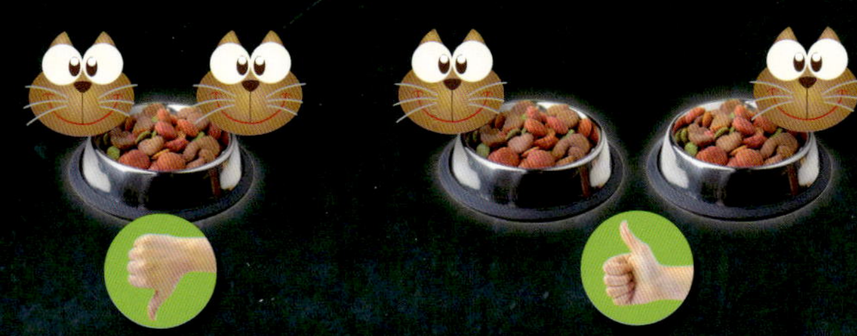

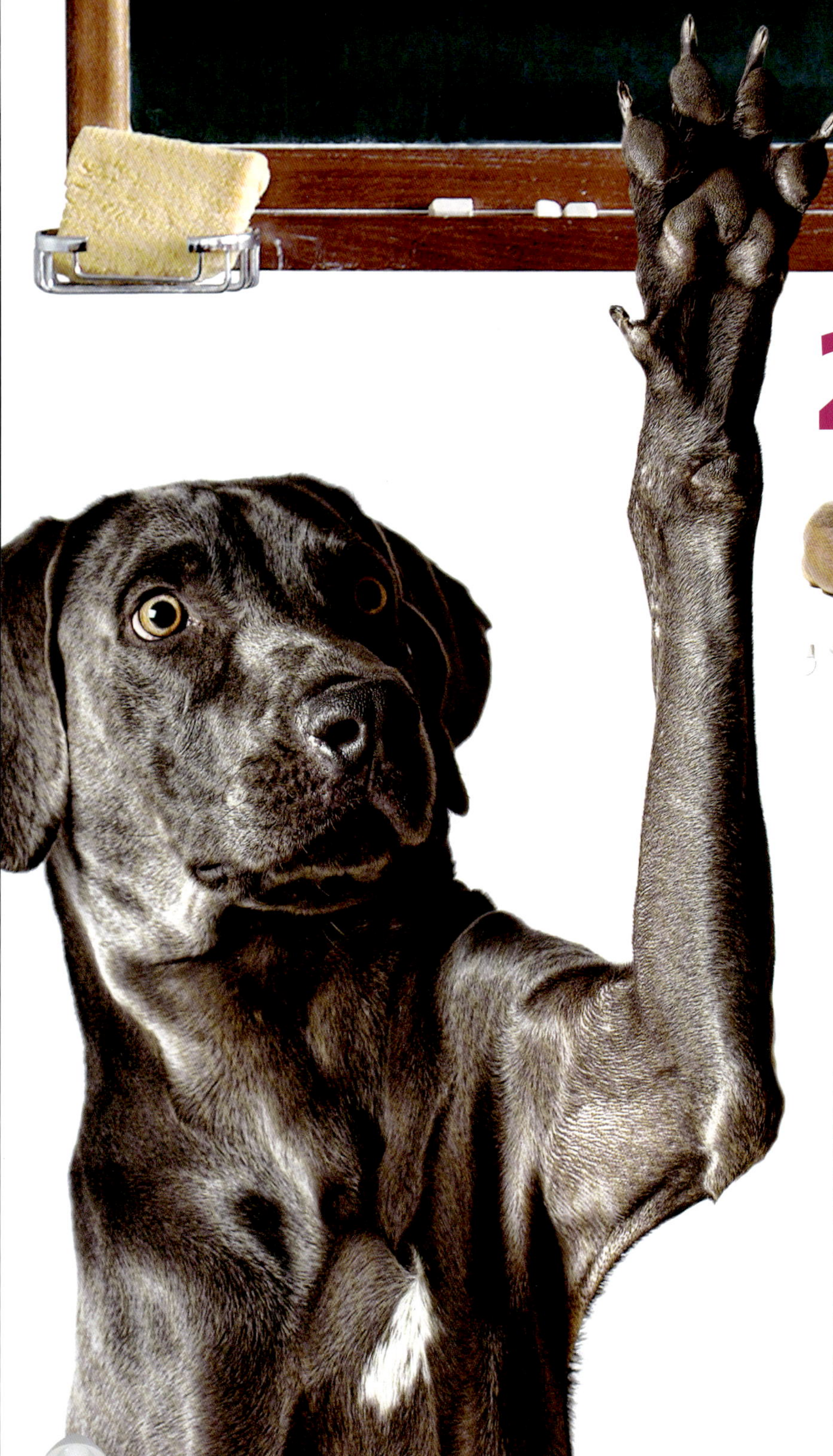

2 Appetite disorders: picky eaters

Our patients are sometimes reluctant to eat certain types of food. Three usual situations are:

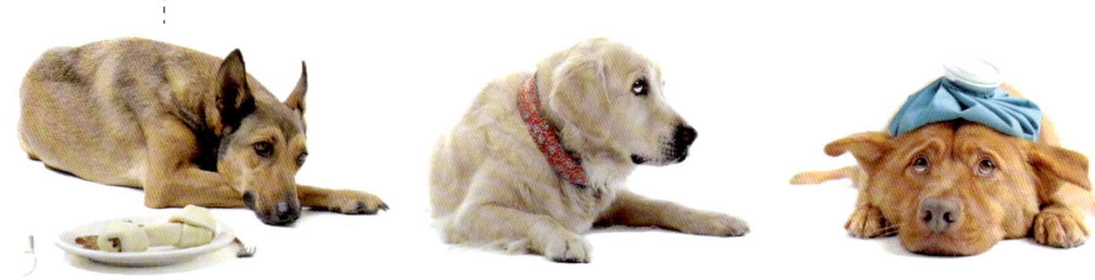

Picky eaters — Senior patients — Sick animals

In the case of old or sick animals it is usually due to a loss of the senses of taste and smell and/or to anorexia-inducing metabolic disorders (because of the disease itself or the treatments used).

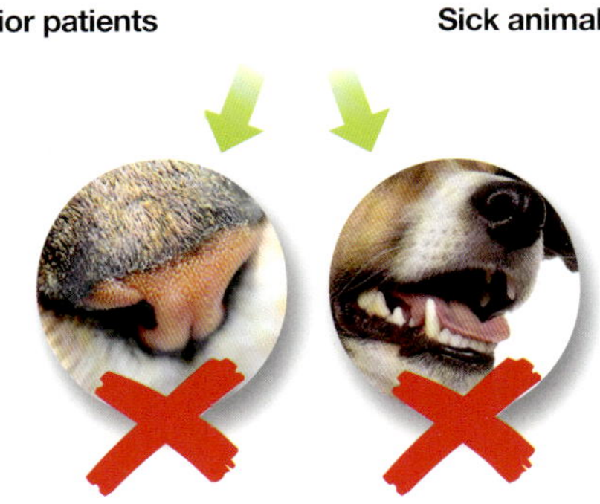

Anorexia

Complete loss of appetite before eating.

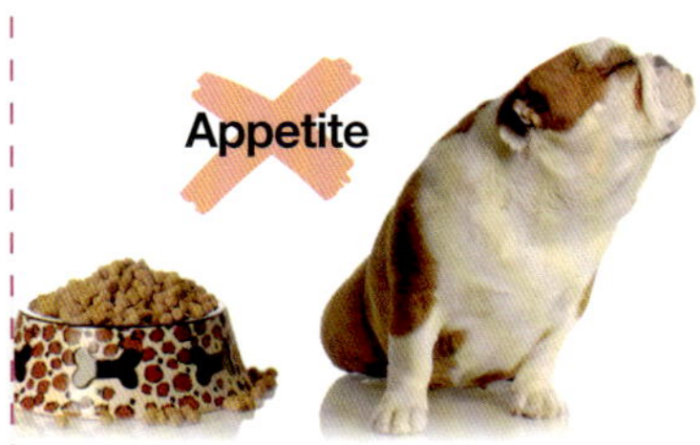

Hyporexia

Decreased appetite for all or certain types of food.

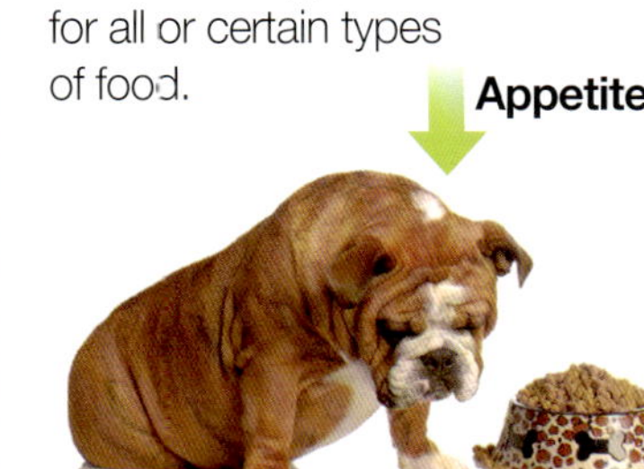

to eat

✔ **With a feeding time protocol:** Cats and dogs should not be fed large meals at the end of the day or immediately after exercising (they should be fed at least an hour after moderate/intense physical activity).

✔ **They should be given a 2-hour rest period after each meal.** Most of the digestive process in the stomach will have taken place by the end of that period. This is an important guideline in cats and dogs with a predisposition to suffer from gastric dilatation-volvulus.

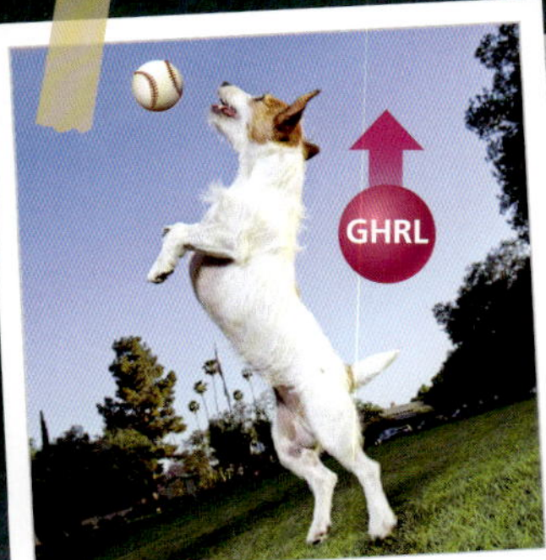

Ghrelin is released when exercising, which increases appetite

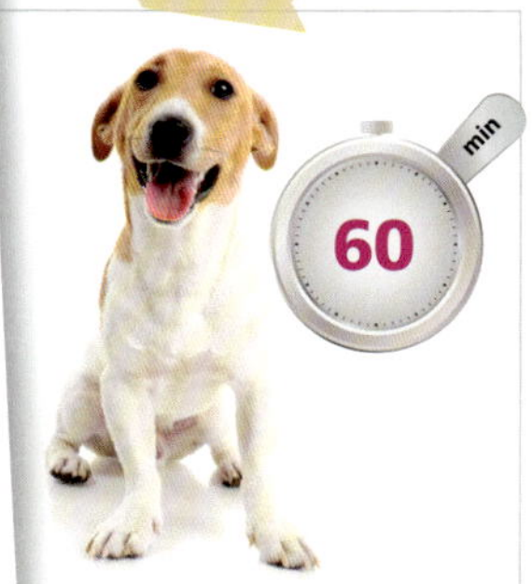

Wait after intense physical exercise

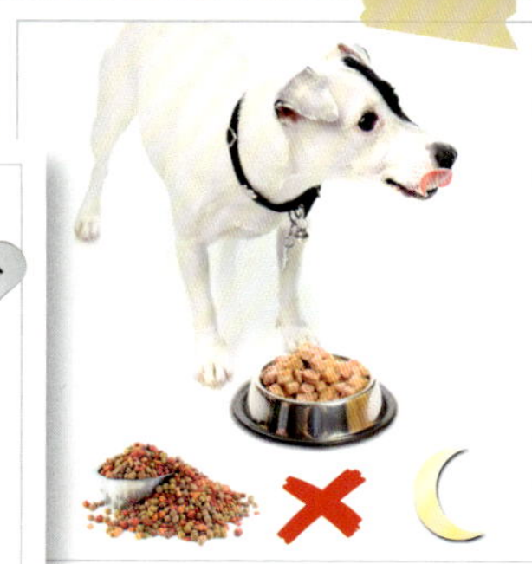

Avoid large meals at the end of the day

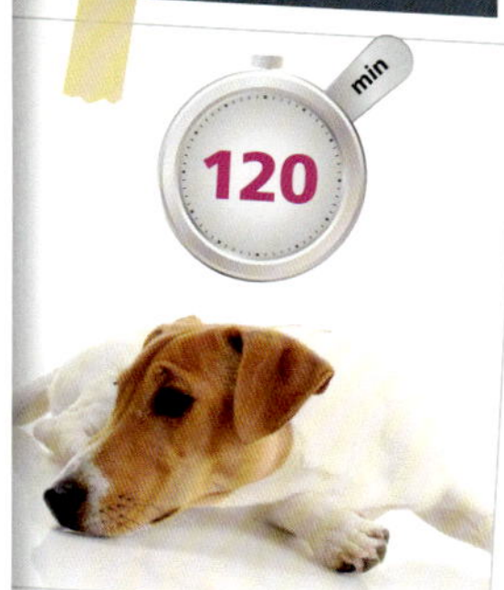

Resting after meals

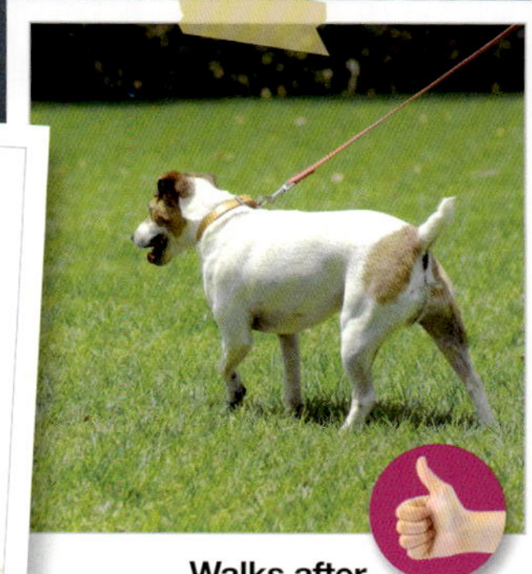

Walks after meals aid digestion

3 Teaching them how and when to eat

✔ **Self-control:** one of the most common mistakes when training a pet, especially a dog, is the lack of discipline and self-control. Training should start before three months of age, to be completed progressively until adult age. Pets must be taught how and when to eat so they can control their desire to eat and not feel frustrated when they are not given any food.

✔ **Training their senses:** with a conditioning process, their senses of taste and smell can be trained to ensure they accept a wide variety of flavors, textures and smells.

✔ **Do not give in:** when pets refuse to eat a complete and balanced diet, we should not be tempted to give them a more appetising type of food, as this is how they will turn into picky eaters.

Many of these pets usually have a dominant behavior at the veterinary clinic, making consultations and procedures more complicated (sometimes risky).

In these cases, there is a hierarchy problem. Although the owner should not be blamed for this behavior, both the pet and the owner will need to be retrained. Healthy animals with a picky appetite will eventually eat the food they are given if managed with common sense.

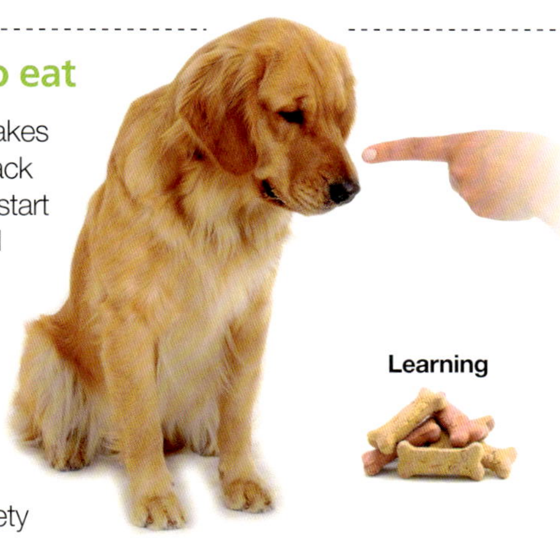

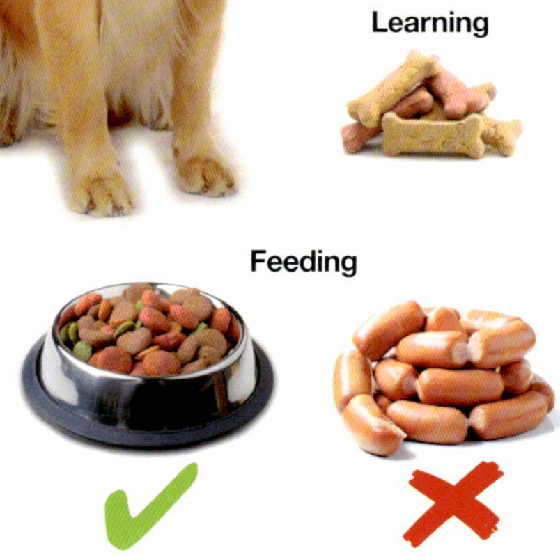

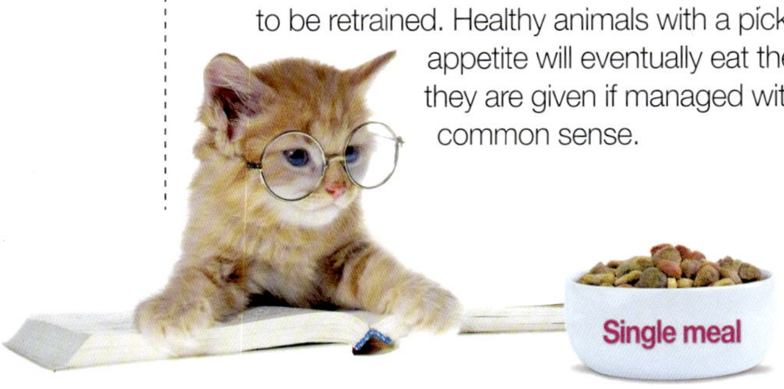

✔ **Cats are the exception to this rule:** they can refuse to eat for long periods of time if the food is not palatable. In this case, it is necessary to study the cause of this refusal. They should not be left more than three days without eating: the effects of fasting on the organism can be lethal (hepatic lipidosis possibly due to the mobilization of fat and the lack of protein to synthesize lipoproteins).

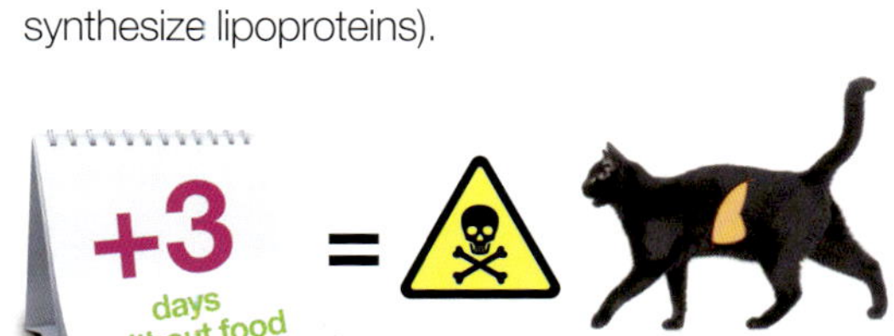

Hepatic lipidosis

✔ **Training tool:** food should be used as a reward for something done but never as a gift. The point is not to limit their access to food but to adjust it. That is why it is important to give them access to food at a set time and for a set period of time (e.g., at 8:00 am for 10 minutes).

Factors involved in appetite loss

The picky appetite of some pets is mainly conditioned by the following factors:

- ✔ Lack of knowledge of the stages of taste development.
- ✔ Poor habits of the owners.
- ✔ Preference or aversion for certain smells or tastes.
- ✔ Moving house or stressful situations.
- ✔ Poor palatability/acceptance of the diet fed.
- ✔ Aging.
- ✔ Diseases and drugs for their treatment.

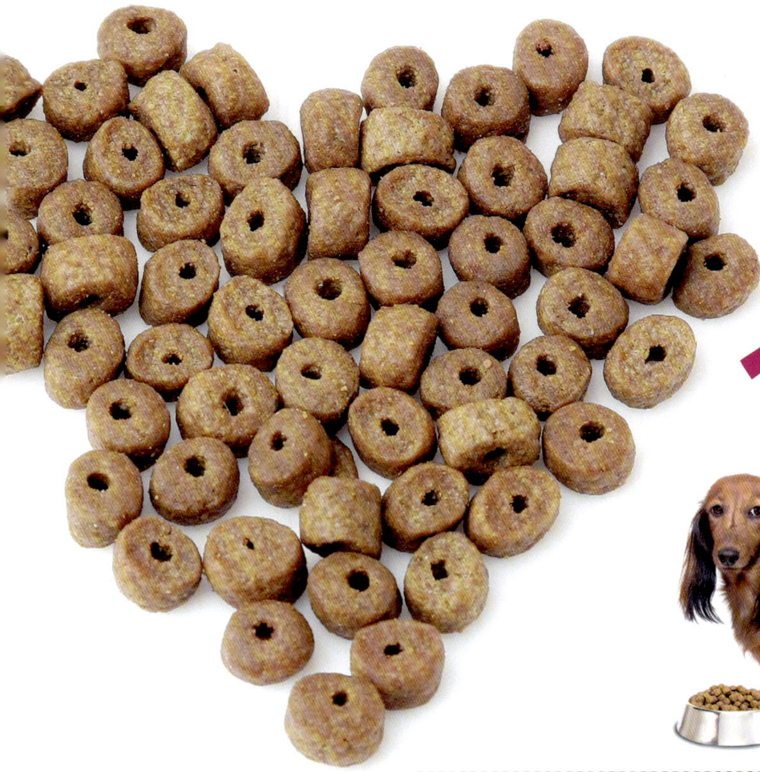

Strategies to

1 Learned behavior

- ✔ Dogs and cats, just like most mammals, receive food from their mothers during the first stages of their lives according to their needs and wishes. However, as they grow, this changes and the animals must start to ingest the same food that their mothers eat. Early separation from the mother sets back this learning.

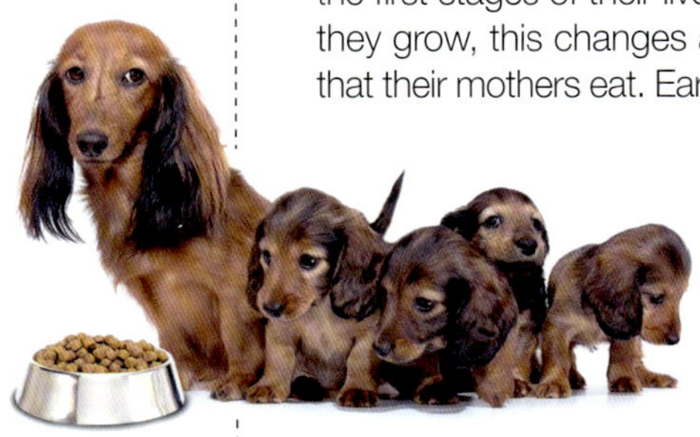

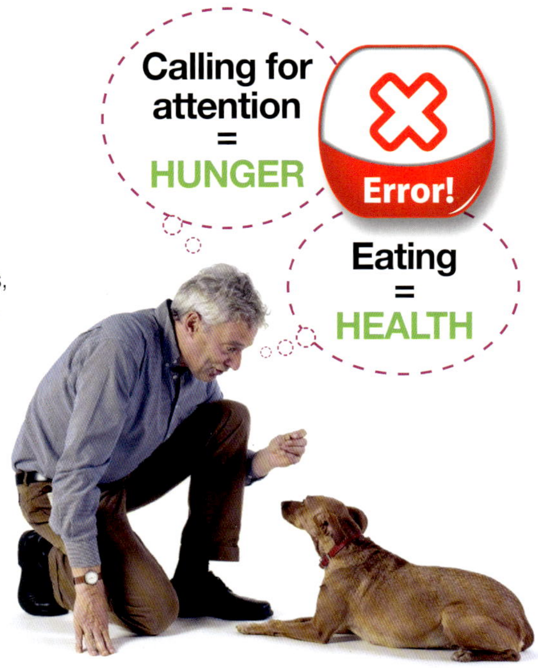
Calling for attention = HUNGER
Error!
Eating = HEALTH

- ✔ Sometimes owners misinterpret the signs of a puppy or a kitten calling for attention as them wanting food. During this entire process, there will be a change and a selection of the palatability of the foods according to the pet's preferences.

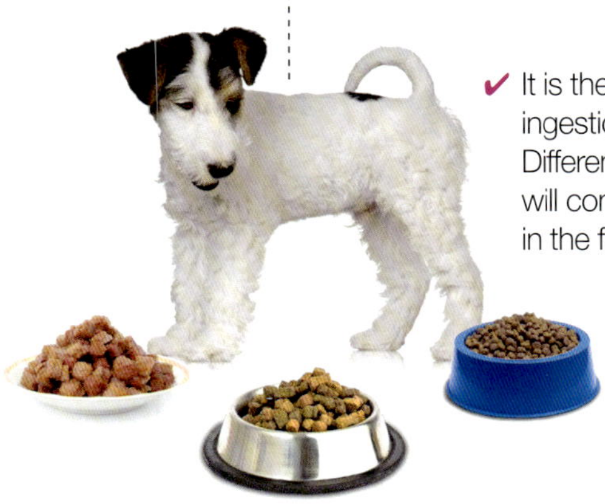

- ✔ It is therefore very important to stimulate an animal's ingestion of different foods from a young age. Different experiences with flavors and textures will condition the acceptance or rejection of foods in the future.

2 Food monotony

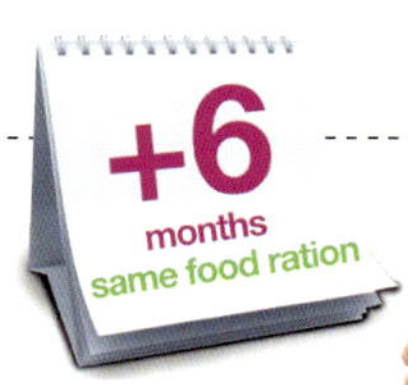
+6
months
same food ration

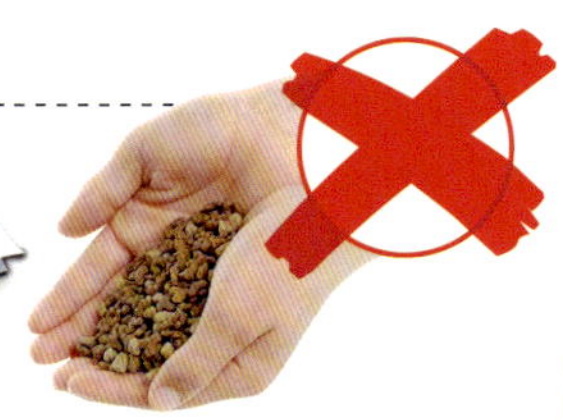

- ✔ It is likely that young animals who have been given the same ration for a period longer than six months will reject a change to their diet.

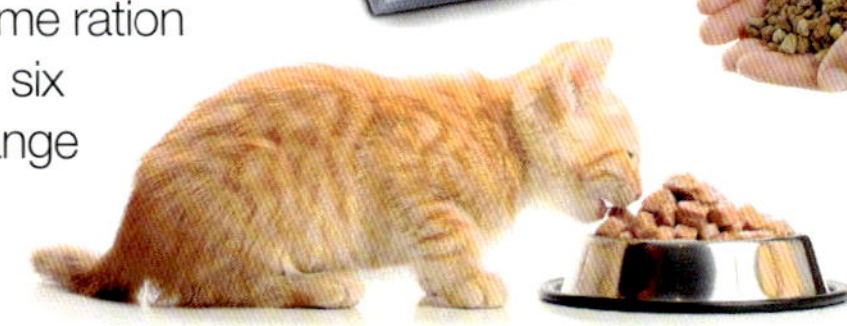

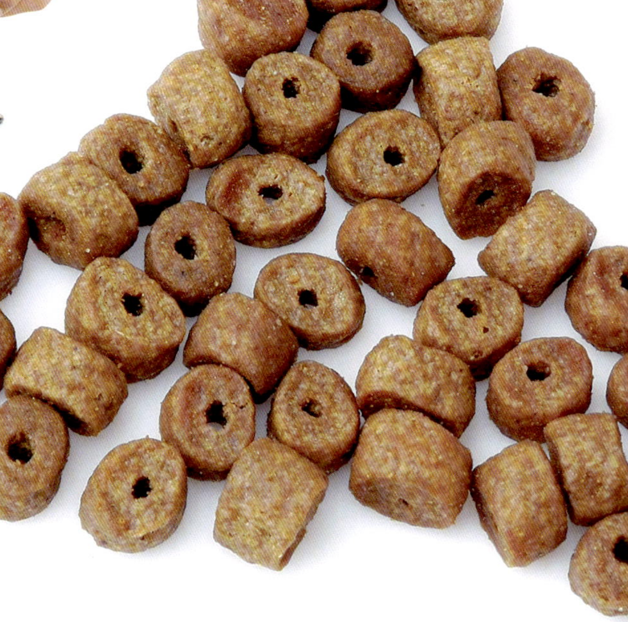

- ✔ When they are adults, the contrary takes place: they show more interest in new flavors and textures than in their previous diet when said diet has been their only food for a long period of time. We could call this food fatigue or monotony. It is important to vary a pet's diet so that they become accustomed to new flavors.

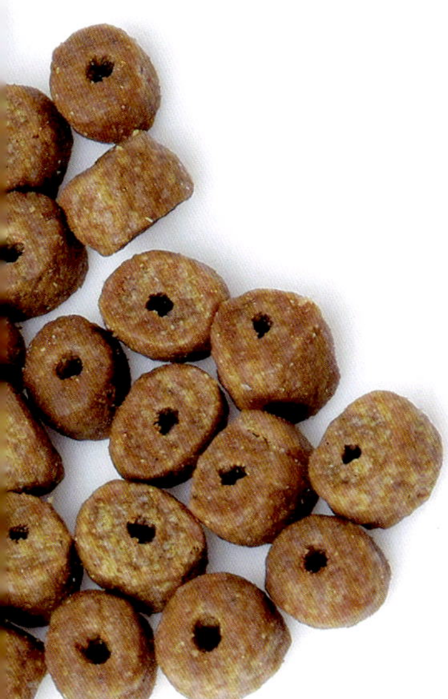

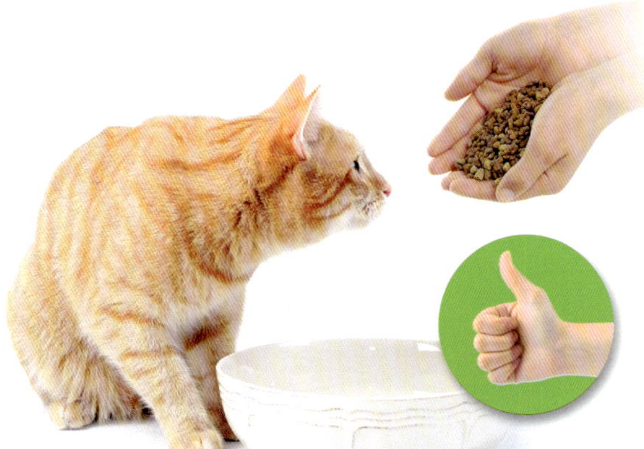

- ✔ Affinity for a diet may occasionally be caused by changing homes or stressful situations. In these cases, formulas to increase voluntary ingestion must be found.

stimulate ingestion (I)

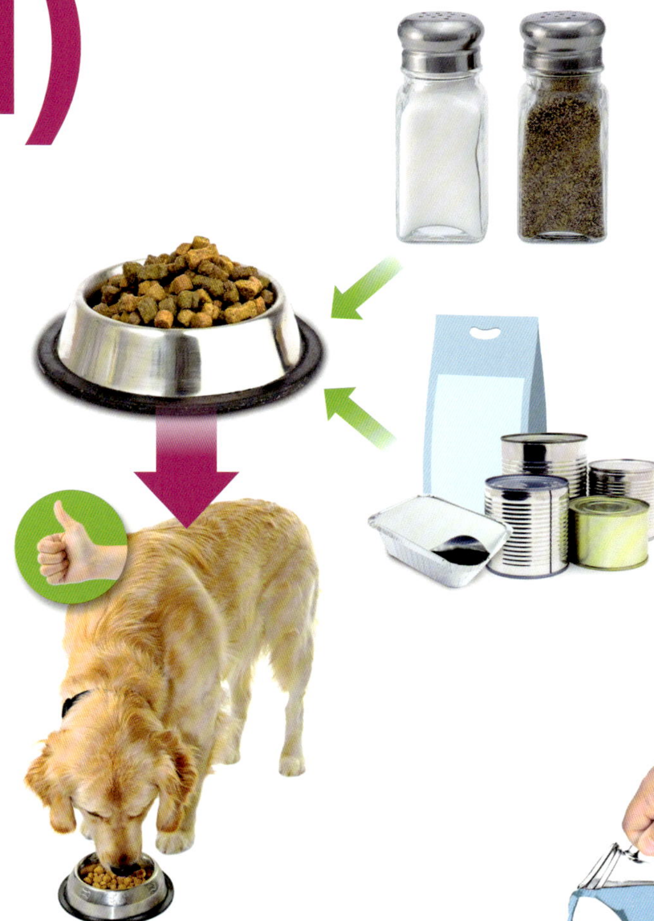

3 Strategies to stimulate consumption in healthy animals

- ✔ In some cases, we can add substances and in others, by varying the form or presentation, we will achieve the desired effect, but we must always respect the pet's nutritional requirements. We must remember that we are trying to modify a poorly learned regime.
- ✔ Having the owner participate in the strategy is highly important, but only as long as they feel deep trust and conviction with the veterinary team. If we can achieve this, success is guaranteed.

4 Improving the palatability of the food ration

- ✔ **Moisture of the food ration:** substituting dry food for canned food (wet) in dogs and cats represents the simplest and most effective technique. This is not only determined by the variations in moisture of the food from 10 % to 75 %, but greater proportions of protein and fat are included in its manufacturing.

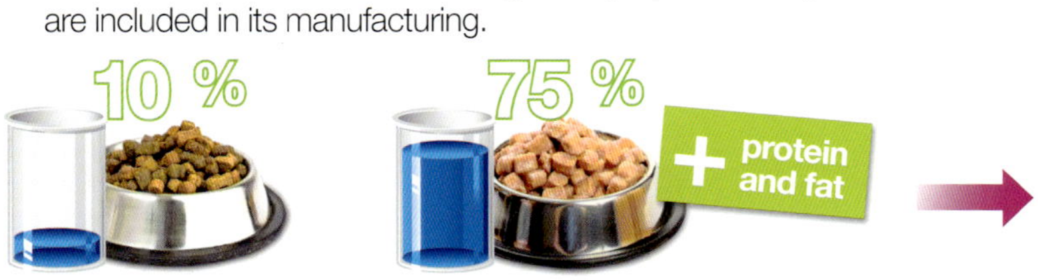

Good results are achieved in some dogs by adding water to their dry food (1/3 or 1/2 of the volume of the food in water).

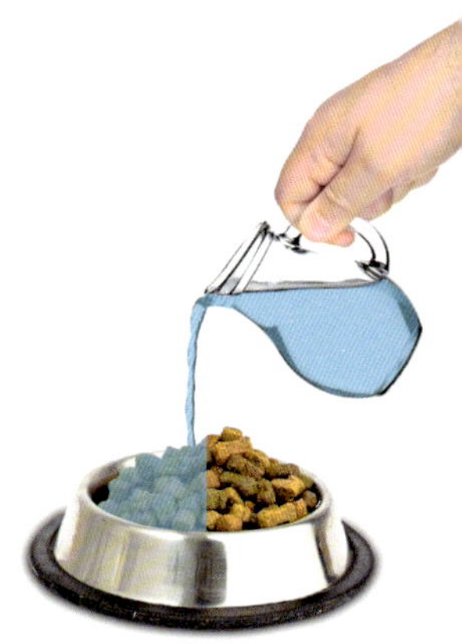

- ✔ **Protein and fat, origin and quality:** proteins, certain protein extracts, some amino acids and animal fat stimulate the consumption of food in both species.

  For cats, there is a high level of acceptance of flavors enriched with fresh meat, liver (with a special preference compared to meat), protein hydrolysates, proline, alanine, lysine, histidine, leucine and animal fat. However, they do not accept medium-chain fatty acids present in coco and palm oils.

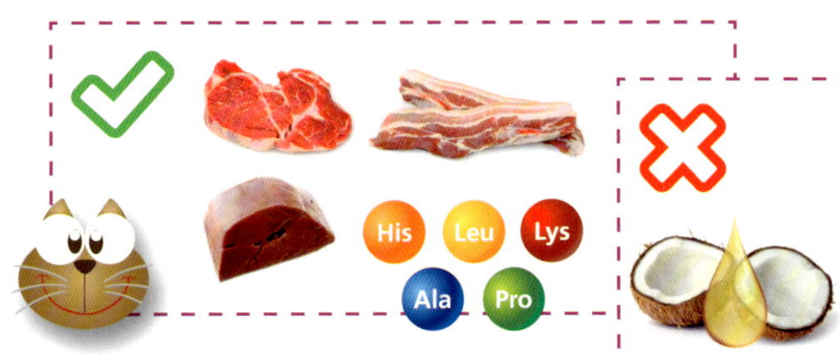

Dogs are not as picky as cats, but they have been known to be selective of meats from different origins, which improves ingestion: they prefer lamb, beef, pork, and horse meat over chicken or liver. Dogs also like certain nucleotides that are generated during the decomposition of cadavers. This selection is more frequently associated with the sense of smell rather than with taste: dogs with anosmia show reduced discrimination between different types of meat.

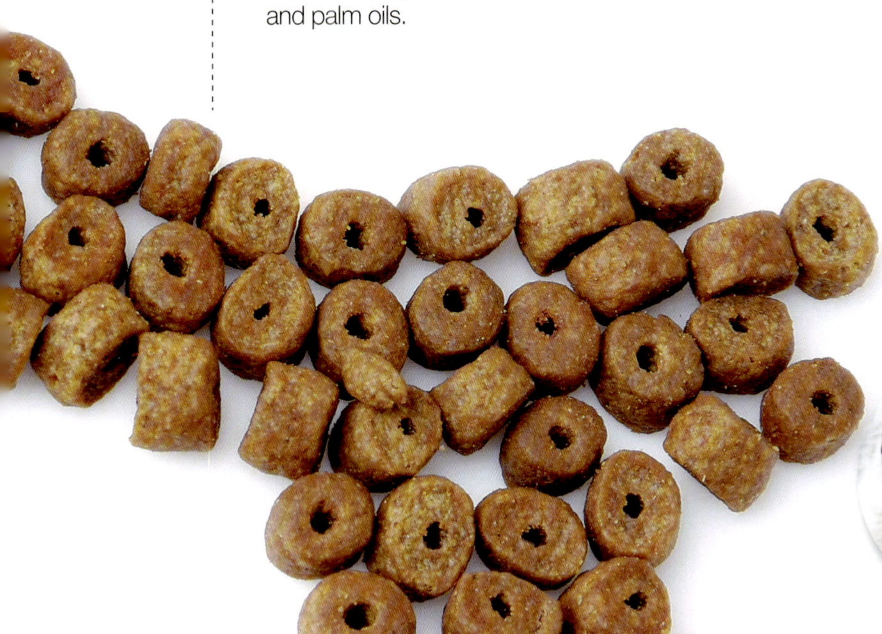

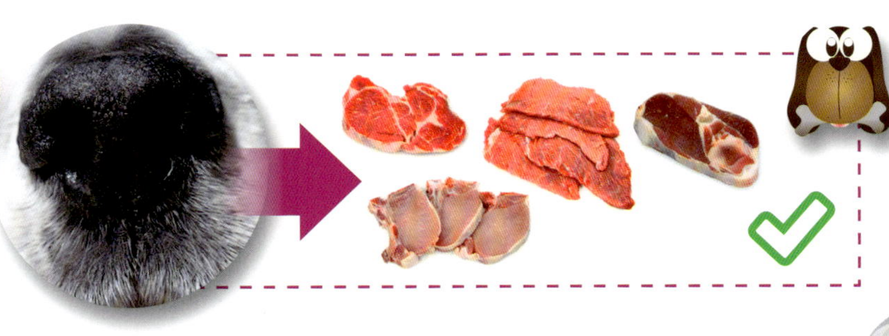

Strategies to

1 Smells

The sense of **smell** and **taste** determine the experience of food ingestion, and therefore, also the processes of affinity or aversion toward said food.
Of all of the organoleptic characteristics of foods, taste is the most complex given that it is a mix of smells and flavor. The importance of the sense of smell for pets to select their food 's greater than that of humans.

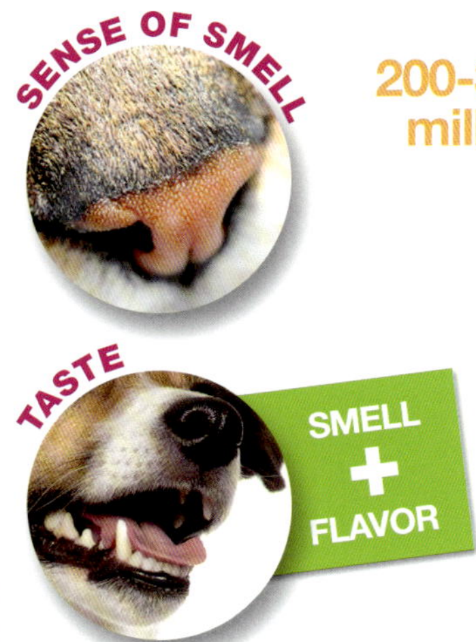

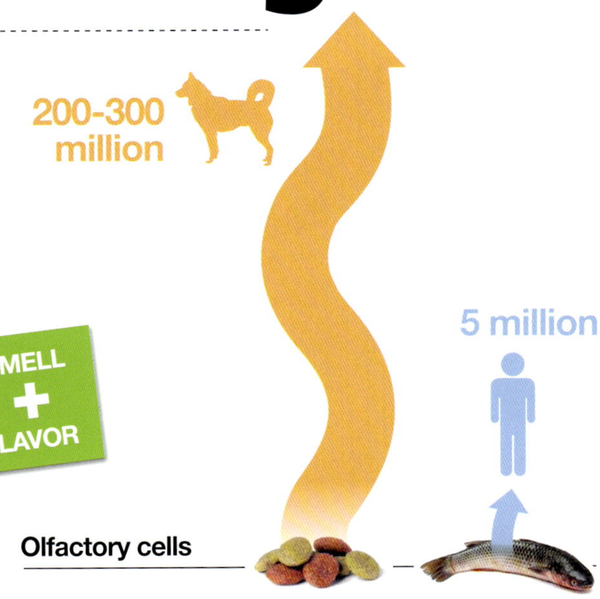

TRICK

✓ Feeding our pets after 30 minutes in an environment where a piece of meat is cooking. The smells produced during the cooking process of certain types of meat stimulate the consumption of food in cats.

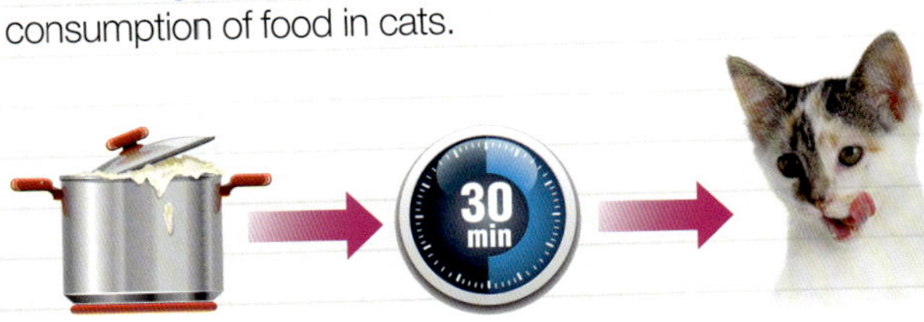

Any substance or extract (meat extracts used in human food, grated cheese) that is similar to the smell and taste of meat can be used to stimulate a pet's appetite.

2 Flavors

Pets' responses to flavors are variable according to their ability to differentiate between different ones, depending on the species.

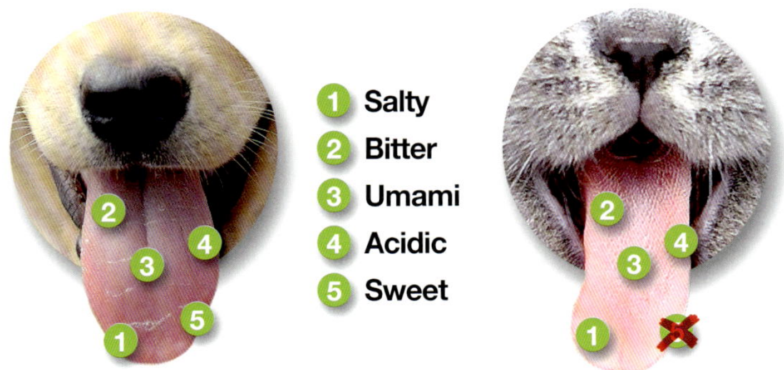

Glutamic acid

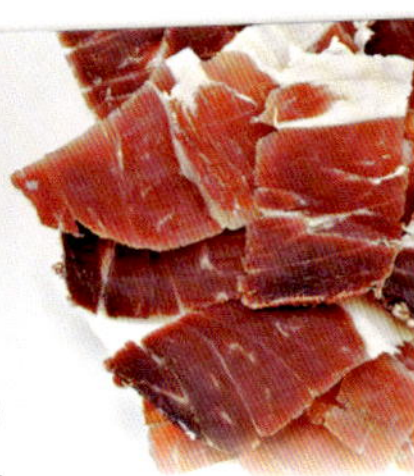

The presence of glutamic acid and its derivatives act as a stimulant for dogs, however, not for cats, who reject this flavor (umami).

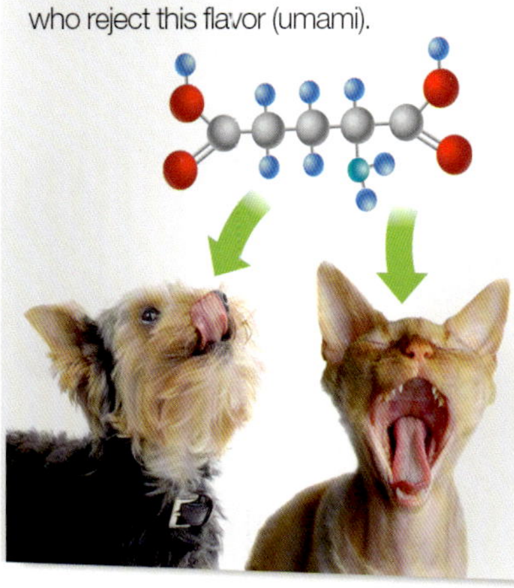

Salt

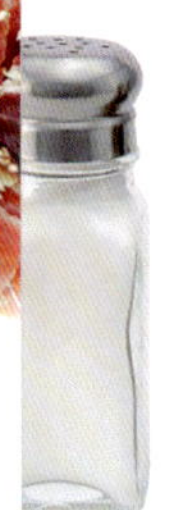

The inclusion of NaCl increases the palatability of food rations for all animals.
In cats, this is based on their preference for foods that do not cause metabolic acidosis: they reject low-sodium diets. Sodium participates in the acid-base balance of the body.

Safe upper limit

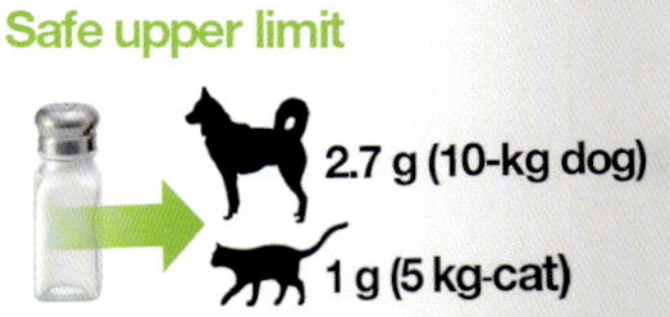

10-25 times the daily requirements

✓ The use of potassium chloride (KCl) is more effective than sodium chloride.

Sugars

Some monosaccharides and disaccharides function properly in dogs, but not in cats (they lack sweet flavor receptors).

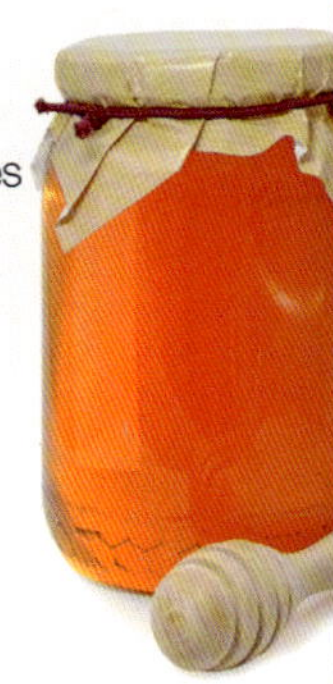

Safe upper limit

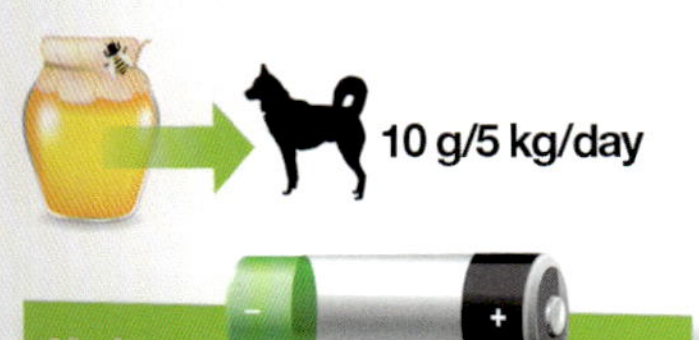

Maximum: 10 % of the calories ingested

Acids

Some organic acids such as phosphoric ("cola" drinks) and citric acid (in fruits) have positive effects on ingestion.

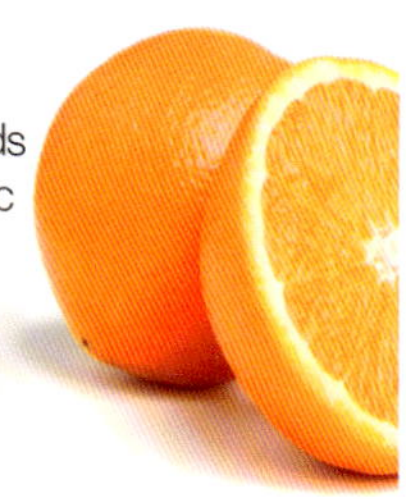

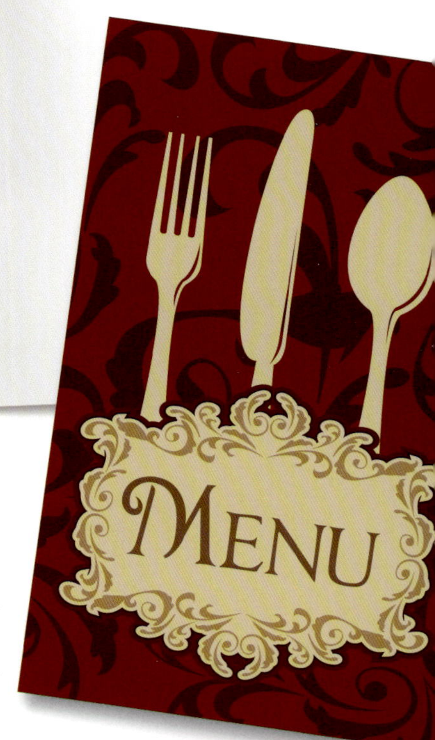

3 Texture

✓ Both species show an elevated preference for textures that imitate pieces of meat. Sticky or powdery foods should be avoided.
✓ Cats also show that they consume foods better when each piece has the same size and form.

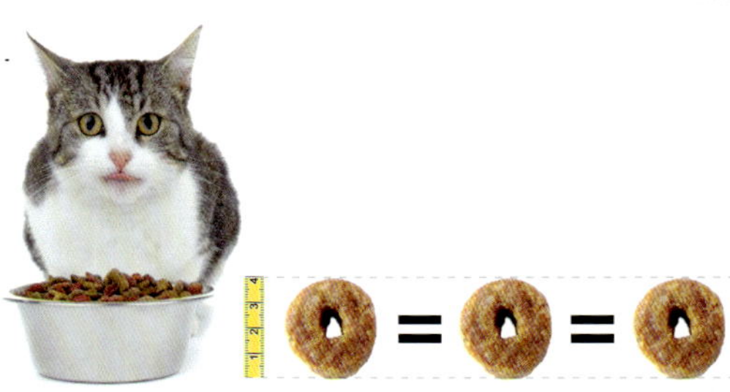

stimulate ingestion (II)

4 Temperature

- ✔ The temperature affects foods with high water content.
- ✔ Heating foods to body temperature has a positive effect on their texture and the sense of smell. Heat releases the volatile compounds present in food.
  - **Refrigerated foods:** 20 % acceptance rate.
  - **Foods at 38.5 °C:** 80 % acceptance rate.
- ✔ Likewise, fresh or recently opened foods stimulate ingestion. The release of aromatic substances is greater. Special attention should be paid to how foods are stored.

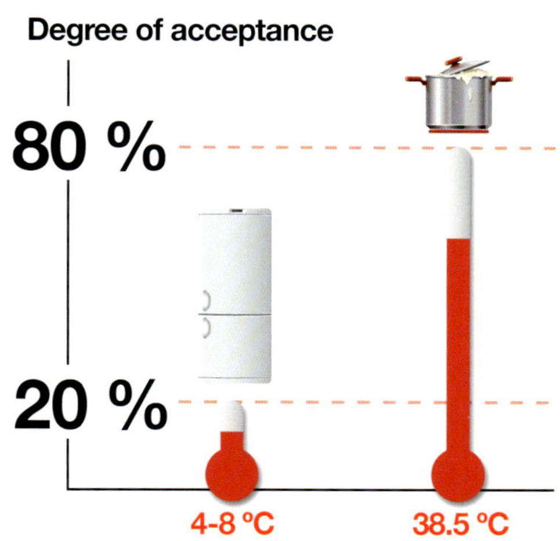

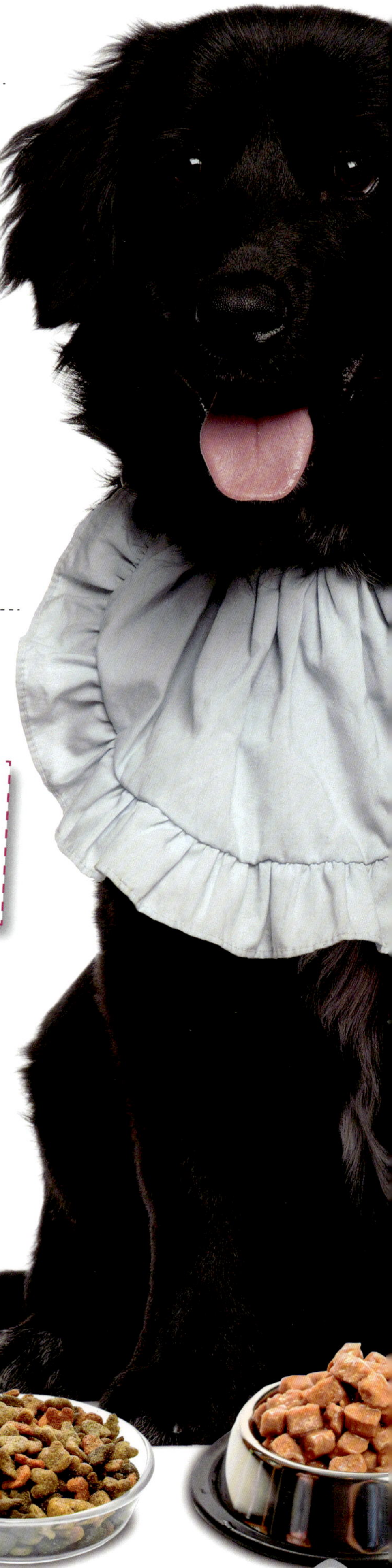

5 Creating an adequate environment

If we use common sense, the same methods that we use for our own meals can be applied to our pets. Most of them are geared toward minimizing stress, such as:

- ✔ A comfortable environment should be created where our pets can eat peacefully. For example: children should be reminded not to bother animals while they eat, voices should be lowered and no electrical kitchen appliances should be used at that time...
- ✔ When pets are kept in confined spaces, their food dishes should be kept away from dirty areas.
- ✔ The animal should not be pushed or frightened when we are offering them food. Preferably, a soft and kind tone of voice should be used.

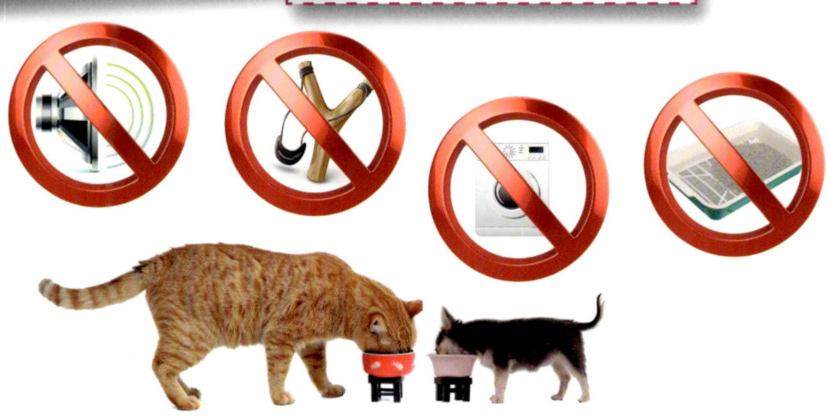

6 Food dishes and feeders

- ✔ **Dish/feeder materials:** materials that do not give off strange smells should preferably be used, such as porcelain, glass or metal.
- ✔ **Dish/feeder design:** occasionally, the surfaces impede correct traction of food.
- ✔ **Dish/feeder cleaning materials:** these may also play a role in the acceptance/rejection of foods.

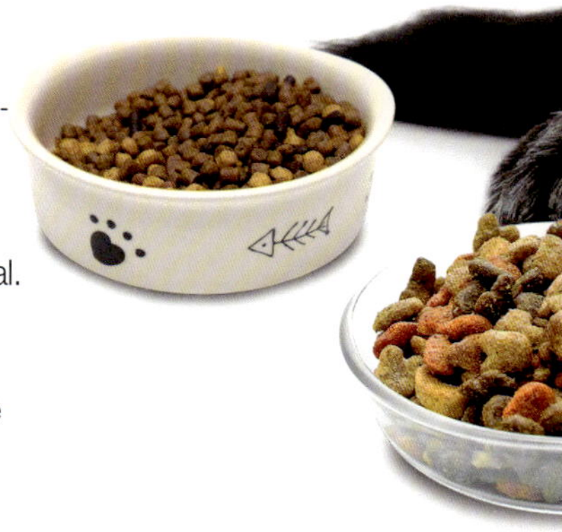

Nutritional management

1 Improving reproductive performance

Improving dog and cat breeds requires the selection of individuals that do not have and cannot transmit malformations to their offspring. Therefore, the objectives are:

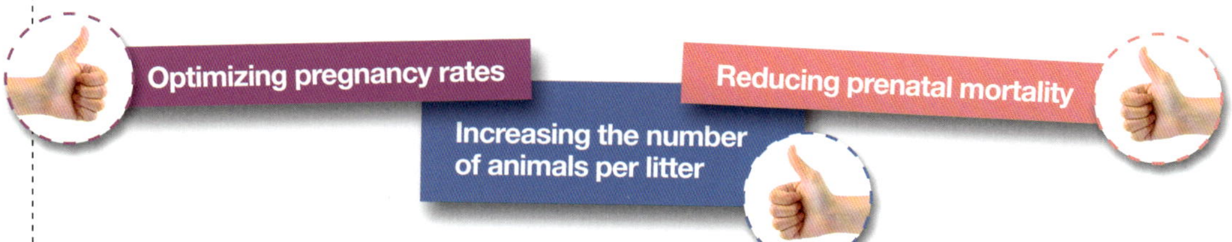

A balanced diet can improve reproductive performance. The following are the main elements influencing reproductive parameters.

- ✔ **The weight** and **body condition score (BCS)** of breeding females.
- ✔ All the factors associated with the diet's **nutritional composition**, e.g., how voluntary intake is affected during estrus and how it can be corrected through the diet's energy content, or the importance of vitamins and minerals on spermatogenesis.

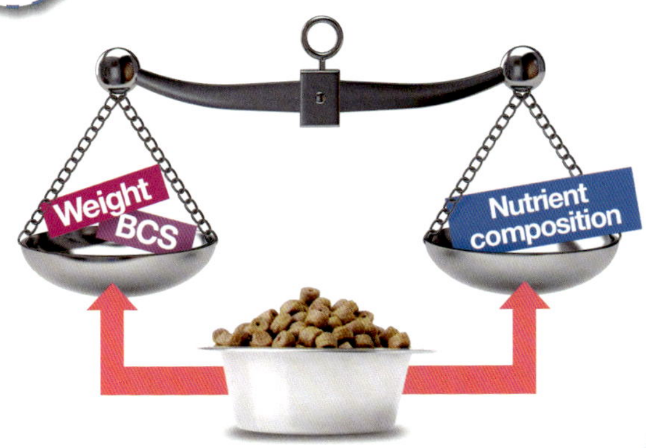

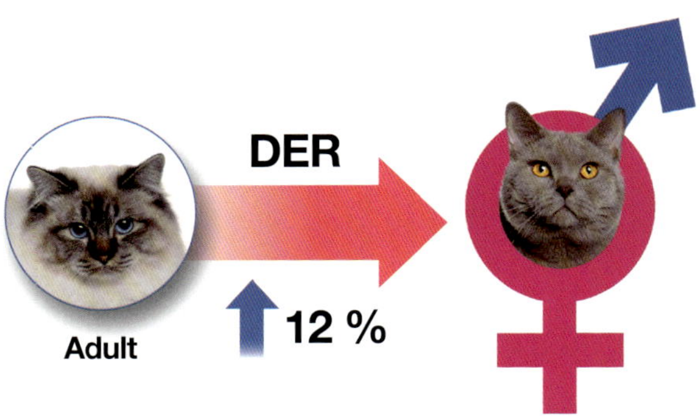

In this regard, it should be highlighted that the daily energy requirements (DER) of breeders are slightly higher than those of adult animals. They are 12 % higher at most.

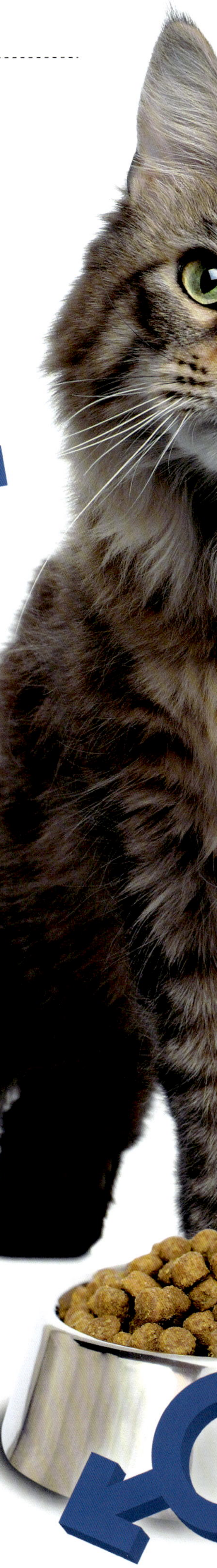

2 An inadequate BCS can affect the estrous cycle

- ✔ Overweight/obese females (BCS ≥ 6/9) and those weighing less than is required (BCS ≤ 4/9) have abnormal estrous cycles.
  It is estimated that females should have a BCS of 5/9 before participating in breeding programs.

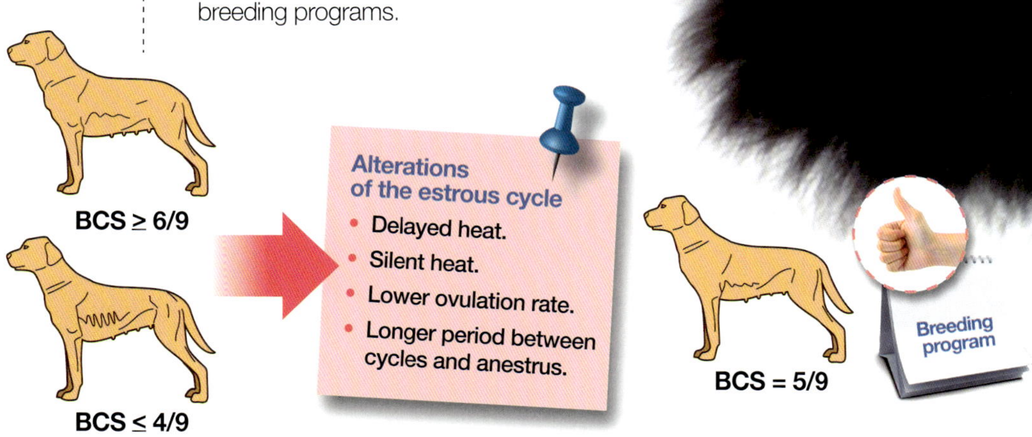

- ✔ Some authors suggest flushing bitches and queens. This practice, used in livestock animals, involves increasing their feed intake during the proestrous period by 5–10 % above the maintenance requirements, and returning to maintenance levels after service. This technique ensures a better development of the reproductive organs and an increased size of the litter. In the cat and dog species, this does not make sense as they usually have a good weight and body condition before the reproductive period.

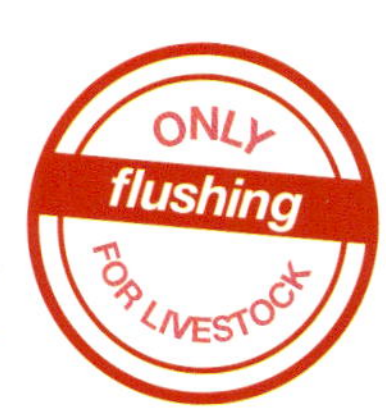

# of breeding animals

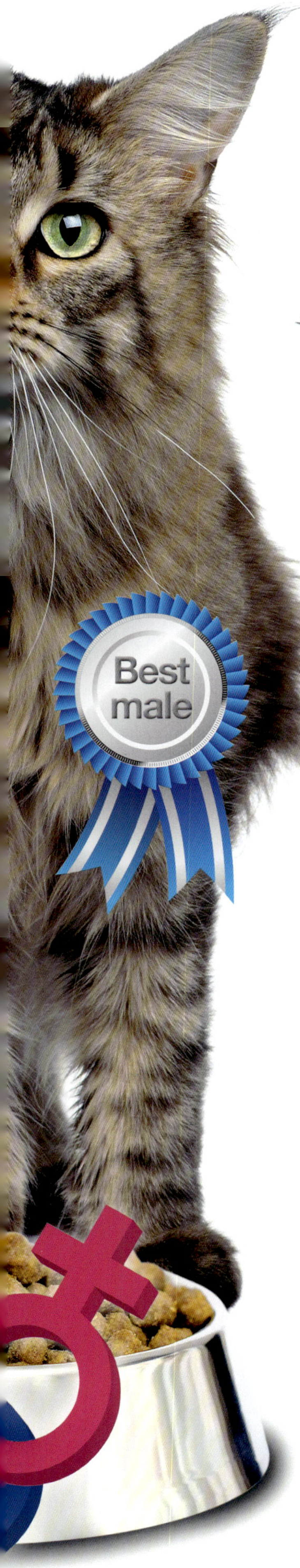

3 Change to a growth/lactation diet

Although their nutritional requirements are similar to those of non-breeding adult females, the diet of future breeding females should be changed to a highly digestible, high-quality growth/lactation diet.

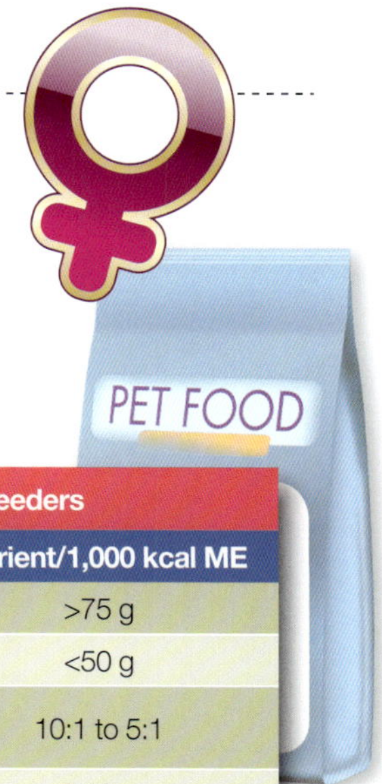

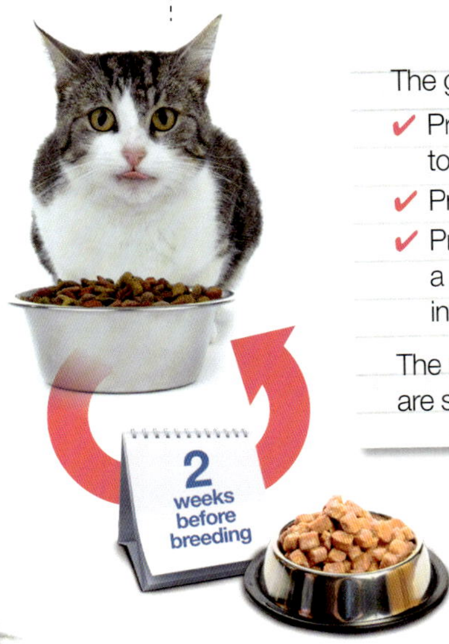

The goals of this dietary modification are to:

- ✔ Prevent digestive disorders due to a sudden change of diet.
- ✔ Prepare the female for lactation.
- ✔ Prevent weight loss due to a lower food intake during estrus: intake is about 20 % lower.

The requirements these diets must fulfil are shown in the table.

Needs of breeders

Nutrient	Nutrient/1,000 kcal ME
Protein	>75 g
Fat	<50 g
Omega-6:omega-3 ratio	10:1 to 5:1
DHA	0.13 g

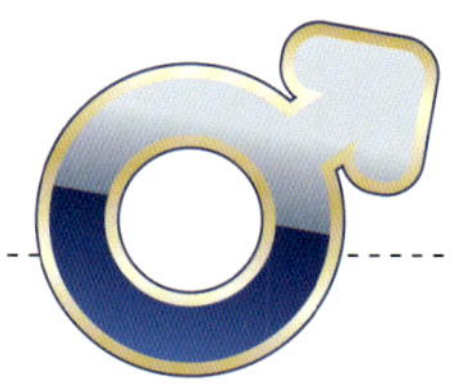

4 Nutritional management of breeding males

✔ There is little information available on the influence of diet in breeding males. Their nutritional needs are the same as those of non-breeding adult males, except for those individuals used as breeders on a regular basis: weight changes and body condition determine the amount of food they must be given.

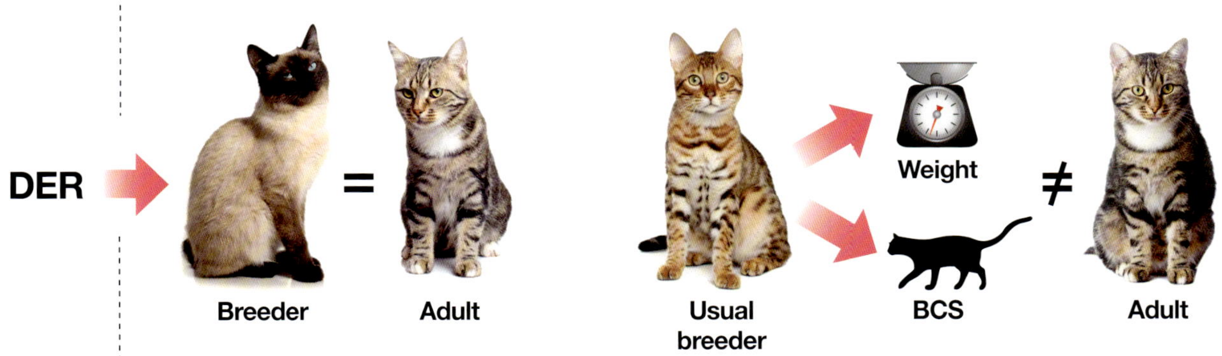

✔ In general, malnutrition characterized by an excessive fat content and a poor content of:

- **Protein**
- **Vitamins** (niacin, pyridoxine and cobalamin)
- **Macrominerals** (imbalances in the Ca:P ratio, with values of 1:15-1:30, manganese)
- **Microminerals** (zinc, sodium, potassium, iron and selenium)

is responsible for alterations in the amount and quality of the semen.

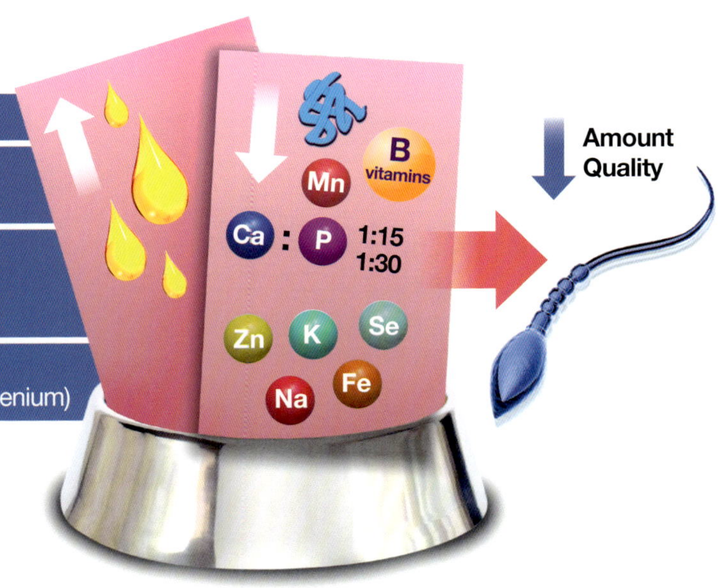

Feeding pregnant

Feeding during this phase is usually the same as for a non-pregnant adult animals until the last trimester of the process. Certain factors should be taken into account that intervene during pregnancy to better understand the food requirements and handling.

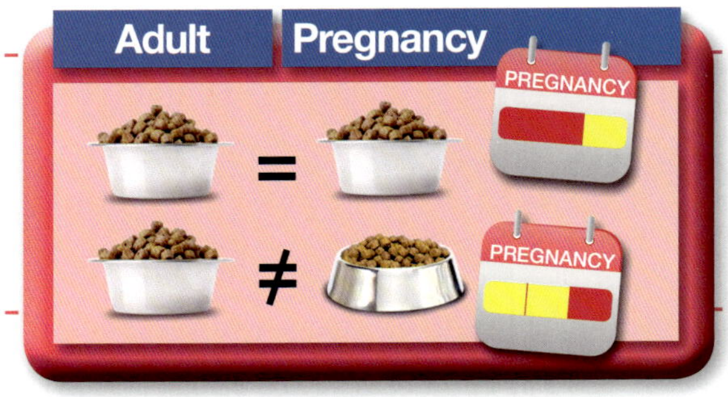

1 Nutrition requirements during pregnancy

Calculating energy

- ✔ The daily energy requirements (DER) of pregnant females increase depending on the stage of pregnancy. This nutrient is considered as the primary limiting factor. In both species, the maintenance requirements must be multiplied by a factor of 1.25 to 1.50 to calculate the DER.
- ✔ In female dogs, we can perform a more precise calculation of the DER taking into account the week of gestation. During the 5th and 9th week, the requirements above maintenance increase by 18 kcal ME/kg of body weight of the female. Coinciding with the exponential growth of the fetuses, the requirements from the 6th to the 8th weeks are increased by 36 kcal ME/kg body weight.
- ✔ As we can see, the requirements vary according to the size of the litter. If the litter is small, the correction factor is 1.30, but when the number of puppies or kittens is higher, the factor can be modified by up to 1.50–1.70.

DER = MER x (1.25 to 1.50)

PREGNANCY 5th week and PREGNANCY 9th week = ↑ 18 kcal ME / kg BW

PREGNANCY 6th week to PREGNANCY 8th week = ↑ 36 kcal ME / kg BW

DER = MER × 1.30

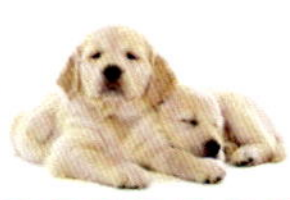

DER = MER × (1.50 to 1.70)

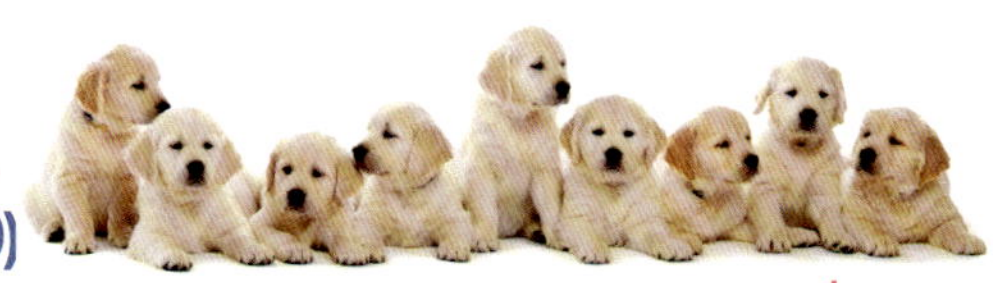

Modifications of MER (kcal/day)			
Gestation week	Female dog's weight (kg)		
	<10 kg	11 to 40 kg	41 to 70 kg
5th to 9th	×1.2	×1.3	×1.4
6th to 8th	×1.4	×1.6	×1.75

Example

What are the DER of a pregnant dog that weighs 25 kg in the 7th week of pregnancy?

$DER_{7th\ week\ of\ pregnancy} = MER + (36\ kcal \times 25)$

$MER = 132 \times 25^{0.75} = 1{,}475.80\ kcal\ ME/day$

$DER_{7th\ week\ of\ pregnancy} = 1{,}475.80 + 900 = 2{,}375.80\ kcal\ ME/day$

Or:

$DER_{7th\ week\ of\ pregnancy} = MER \times 1.6 = 2{,}361.28\ kcal\ ME/day$

With a difference smaller than 1 % regarding the previous calculation.

Are the DER adequate?

Checking the female animal's weight progress is sufficient for evaluation of the DER.

In female cats, there is an approximate weekly increase of 5 % from the 2nd week of pregnancy. There is an equation that allows us to determine the average weight gain during this stage depending on the number of fetuses (nf):

Weight gain (g) = 888.9 + (106.5 × nf)

In female dogs the weight variations are not noticeable until the 5th week of gestation. Between the 5th and 7th week, 75 % of the growth of the fetus takes place. From this moment until birth, the average weight gain is approximately 6.25 % weekly.

Evaluation of total proteins in plasma. Although there are variations in the concentrations of urea in blood, the protein concentrations remain constant; a decrease indicates sub-nutrition.

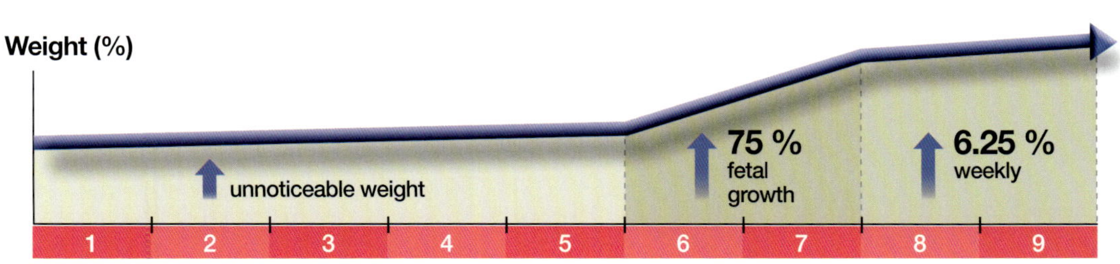

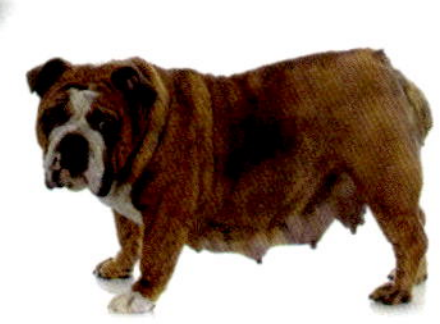

Gestation week

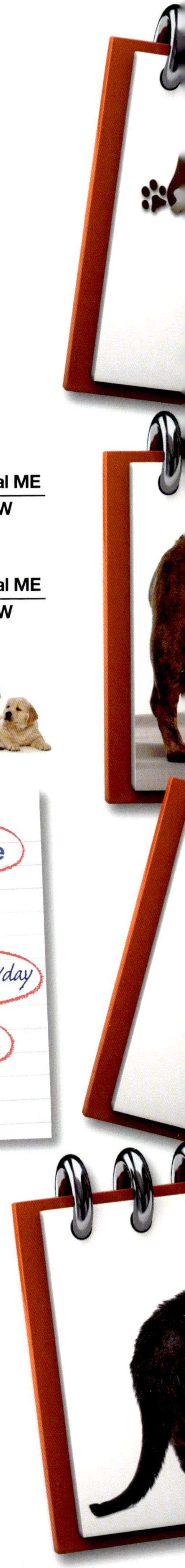

females

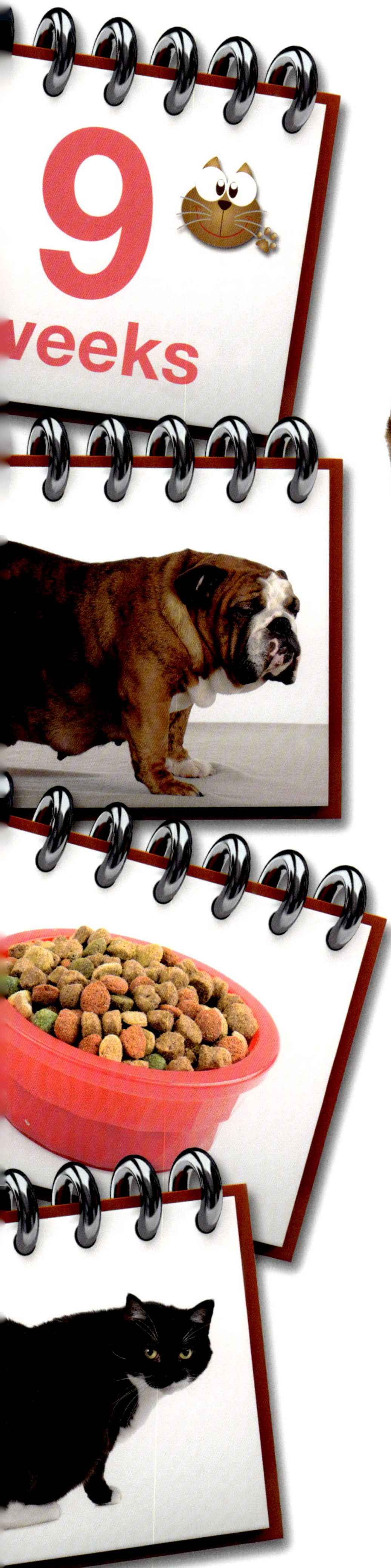

2 How do the estrous cycle and pregnancy affect feeding?

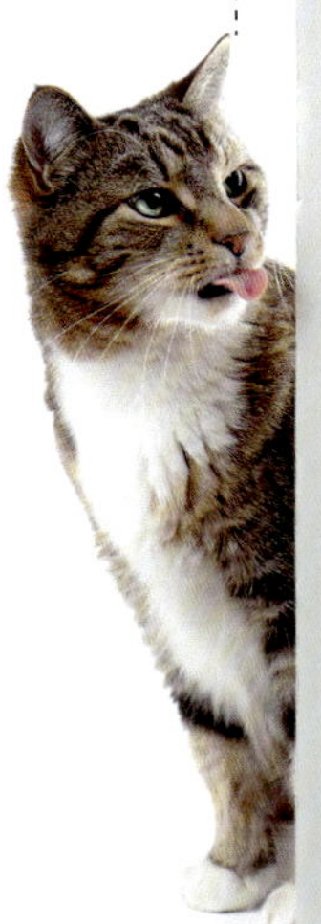

	Female dog	Female cat
Puberty	6-9 months	5-9 months
Reproductive age	2 to 7 years	
Type of estrus	Seasonally monoestrous (Spring and Autumn)	Seasonally polyestrous (January and September)
Repeated estrus	No	Yes, every 2-19 days (average of 8)
Receptiveness of male	7 days	7 to 9 days
Ovulation	Day 9-11 from the start	Induced
Hyporexia during estrous	Yes	No
Pregnancy	63 ± 2	63 ± 5
Gestational weight gain	From the 4th-5th week	From the first day
Weight gain	15 to 25 %	12 to 40 %
Maximum fetal growth (%)	5th to 7th week (75 %)	Not available
Tissue growth	Fetuses and appendages	Fatty tissue, fetuses and appendages
Increase in the daily energy requirements	From the 5th week	From the 2nd week
Increase in the maintenance requirements	25 to 50 %	
Gestational hyporexia (fetal implantation)	Brief, at 3 weeks	2 weeks
Pre-partum anorexia	12 hours before	7 days before
Post-partum weight loss	95 %	40 %

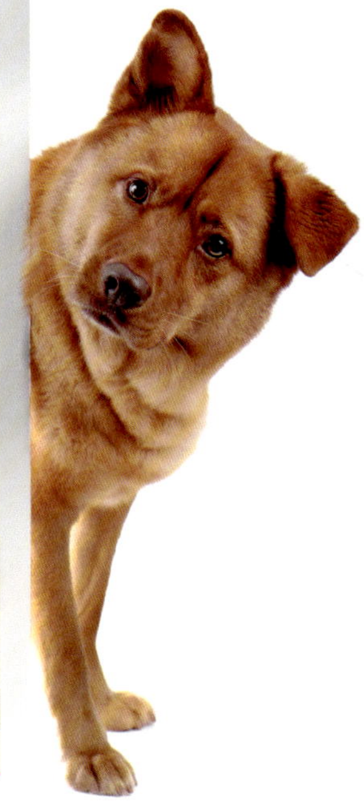

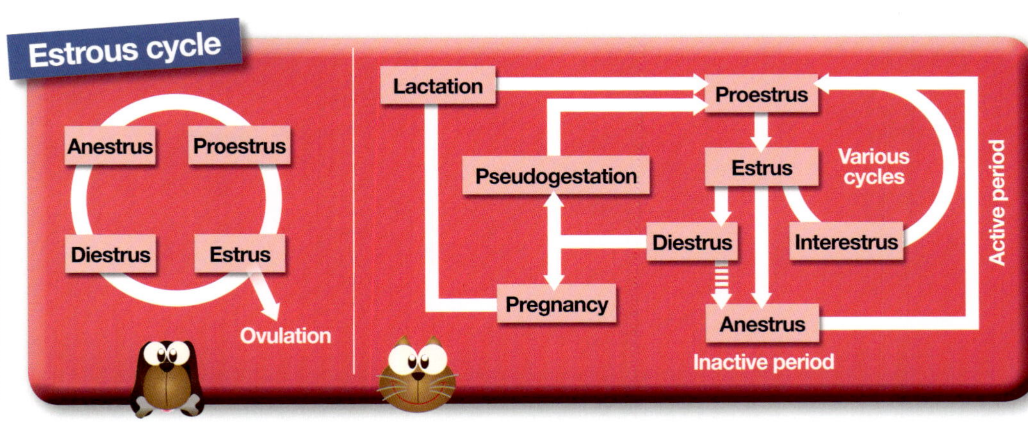

3 Carbohydrates during pregnancy

No absolute recommendations have been proven regarding carbohydrates in cats. However, in female dogs, the use of rations free of hydrates determines the following:

- ✔ Decrease in the ingestion of food.
- ✔ Weight loss.
- ✔ Hypoglycemia.
- ✔ Gestational ketosis.
- ✔ Low birth weight of puppies.
- ✔ Premature births.

The explanation is based on the fact that more than half of the energy needs of fetuses depend on glucose.

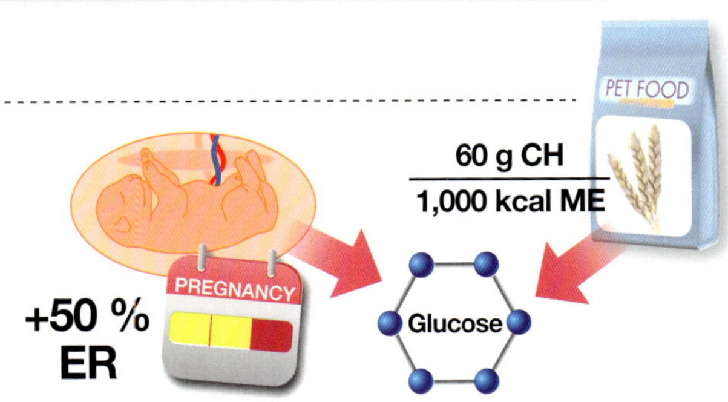

They are especially sensitive to this effect during the last third of the pregnancy. If we provide approximately 60 g of digestible carbohydrates/1,000 kcal ME, we avoid the effects of deficiencies.

When using rations without a sufficient amount of carbohydrates, we must modify the protein levels in the rations.

Fats and proteins

1 Fat and fatty acid requirements

The total fat requirements vary among different species

In female cats, there are no differences between maintenance and pregnancy regarding the recommendations. However, in dogs, there is an increase of 55 % between both states. In both cases, the total ingestion of fat is increased as a consequence of the increased energy requirements.

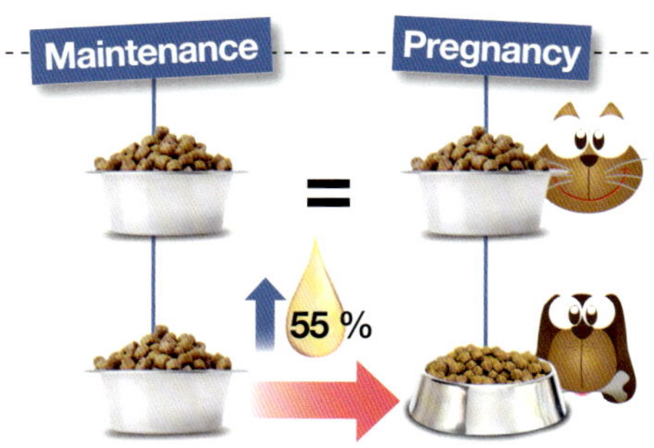

The proportion of fat is greater for larger litters or giant breeds

Similar to that which occurs with other nutrients, there are many factors that modify the requirements, especially the ingestion of food (which is found to be decreased).

In this sense, the recommendations of total fat for pregnant dogs with larger litters (in the last third of the pregnancy) or for giant breeds are, as a minimum, 50 g/1,000 kcal ME.

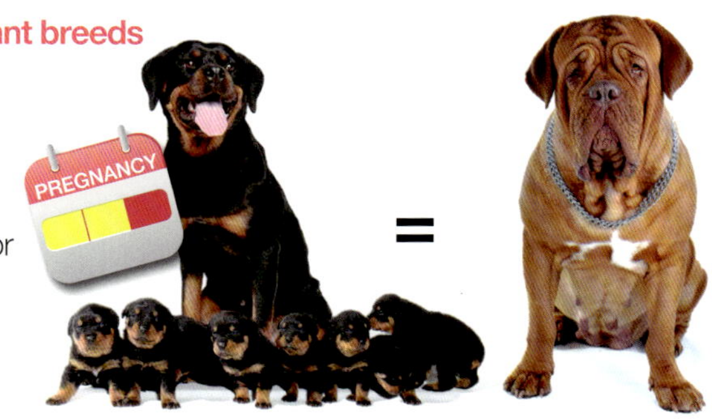

50 g/1,000 kcal ME

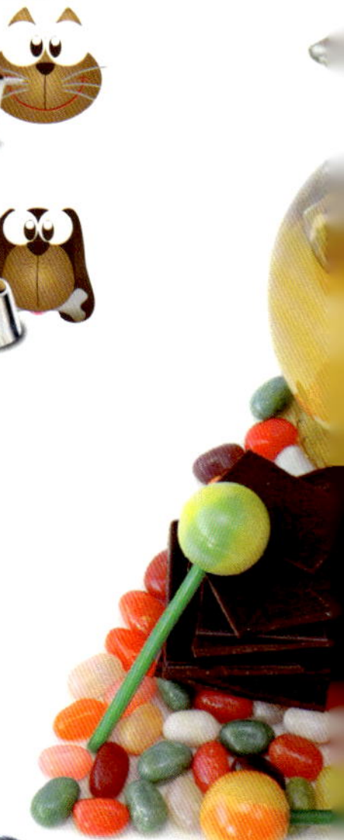

2 Protein requirements

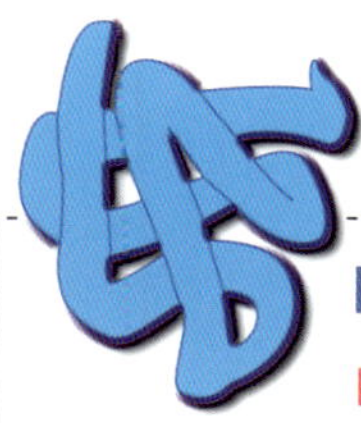

Protein requirements increase in the 2nd half of the pregnancy

The protein requirements only begin to increase after the first half of the pregnancy, when the fetal growth and development are maximum. The variations regarding a non-pregnant female are between 40-70 % above maintenance.

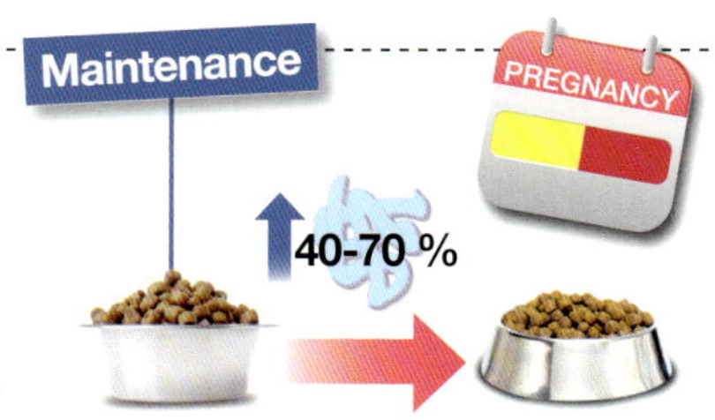

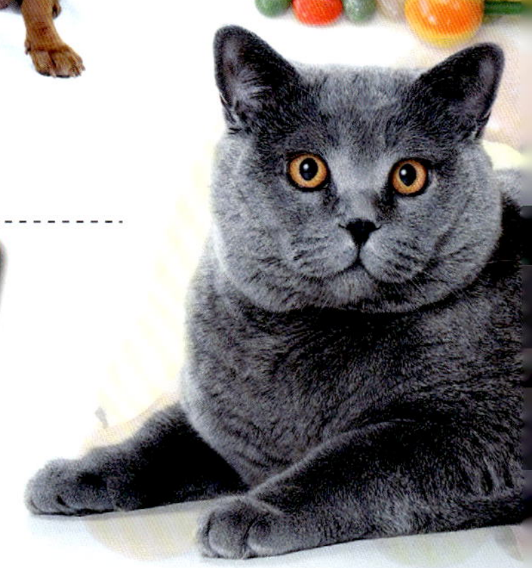

Official recommendations

The table summarizes the protein recommendations according to the NRC 2006, FEDIAF and AAFCO.

AAFCO Association of American Feed Control Officials

NRC The National Research Council

fediaf

	Protein (g)/1,000 kcal ME	
	Female dog	Female cat
NRC 2006	50	53
FEDIAF and AAFCO	56.25-78	70-110

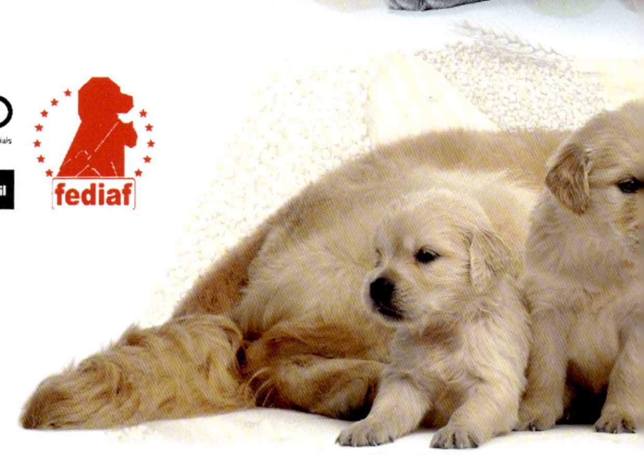

A deficiency in protein is detrimental to the offspring

A protein deficiency during pregnancy has undesirable effects on the offspring:

- ✔ Greater neonatal mortality
- ✔ Locomotive abnormalities
- ✔ Lack of response to stimuli
- ✔ Lower litter weight
- ✔ Disorientation
- ✔ Lack of immune system response

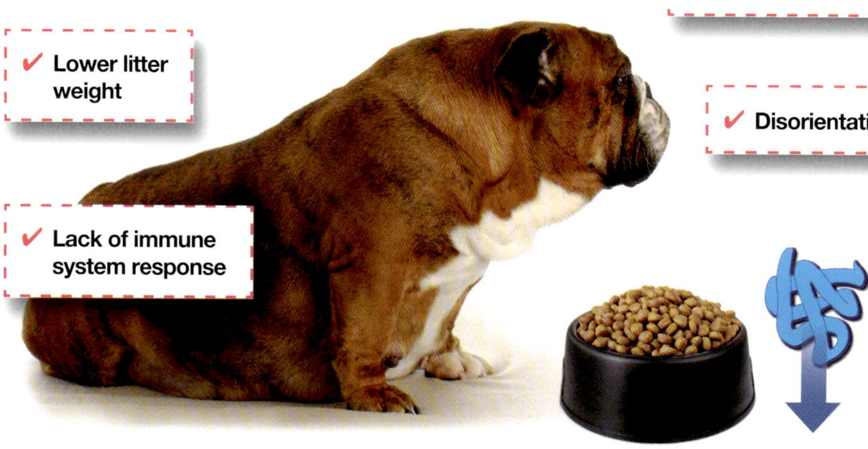

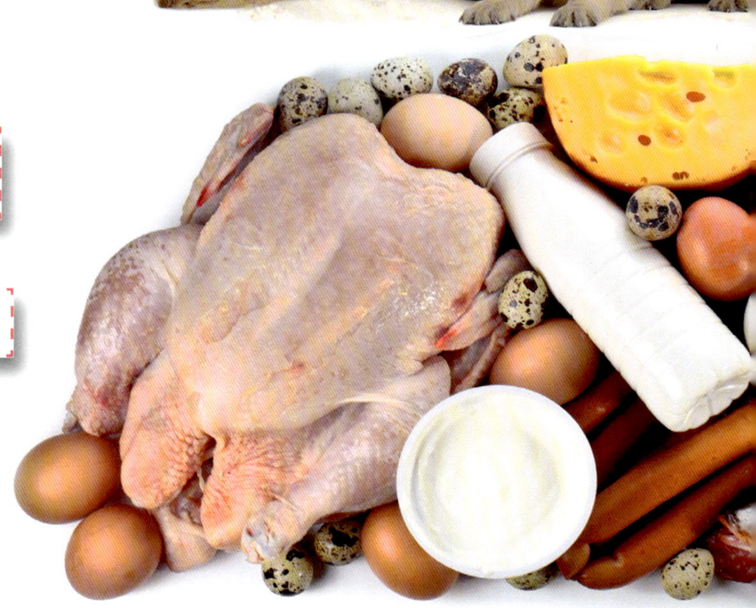

during pregnancy

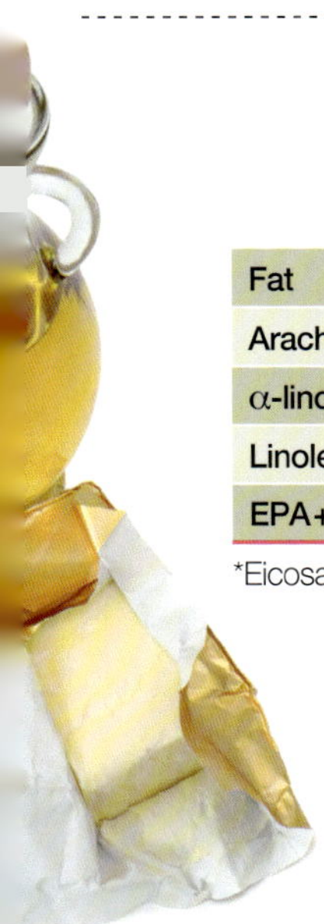

	Nutrient (g)/ 1,000 kcal ME			
	Female dog	× MER	Female cat	× MER
Fat	21.3	1.54	22.5	1
Arachydonic acid	Not needed		0.05	3
α-linolenic acid	0.2	1.82	0.05	-
Linoleic acid	3.3	1.18	1.4	1
EPA+DHA*	0.13	1.18	0.025	1

*Eicosapentaenoic+docosahexaenoic.

EFA recommendations

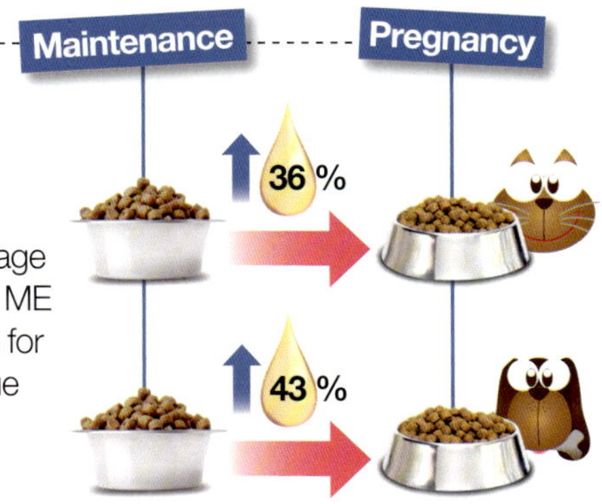

- ✔ Evaluating the different EFAs, and based on the WHO indications (FAO-WHO), the recommendations for fetal growth and appendage tissues should represent between 1-2 % of the ME consumed. Accordingly, the recommendations for EFAs are increased to 36 % as an average value compared to maintenance, which are higher in female dogs (≈ 7 %) than in female cats.
- ✔ In the case of female cats, a prolonged deficiency in the arachydonic acid (AA) time determines the delivery of stillbirths. The NRC, FEDIAF and AAFCO recommendations are very similar. The table summarizes the requirements in both species.

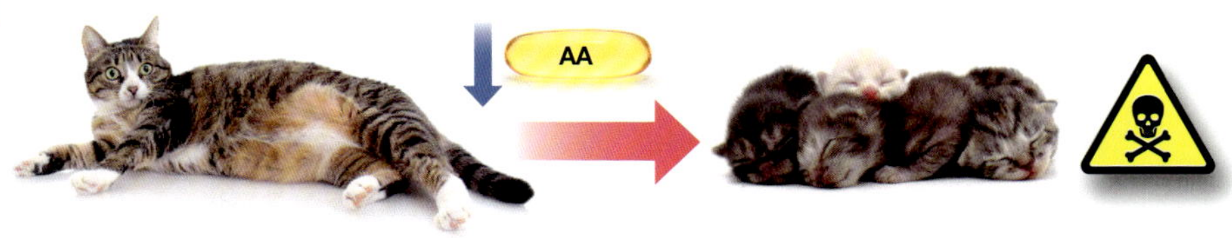

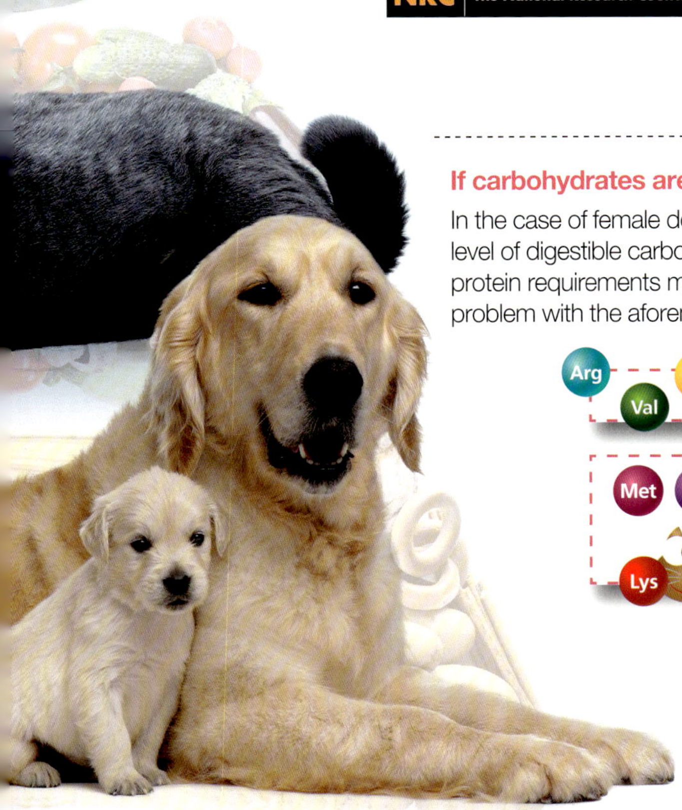

If carbohydrates are decreased, proteins must be increased

In the case of female dogs, the protein recommendations are determined by the level of digestible carbohydrates. If we do not provide carbohydrates in the rations, the protein requirements must be double the recommendations: 100 g/1,000 kcal ME. One problem with the aforementioned is that the stool becomes soft, sticky and foul-smelling.

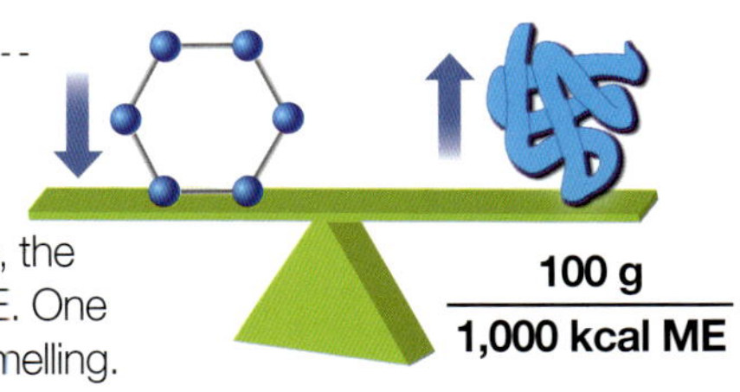

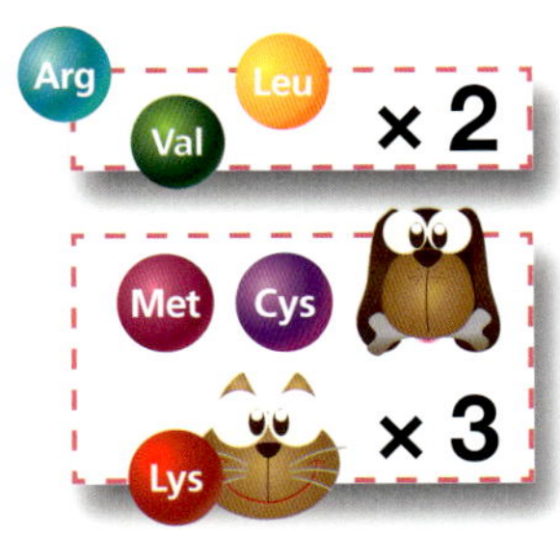

Double or triple essential amino acids (EAs)

Regarding EAs, there is not enough information to determine which are the minimum recommendations during pregnancy in both species. The variations will depend on the quality of the protein and the factors that modify it. Generally, the recommendations for EAs is to double them (although in the case of methionine-cysteine in female dogs and lysine in female cats, the recommendations are tripled).

Taurine in cats

Taurine is an essential amino acid for feline reproduction and fetal development. A deficiency during pregnancy causes the following:

- ✔ Abortion.
- ✔ Elevated neonatal mortality.
- ✔ Embryonic death.
- ✔ Fetal malformations (abnormal development of the hind legs, hydrocephaly, and anencephaly).

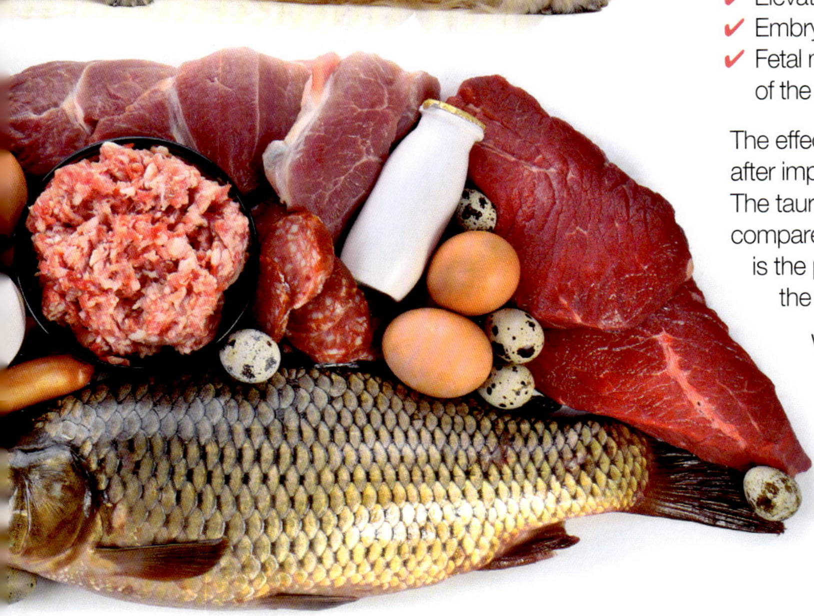

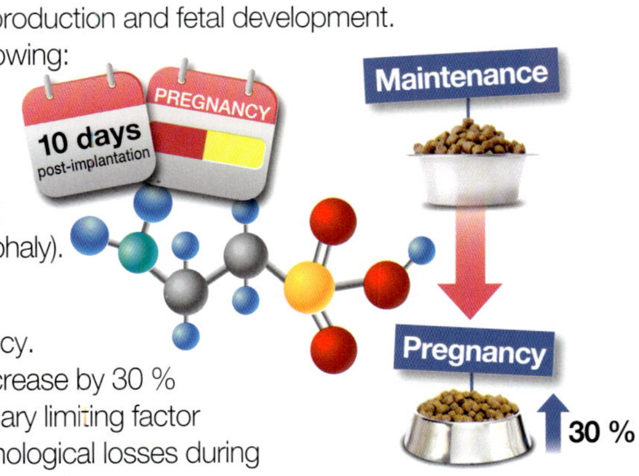

The effects take place in the first 10 days after implantation or halfway through pregnancy. The taurine requirements during this stage increase by 30 % compared to maintenance, although the primary limiting factor is the presentation of food, due to the technological losses during the manufacturing process (high temperatures).

Wet foods should include double (or even up to 2.5 times more) taurine when compared with dry foods. The recommendations for dry foods vary from 0.13 to 0.25 g/1,000 kcal ME.

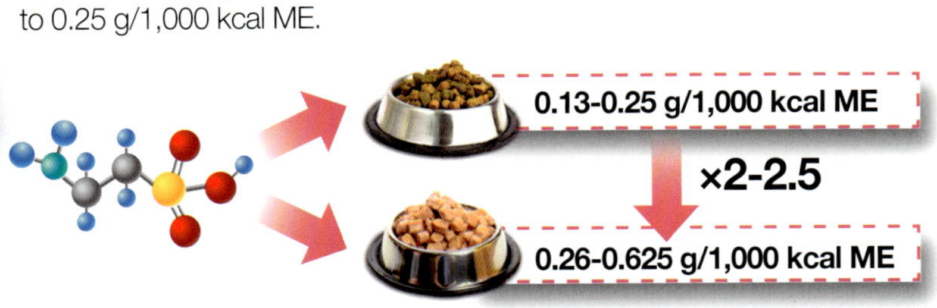

In general, most mineral and vitamin requirements during this period are increased by more than 60 % with respect to maintenance requirements, and may even double these values.

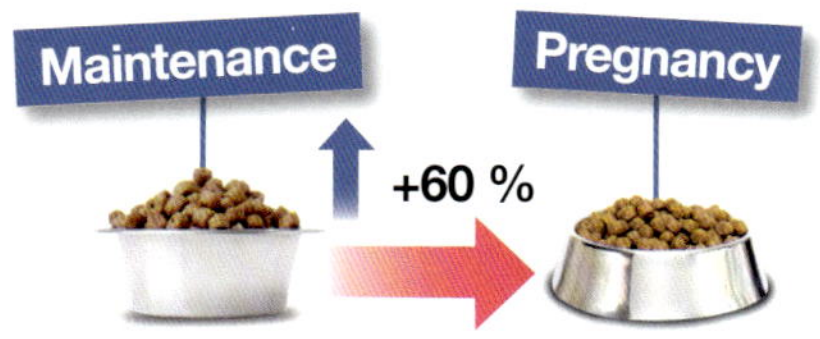

Minerals in pregnancy

1 Iron and copper

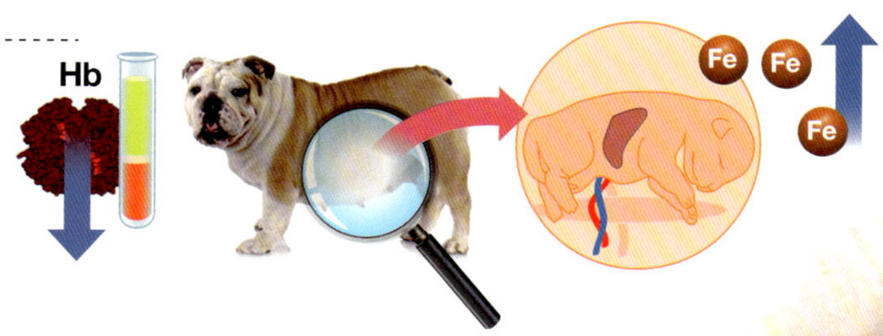

- ✔ It has been reported that term-pregnant females show slight iron-deficiency anemia: hematocrit, hemoglobin and plasma iron values are reduced. This is due to the accumulation of iron that takes place in the liver of fetuses.
- ✔ To prevent these situations, it is necessary to ensure the diet contains adequate iron and copper levels (component of ferroxidases that participate in hematopoiesis). Dietary requirements for both these minerals are twice those of adults.

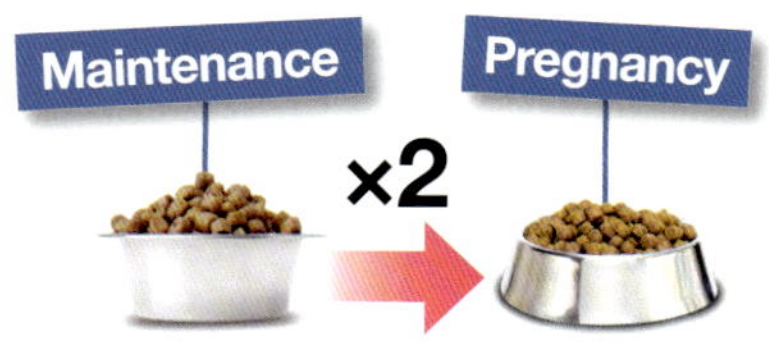

- ✔ In the case of **iron**, due to its low bioavailability (it is calculated to be 30 % in dry food) and to variations in food intake, recommendations for pregnancy are 17-20 mg/1,000 kcal ME.

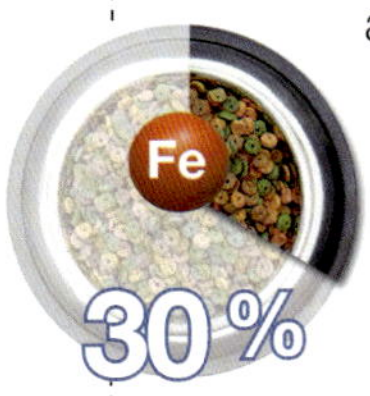

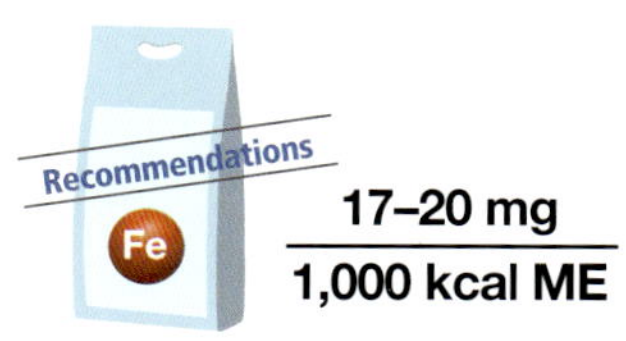

- ✔ The bioavailability of this mineral may vary from nearly 100 % to less than 10 % and depends on:

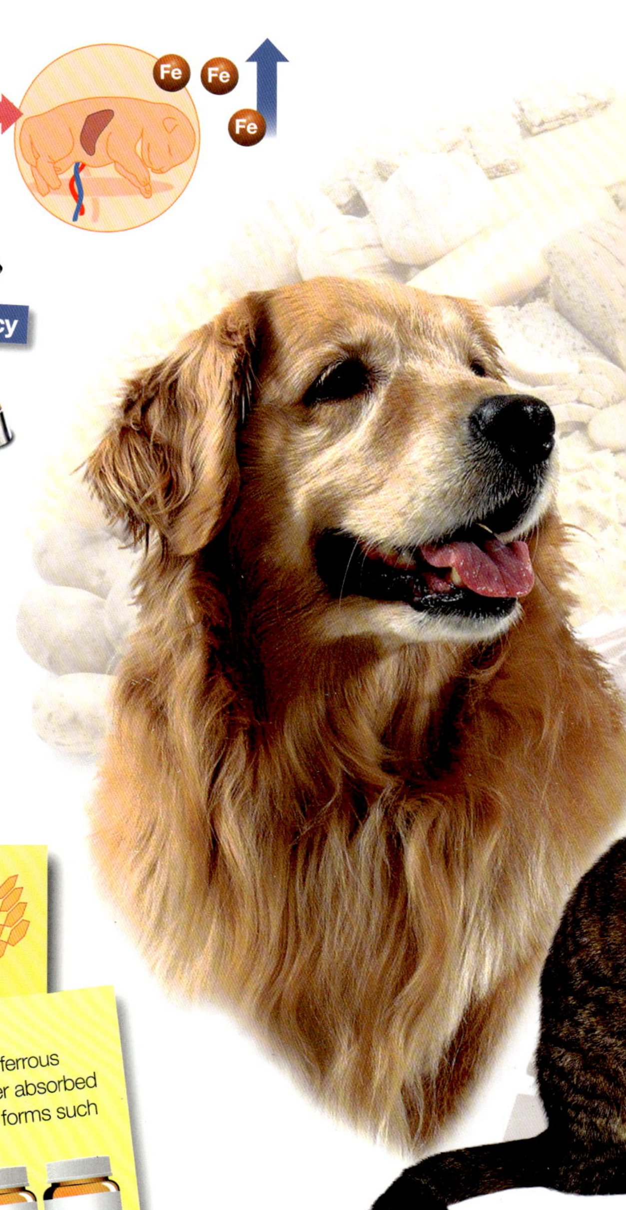

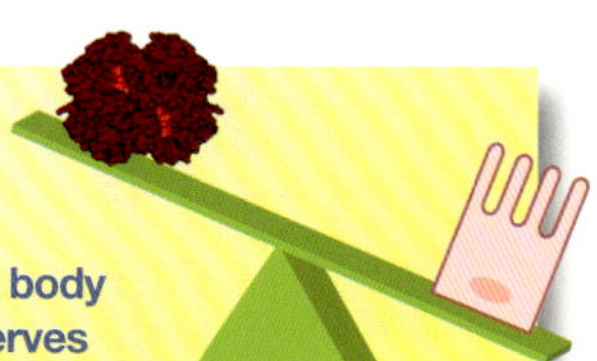

Iron body reserves
Intestinal absorption is lower as organic iron reserves (in the form of heme) increase.

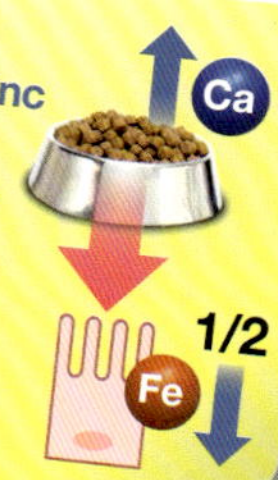

Calcium, phosphorus, zinc and copper concentrations in the diet
For example, iron uptake can be reduced by half by calcium supplements.

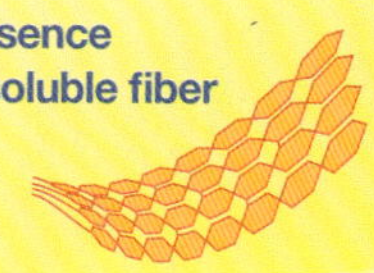

Presence of soluble fiber

Types of supplements
Some supplements, e.g., iron in ferric form, ferrous chloride and ferric pyrophosphate, are better absorbed (bioavailability higher than 60 %) than other forms such as ferric oxide and carbonate.

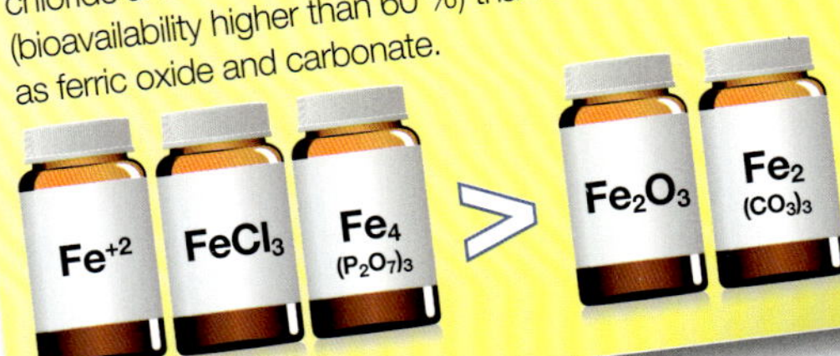

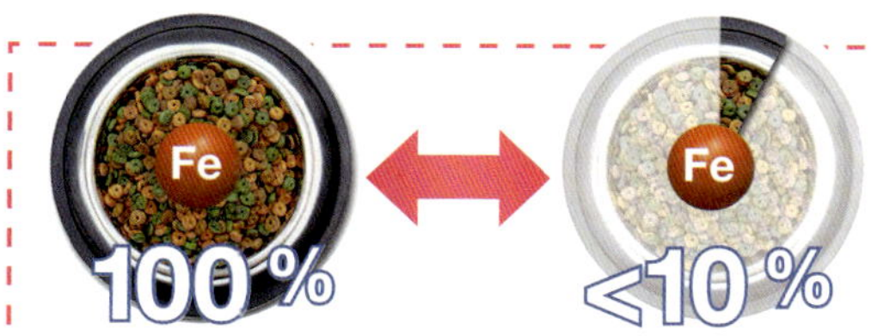

- ✔ The body concentration of **copper** is very low; the main body reserve is bound to proteins in the liver. It is a cofactor of several enzymes that participate in oxidation reactions.
- ✔ As in the previous case, its bioavailability depends on several factors and varies from 30 % to 75 %.

A deficiency in copper causes abortions, fetal malformations (syndactyly and craniofacial deformations) and cerebral dysgenesis.

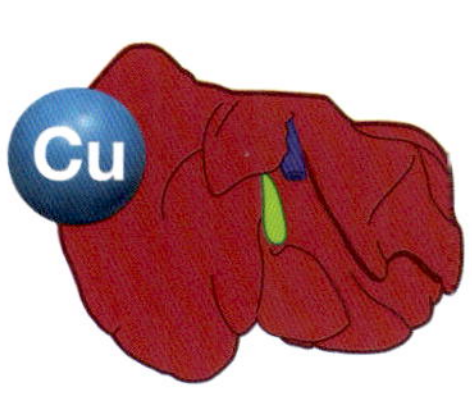

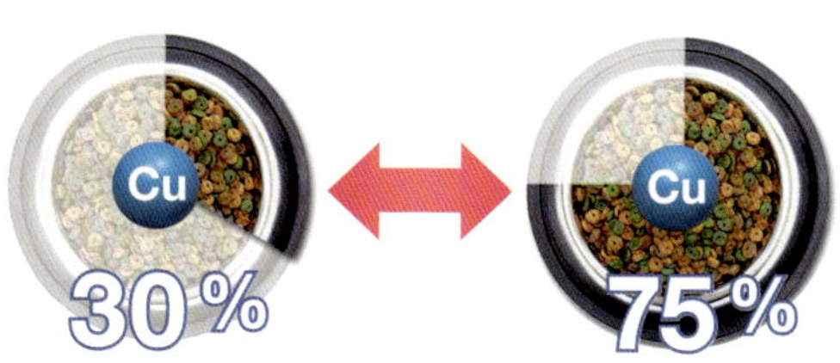

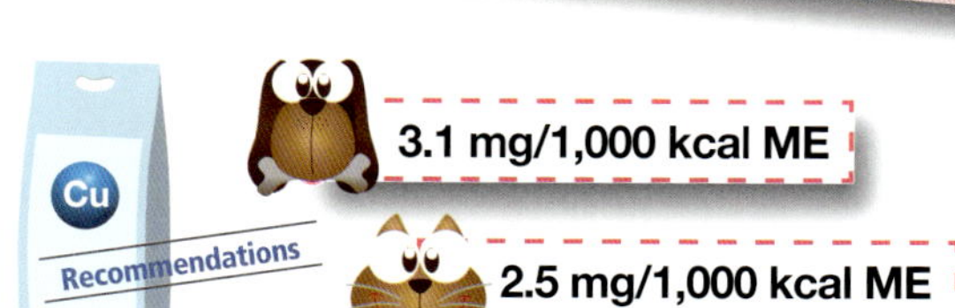

and vitamins

2 Calcium and phosphorus

Calcium and phosphorus requirements only vary in the last third of pregnancy due to fetal bone development. It is very important to avoid diets containing excessive calcium during pregnancy (prevention of peripartum preeclampsia). That is why a calcium:phosphorus ratio of 1:1 to 1.5:1 must be ensured.

Ca Recommendations
- Dog: 1.9–2.5 g/1,000 kcal ME*
- Cat: 1.9 g/1,000 kcal ME

P Recommendations
- Dog: 1.2–2.25 g/1,000 kcal ME*
- Cat: 1.2 g/1,000 kcal ME

*Including giant breeds.

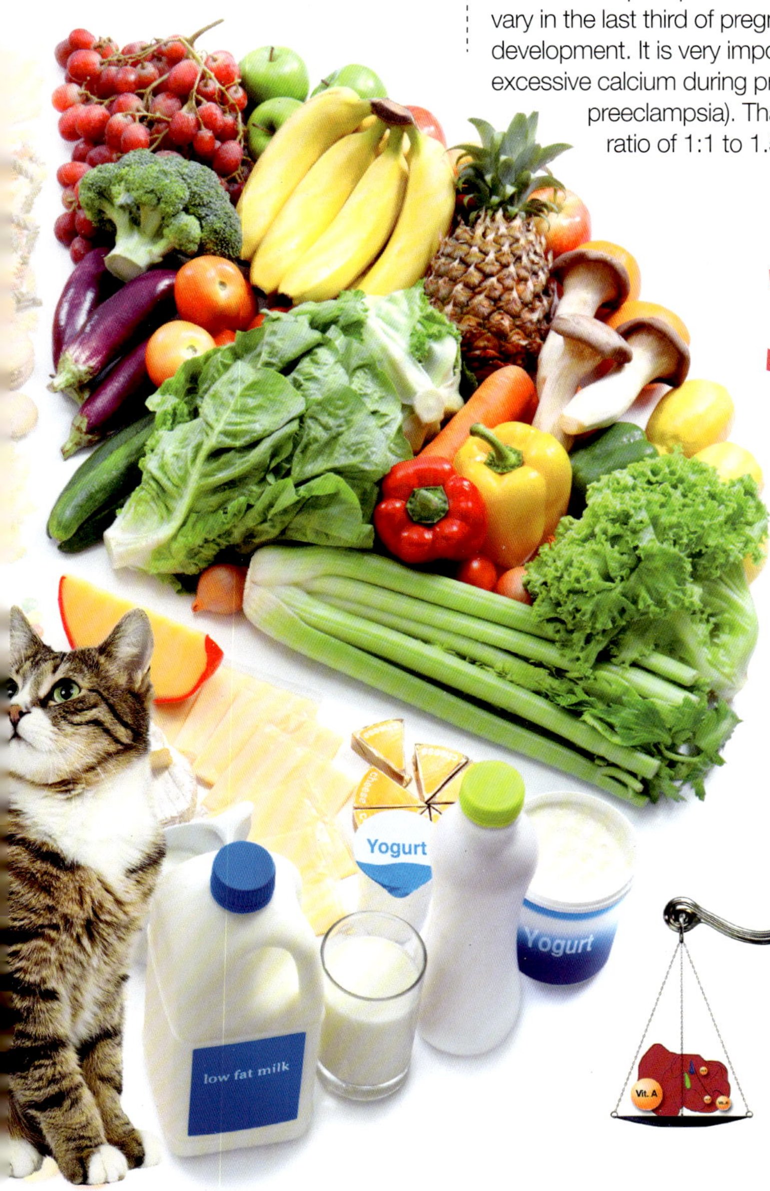

3 Vitamin A

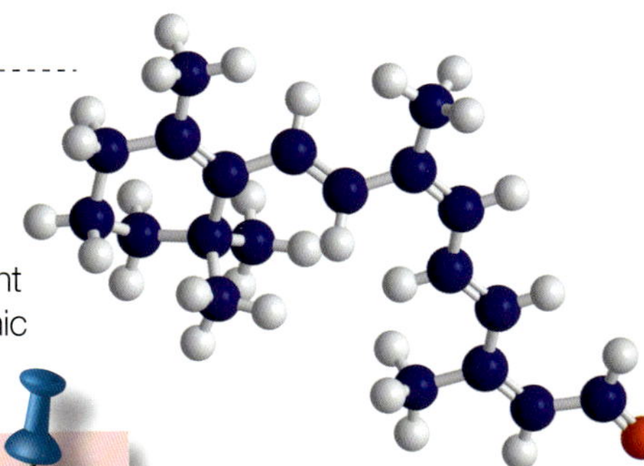

✔ Vitamin A is one of the nutrients that plays a major role in morphogenesis, as there are many vitamin A-dependent receptors and proteins in the embryonic tissue.

Be careful with vitamin A excesses!

Taking into account that it has a high digestibility (80–90 %) and that it is stored in high concentrations in the liver (30–60 % of the vitamin A absorbed is stored), an excessive intake of this vitamin during pregnancy causes teratogenic abnormalities.

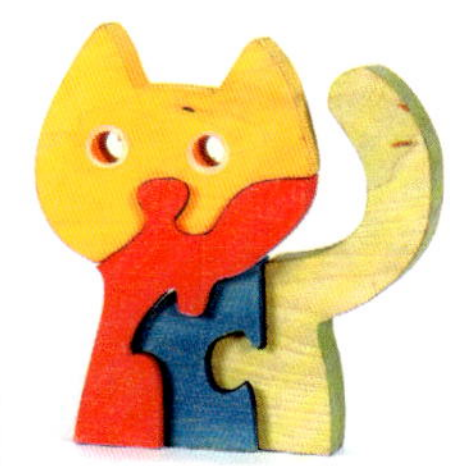

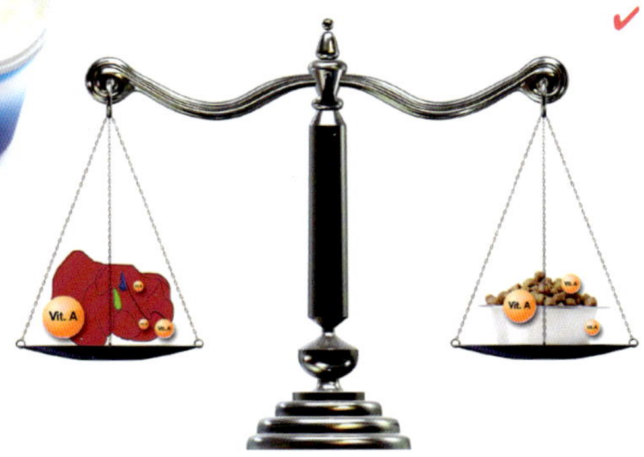

✔ The requirements for this vitamin are determined by the balance between vitamin A reserves in the liver and its presence in the diet. Although no quantitative studies on this vitamin are available, 300-500 µg in queens and 379 µg in bitches (per 1,000 kcal ME) seem appropriate for pregnancy. The safe upper limit for this vitamin is 10 times higher than the recommendations.

Vit. A Recommendations
- Dog: 379 µg/1,000 kcal ME
- Cat: 300–500 µg/1,000 kcal ME

4 Vitamin and mineral requirements

The following table summarizes the requirements (according to the NRC, AAFCO and FEDIAF) of some minerals and vitamins during pregnancy. The requirements for those that do not appear are similar to those of adult animals in maintenance.

	Nutrient/1,000 kcal ME		
	Unit	Bitch	Queen
Calcium	g	1.9	2.5–2.7
Phosphorus	g	1.2	1.9–2.1
Sodium	g	0.5	0.4–0.67
Chloride	g	0.75	0.75–1
Magnesium	g	0.15	0.125
Copper	mg	3.1	2.2
Iodine	µg	220	450
Vitamin A	µg	379	500–675
Vitamin D	µg	3.4	1.75–4.68
Vitamin B_6 (pyridoxin)	mg	0.375	0.625–1.0

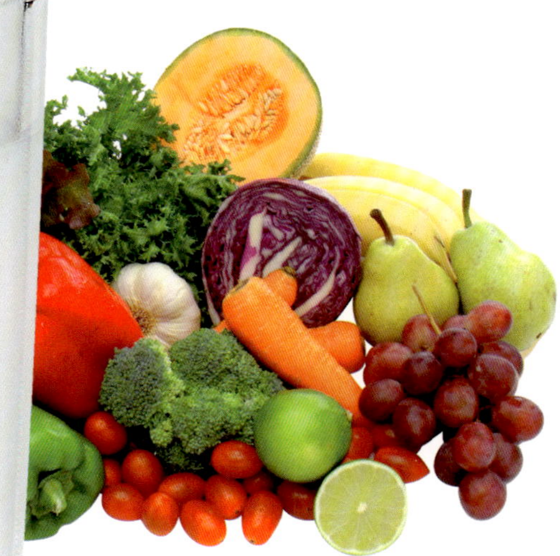

Feeding management for pathologies

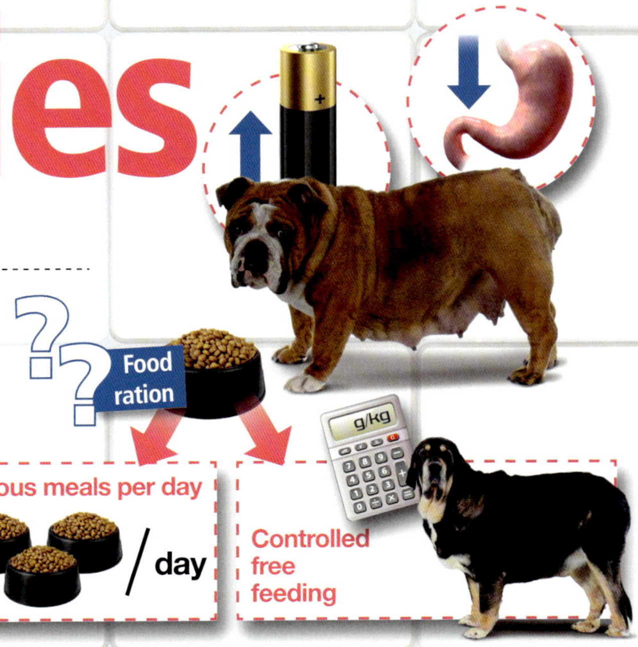

1 Feeding system

Two factors determine the feeding system for pregnant females:

- ✔ **Increase in the daily energy requirements.**
- ✔ **Decrease in the storage capacity of the gastrointestinal system** as a consequence of the development of fetuses and appendages.

For this reason, once the daily ration is calculated, there are two options:

- ✔ **Offer various meals throughout the day:** 2 to 3 daily meals.
- ✔ **Controlled free feeding.** This option is ideal for giant breed dogs (for example: Great Danes).

Incorrect practice can result in pathologies

Some incorrect practices in food management may cause certain pathologies in pregnant or lactating females. This involves two processes: **peri-partum hypoglycemia** and **pre/post-partum eclampsia**.

Gestational hypoglycemia

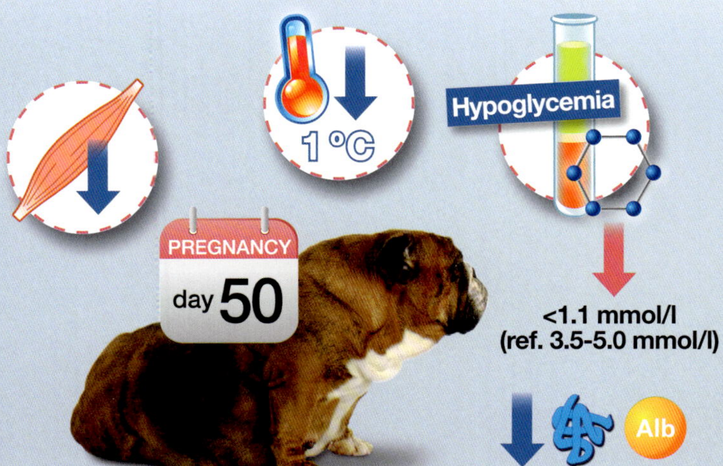

Symptoms

- ✔ Infrequent acute process described in full-term female dogs (after day 50).
- ✔ Neurological symptoms: muscle weakness 48 hours before the clinical condition appears, lack of response to stimuli, clonic spasms (especially of the jaw) and general collapse.
- ✔ The body temperature reduces by one degree. There are no changes to the respiratory or heart rates.
- ✔ It is sometimes confused with eclampsia and treated as such, but the results are not satisfactory.
- ✔ Blood values: marked hypoglycemia, with rates under 1.1 mmol/l (reference 3.5-5.0 mmol/l) and ketonemia. Also hypoproteinemia and hypoalbuminemia. The rest of the biochemical and electrolyte values are normal.

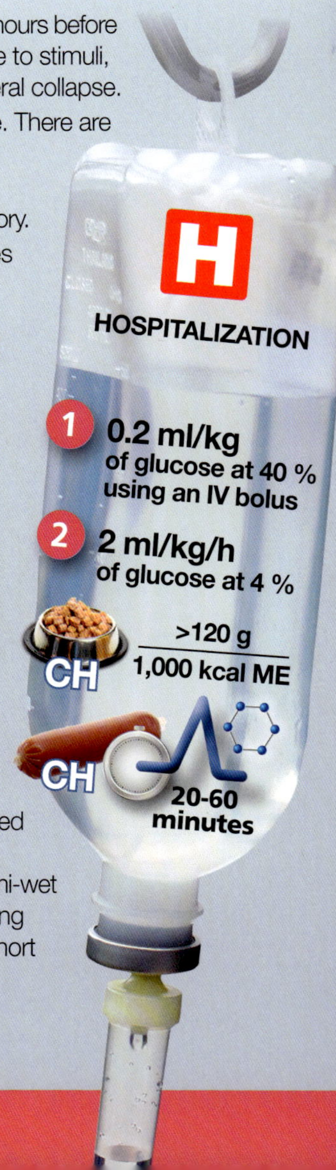

Possible causes

The possible causes are not well defined, but various hypotheses have been proposed:

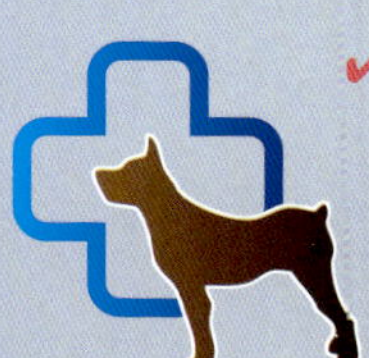

- ✔ Poor management of the pregnant female's diet:
  - Changes to the frequency of feeding.
  - Inadequate diets: high energy foods, rich in fat and poor in carbohydrates (without compensating with protein).
- ✔ Poor body condition during pregnancy.
- ✔ Uterine atony.

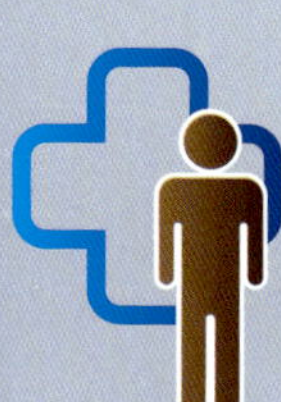

Other options are offered in human medicine as well: forced fasting, fatty liver degeneration, insulinoma, and hyperadrenocorticism.

Treatment

- ✔ This is an urgent condition that requires hospitalization.
- ✔ As a first step, we can administer 0.2 ml/kg of a glucose solution at 40 % in an IV bolus. The muscular condition improves in a few minutes. Afterwards, we can use saline solution with 4 % glucose at a velocity of 2 ml/kg/hour, monitoring glycemia levels.
- ✔ Wet, carbohydrate-rich food can then be offered with values greater than 120 g/1,000 kcal ME (for example, foods for hepatic diseases), or semi-wet food, as it uses simple carbohydrates as binding elements and produces a glucose peak in a short period of time (20-60 minutes).

pregnant pets and possible

2 Nutritional profile

- A complete and balanced food for maintenance is valid the first 4 weeks of pregnancy, but after this time, one that is specific for pregnancy should be used. These goods do not exist on the market as such (they are not recognized by legislation) and thus we must use a food meant for growth periods.
- The energy density should be greater than 4.3 Mcal/kg DM, with a high digestibility.
- The use of vitamin or mineral supplements, or calcium-rich raw materials (cheese or powdered milk) is not recommended.
- The palatability of the ration may need to be increased at times along with improving the ingestion of the food to counter any hyporexia/anorexia in females.
- Fresh and clean water should be available at all times.

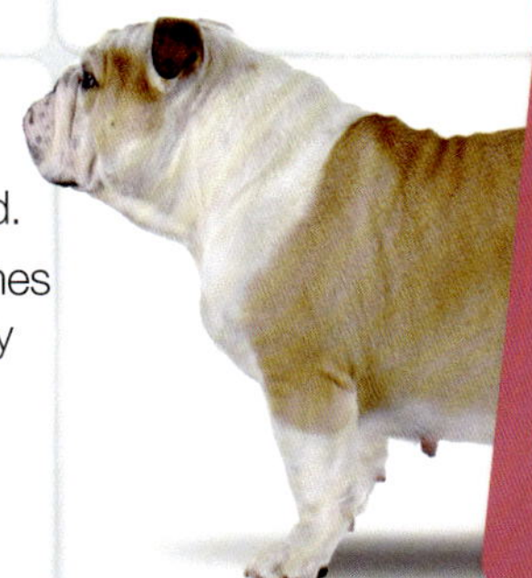

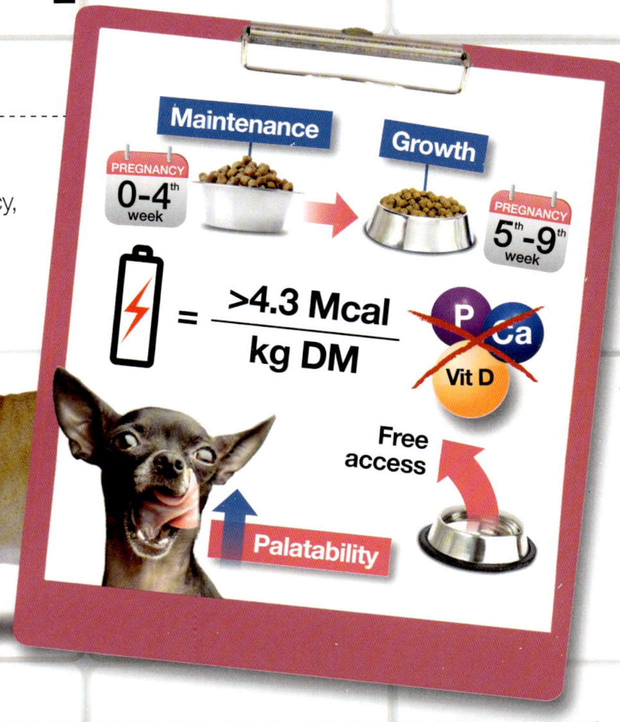

Puerperal eclampsia adasd

- Puerperal eclampsia is an acute, life-threatening process that affects female dogs in the 3rd-4th weeks of lactation, and in female cats during the last 2 weeks of pregnancy. Small-breed female dogs and large litters are predisposing factors. The table summarizes the clinical condition:

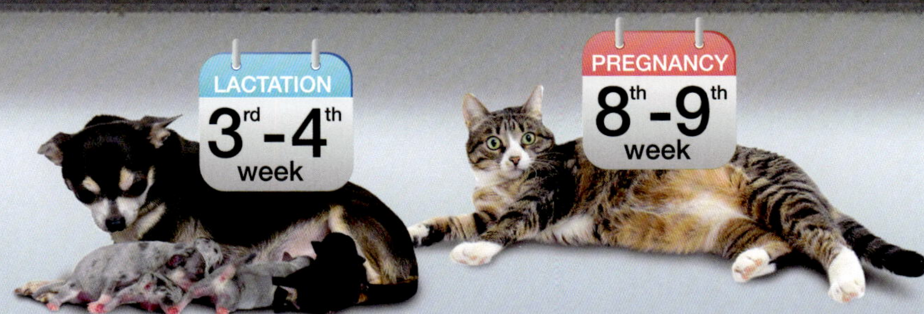

Presentation	Common	Rare
Moment	Lactation peak	Full-term pregnancy
Diagnosis: total calcium	<6.5 mg/dl	<6 mg/dl
Diagnosis: ionized calcium	<0.8 mmol/l	0.77-1.27 mmol/l
Nervous system	Excitation, aggressiveness, epilepsy	Lethargy, weakness
Cardiovascular	Tachycardia	Bradycardia
Respiratory	Panting	Dyspnea
Temperature	Hyperthermia	Hypothermia
Glycemia	Normal	Hypoglycemia

Treatment			
Emergency		Diazepam (1-5 mg IV). 0.22-0.44 ml calcium gluconate at 10 % IV for 10-30 minutes. Do not use corticosteroids.	
Stable patient	Phase I	0.5-1.5 ml solution 10 % Ca/kg IV every 6-8 h	2.5 ml solution 10 % Ca/kg IV every 6-8 h
	Phase II	50 % of calcium gluconate solution at 10 % + SS at 0.9 %, administered subcutaneously, three times per day. Calcemia monitoring	
Preventive		25-55 mg Ca/kg/day	50-100 mg Ca/kg/day
		Some cases require vitamin D: 10,000-20,000 IU/day	

- Muscular irritability is due to an ion imbalance: the lack of calcium increases sodium permeability in the nerve cells, altering the action potential.

Possible causes

- Calcium and vitamin D supplements during pregnancy.
- Low-calcium diets or those with a calcium imbalance: meat-based supplements (rich in phosphorus and low in calcium).
- Loss of calcium during ossification of the fetuses.
- Large losses through lactation to the puppies or kittens.

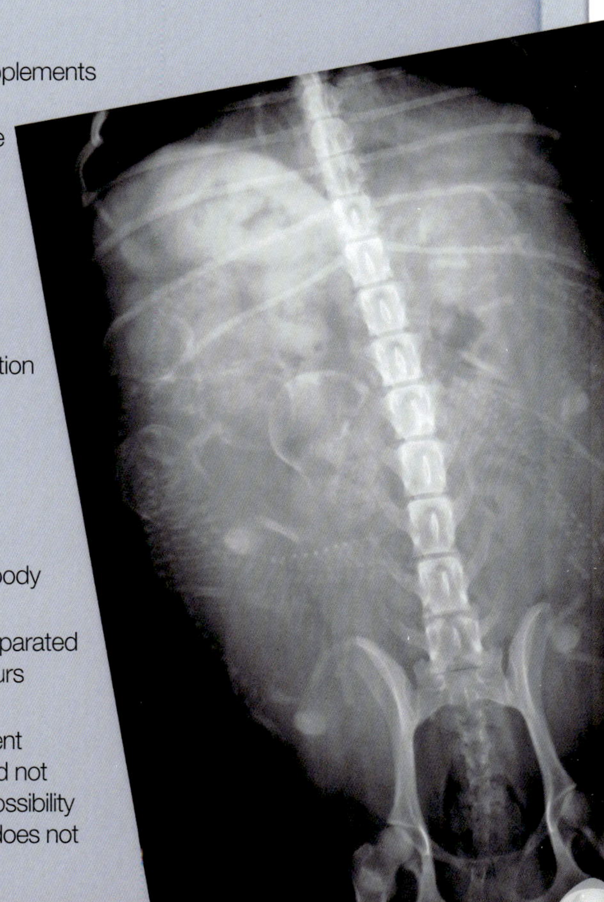

Treatment

- Urgent clinical treatment must be initiated, with electrocardiographic and body temperature monitoring.
- The entire litter must be separated from the mother for 48 hours or indefinitely.
- The female dogs that present this type of condition should not reproduce given that the possibility of recurrence is high. This does not happen in female cats.

Females in lactation:

Lactation is one of the processes that requires most nutrients. It is comparable to growth and is only exceeded by specific sports situations. At this stage, a female's dietary requirements depend directly on her milk production, which, in turn, depends on the size of the litter.

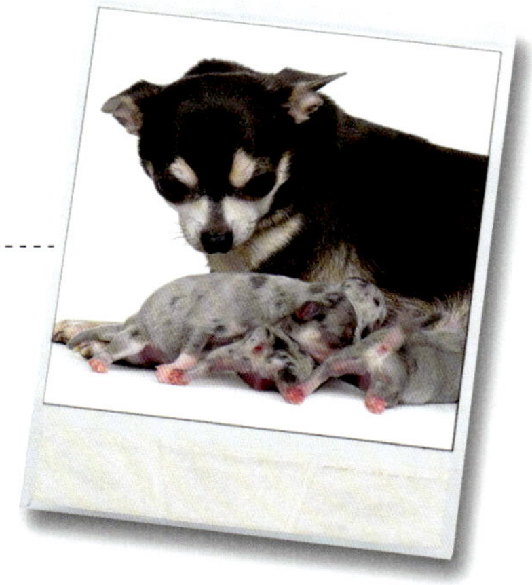

1 Colostrum

- The secretion of colostrum, which is very important for newborn animals, occurs in the first 36–72 hours postpartum.
- Its composition is different from that of milk: it has a higher dry matter and protein content (especially immunoglobulins and in particular IgG, with a concentration of 3.2 g/100 ml) and also contains more fat, non-fatty solids, vitamins and minerals.
- Ig are absorbed in the jejunum by endocytosis and released entirely in the lamina propria. This only lasts for 12–24 hours.
  The period of immunoglobulin absorption is shorter in cats than in dogs.
  There are currently no good colostrum replacers available as their IgG content is usually very low.

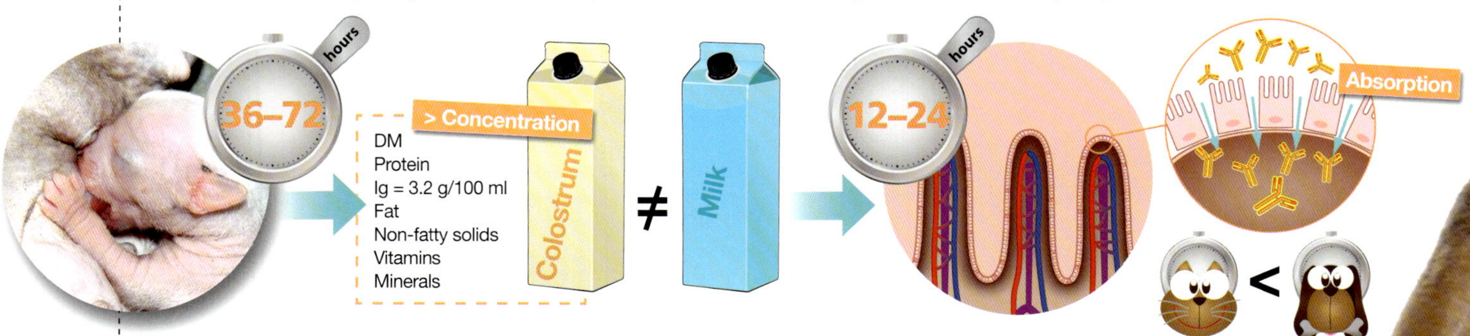

- The functions of colostrum can be summarized as:

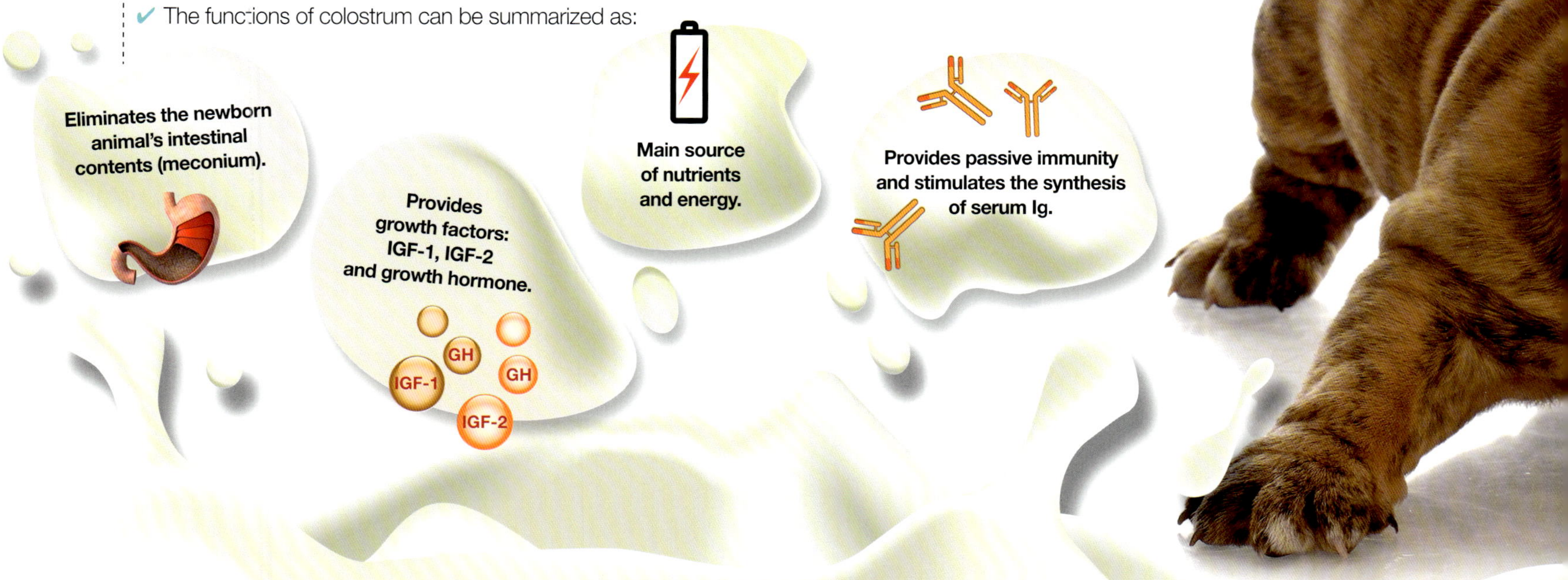

3 Energy requirements during lactation

- As in pregnant females, energy is considered as the main limiting factor.
- Bitches increase their food intake to meet the requirements of lactation.
  Giant dog breeds are particularly sensitive to poor nutrition at this stage.
  Queens use the body reserves they have accumulated during pregnancy.

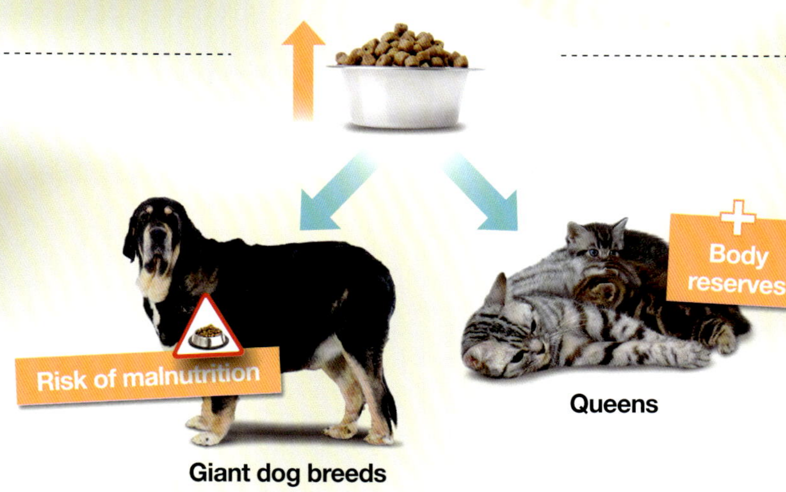

colostrum and milk

2 Mother's milk composition

- After colostrum, the composition of the dam's milk is stable, and its quantity and quality depend directly on the composition of the diet and lactation curve.
- The lactation period lasts about 7 weeks in queens and bitches, with a peak at weeks 3 and 4.

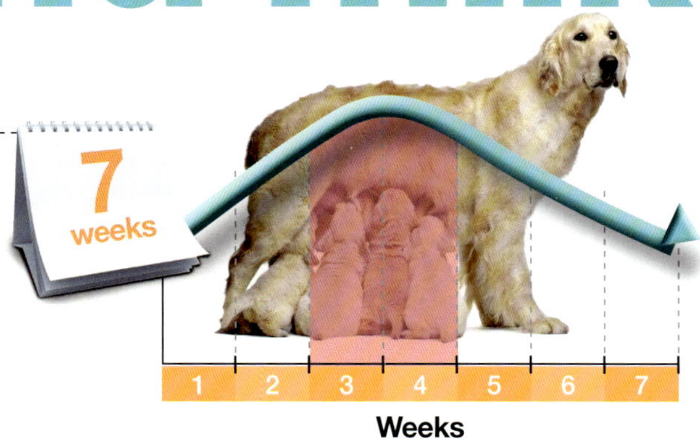

Milk production depends on the dam's body weight.

	Composition of milk (as food)			
	DM	Protein	Fat	Energy (kcal/100 g)
Cow	12.3	3.3	3.5	74
Bitch/queen	21–23	7.5	9	146

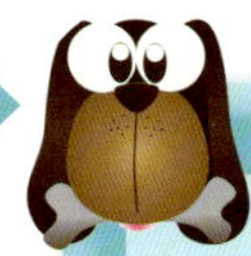

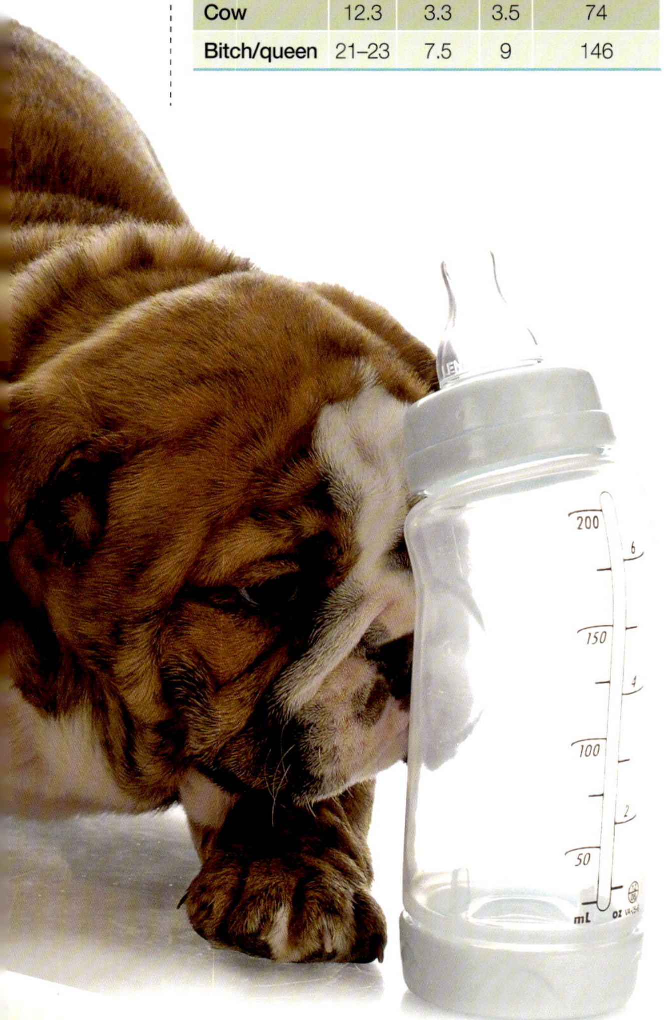

Milk production is equivalent to 3 % of the dam's weight in the first weeks, but it reaches 8 % of her weight during peak lactation, the same value as in cows. This means a 12-kg bitch will produce approximately 0.9 litres/day at peak lactation.

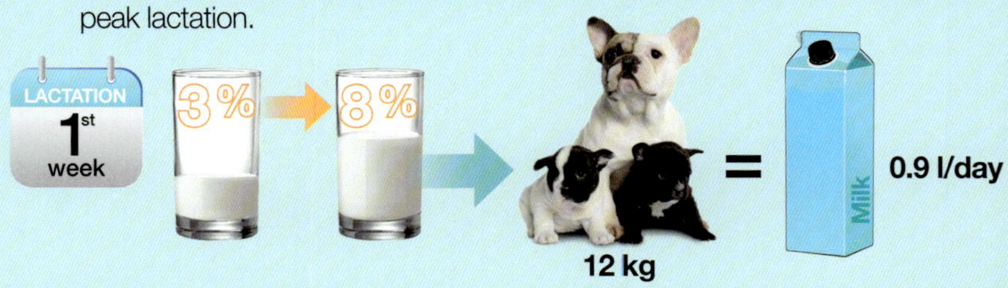

However, the time necessary to double the weight of the newborn animal is 50 days in cows, but 9 days in cats and dogs. This indicates that milk does not have the same composition depending on the species (see table on the left).

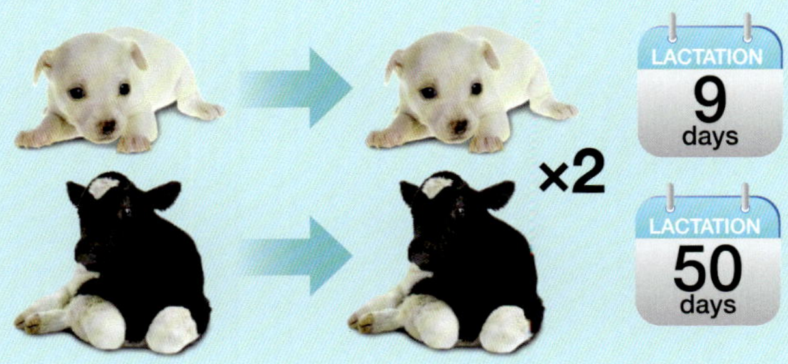

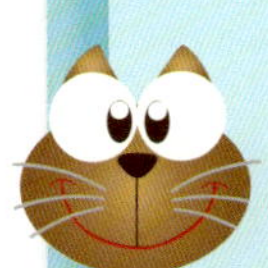

In the first week of lactation, milk production is equivalent to approximately 1–3 % of the queen's weight. It then increases to reach 6 % at peak lactation, when it starts to decline until weaning.

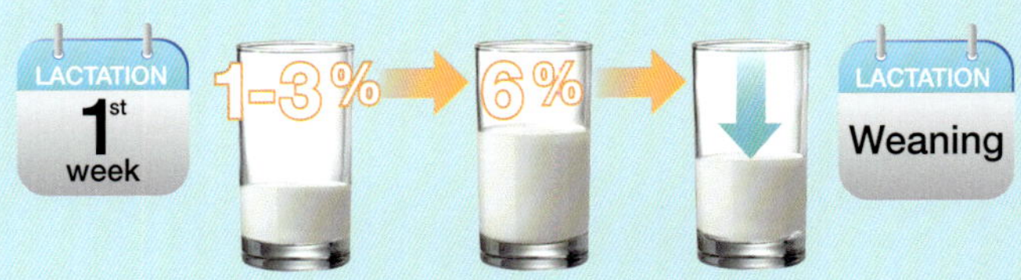

- Energy needs during lactation progressively increase, and reach a peak in the **3rd–5th** week, when the DER are twice or three times the maintenance needs. Production decreases from the 5th week on. In general, and taking MER as a reference, energy needs vary with each week of lactation as shown in the table below.

	Week of lactation							
	1st	2nd	3rd	4th	5th	6th	7th	8th
	× MER							
Bitches	×1.5	×2	×3	×3	×3	×2.5	×2	×1.25
Queens	×1.76	×2	×2.15	×2.2	×3	×3.5	×2	×1.25

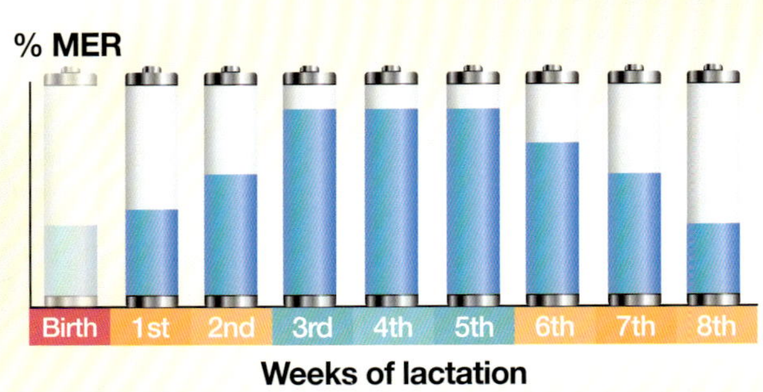

- Dietary requirements at this stage can be determined more precisely. They are divided by species in the following pages.

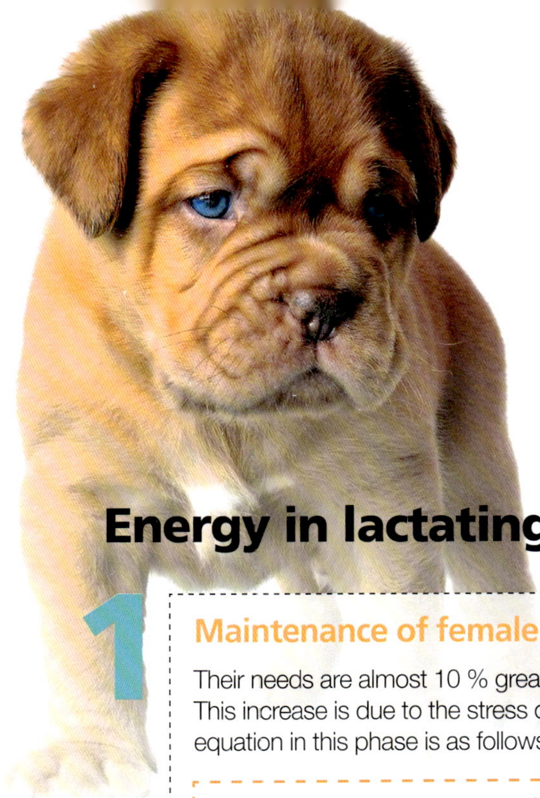

Energy during lactation (I)

Energy in lactating female dogs

1 Maintenance of female dogs during lactation

Their needs are almost 10 % greater than those of maintenance (MER). This increase is due to the stress caused by raising their litter. The prediction equation in this phase is as follows:

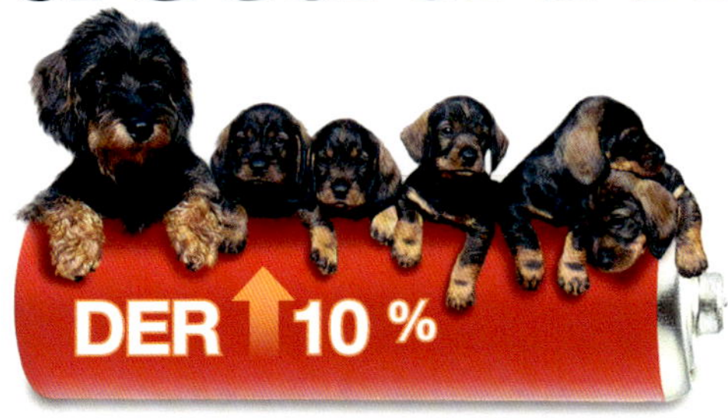

$$DER_{\text{maintenance during lactation}}\ (\text{kcal ME/day}) = 145 \times BW\ (\text{kg})^{0.75}$$

Or similarly:

$$DER = MER \times 1.1$$

2 Requirements for the production of milk

The requirements are conditioned by the quantity and composition of the milk, lactation week, the number of puppies and the weight of the female.

There are three options:

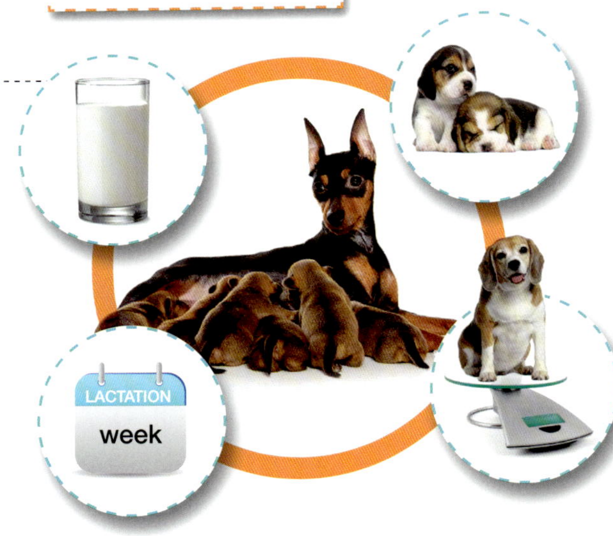

Method 1 In this case, we take into account the **number of puppies** and the **lactation week**.

$$DER_{\text{milk production}}\ (\text{kcal ME/day}) = BW \times (24\,n + 12\,m) \times LW$$

Where:

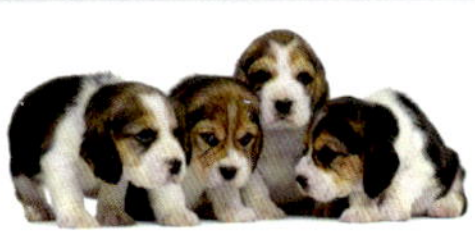

n = no. of puppies up to 4 (inclusive).

m = no. of puppies from 5 to 8 (inclusive) but with the previous sum of n. For example, 7 puppies is n = 4 + m = 3.

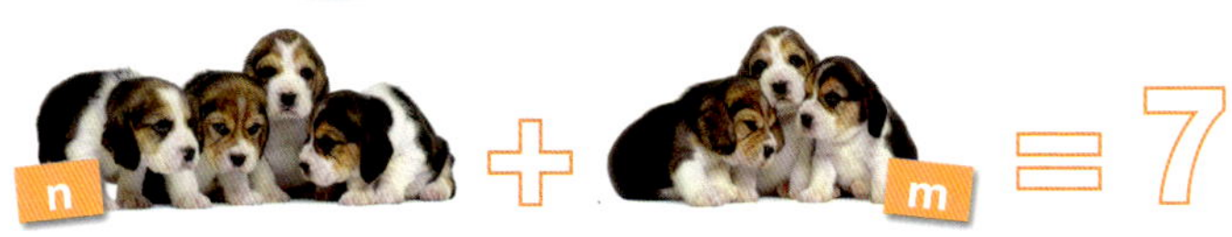

LW = correction factor regarding the lactation week. The LW values vary with the week:

1st week	2nd week	3rd week	4th week
0.75	0.95	1.1	1.2

Method 2 We estimate that the requirements for the production of milk represent a **25 % increase for every puppy of the litter** over the maintenance requirements of the mother.

↑ 25 %/ puppy

$$DER_{\text{milk production}} = DER_{\text{maintenance during lactation}} + 25\,\%\,n$$

n = number of puppies.

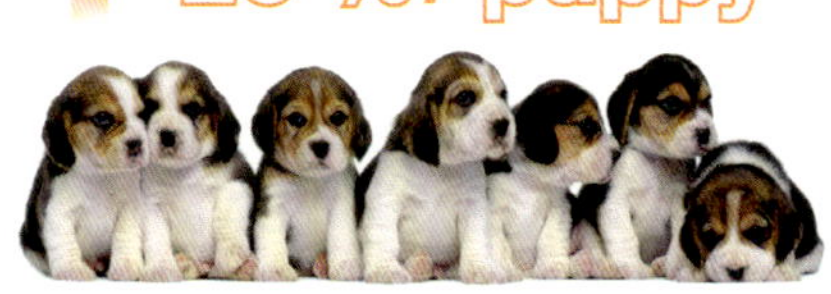

Method 3 We calculate the liters of milk produced in the curve (MP), taking into account the body weight of the female dog, the number of puppies and the phase of the lactation curve. Once we have calculated this, we estimate its energy concentration. The equations is as follows:

$$MP_{\text{up to day 45}}\ (\text{liters}) = (BW\ (\text{kg}) \times K) + [(n - 4) \times (0.1 \times BW)]$$

$$MP_{\text{production peak (3rd to 4th week)}}\ (\text{l/week}) = (MP_{\text{up to day 45}} \times 0.04) \times 7$$

n = no. of puppies.

K = correction factor for the breed (size) of the female.

Take three values: K = 1.6 in females <8 kg. K = 1.8 in females from 8 to 25 kg. K = 2 in females >25 kg.

Energy requirements in lactating female dogs

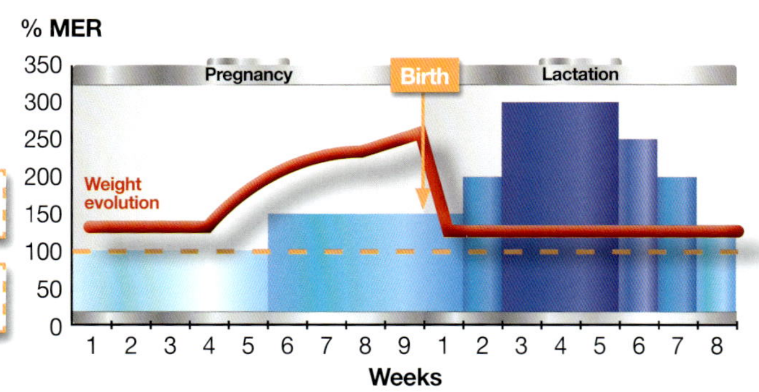

requirements

Examples

What are this animal's energy requirements?

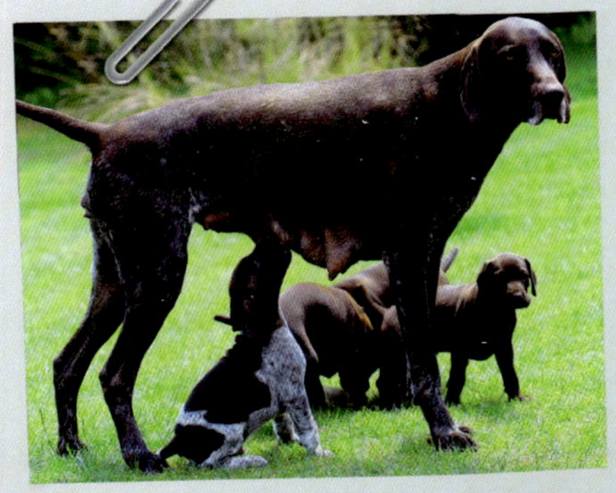

German short hair

Weight: 32 kg after delivery
Lactation: 3rd week
Litter: 5 puppies

1 Requirements for maintenance during lactation

$$DER_{maintenance\ during\ lactation}\ (kcal\ ME/day) = 145 \times BW\ (kg)^{0.75}$$

$$DER_{M\ during\ lactation} = MER \times 32^{0.75} = 1{,}950.88\ kcal\ ME/day$$

2 Requirements for the production of milk

Method 1

$$DER_{milk\ production}\ (kcal\ ME/day) = BW \times (24\ n + 12\ m) \times SL$$

$$DER_{milk\ production} = 32 \times (24 \times 4 + 12 \times 1) \times 1.1 = 3{,}801.60\ kcal\ ME/day$$

$$DER_{lactation} = DER_{M\ during\ lactation} + DER_{milk\ production}$$

$$DER_{lactation} = 1{,}950.88 \times 3{,}801.60 = 5{,}752.48\ kcal\ ME/day$$

Method 2

$$DER_{milk\ production} = DER_{maintenance\ during\ lactation} + 25\ \%\ n$$

$$DER_{milk\ production} = 1{,}950.88 + 487.72 \times 5 = 4{,}389.48\ kcal\ ME/day$$

Method 3 Based on the total production of milk

$$MP_{up\ to\ day\ 45}\ (liters) = (BW\ (kg) \times K) + [(n - 4) \times (0.1 \times BW)]$$

$$MP_{production\ peak\ (3rd\ to\ 4th\ week)}\ (l/week) = (MP_{up\ to\ day\ 45} \times 0.04) \times 7$$

$$MP_{until\ day\ 45} = (32 \times 2) + [(5 - 4) \times (0.1 \times 32)] = 67.2\ liters$$

$$MP_{production\ peak\ (3rd\ to\ 4th\ week)} = (67.2 \times 0.04) \times 7 = 18.82\ liters$$

$$MP_{total} = 86.02\ liters$$

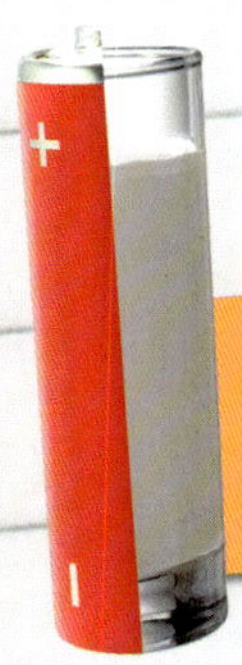

$$DER_{lactation} = 1{,}950.88 + 4{,}485 = 6{,}436\ kcal\ ME/day$$

Energy from the milk = 1,460 kcal/liter
Energy from the milk (kcal/day) = 1,460 kcal/l × 86.02 l/28 days*
Energy from the milk (kcal/day) = 4,485 kcal/day

*Lactation peak, calculated with the maximum production.

As we can see, the differences between one and the other are relatively large. The first of the three methods is the most reliable as it takes into account the week of lactation and the number of puppies in the litter.

Energy during lactation (II)

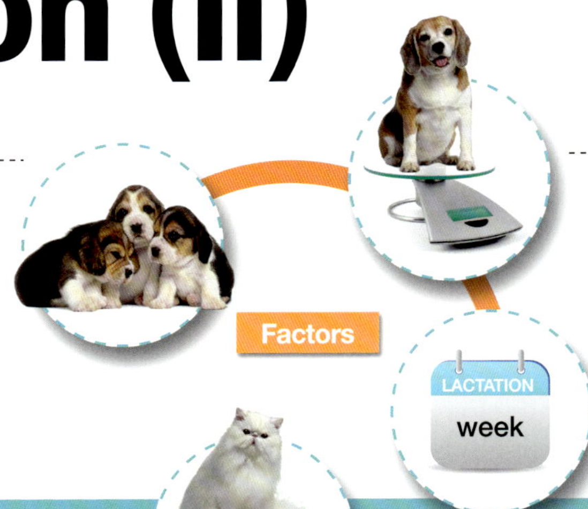

1 Simple method to calculate energy for female dogs

The simplest method to evaluate the energy requirements for female dogs is based on the modifications to the MER. The table summarizes the recommendations. Factors including the female's weight, the week of lactation, and the size of the litter have been taken into account to create the table. Its calculation may not be precise, but its purpose is useful for daily clinical practice.

Energy in lactating female cats

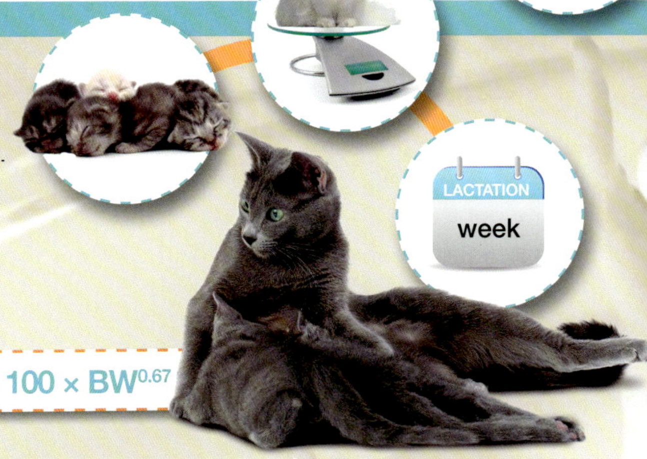

2 Calculation and example

The daily energy requirements in lactating female cats depends on the body weight at the time bred, the number of offspring and the lactation week, and they can be calculated using the following equation.

$$DER_{lactation}\ (kcal\ ME/day) = MER + nK \times BW \times LW$$

$$MER = 100 \times BW^{0.67}$$

Where:

LW Take different values depending on the lactation week:

1st-2nd week	3rd-4th week	5th week	6th week	7th week
0.9	1.2	1.1	1.0	0.8

nK Take different values depending on the number of offspring:

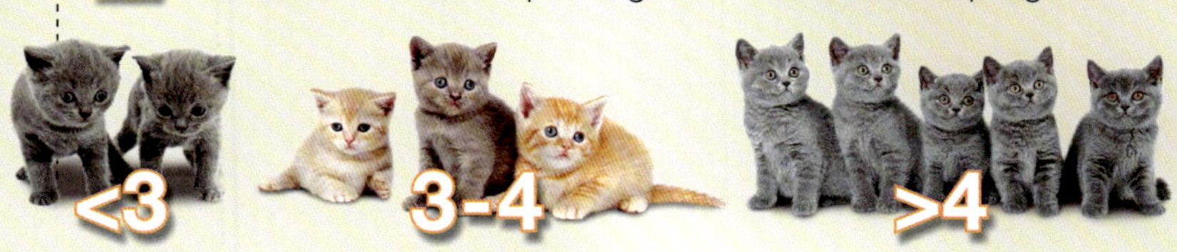

nK = 18 | nK = 60 | nK = 70

Energy requirements in lactating female cats

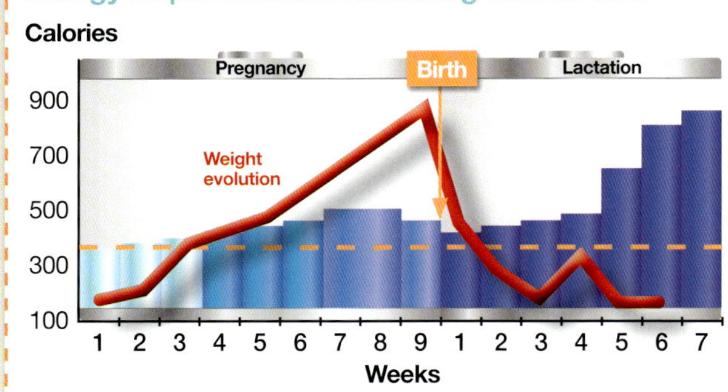

3 Various meals per day

- As the calorie requirements during this stage are very high and the digestive capacity is limited, it is recommended that several meals, preferably more than four (4-6 times per day), be provided each day.

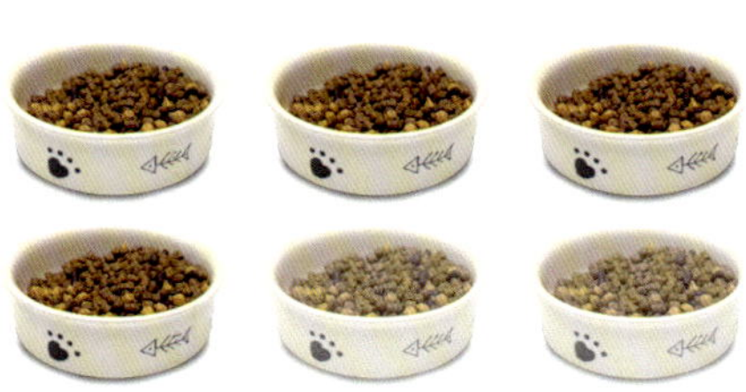

/day

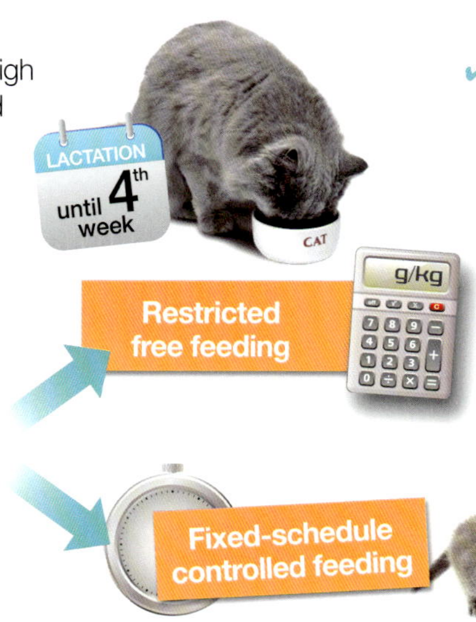

- Restricted free feeding or fixed-schedule controlled feeding systems can be used. The first can be used until the offspring start to show interest in the solid food (at approximately 4 weeks of life): from this moment on, there is competition for the food ration.

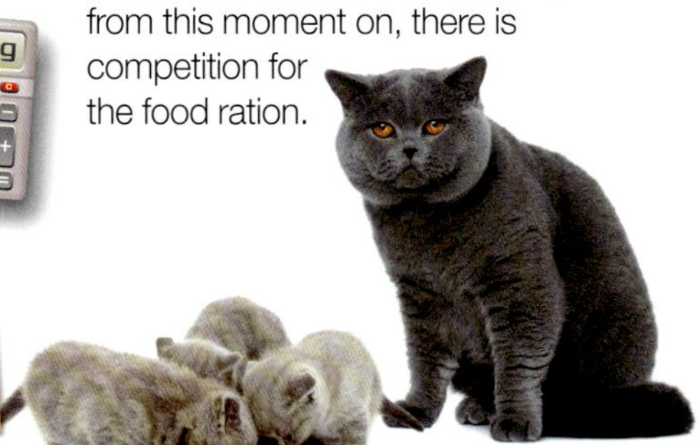

requirements

Week	1st-2nd				3rd-4th			
No. of puppies	2	4	6	8	2	4	6	8
Female dog's weight (kg)	× MER							
<10	1.5	2	2.3	2.6	1.6	2.3	2.8	3.1
10-20	1.5	2.1	2.5	2.8	1.7	2.5	3	3.5
20-30	1.6	2.3	2.7	3	1.8	2.7	3.3	3.8
30-40	1.7	2.4	2.9	3.2	1.8	2.9	3.5	4
40-50	1.7	2.5	3	3.4	1.9	3	3.7	4.2
<50	1.7	2.6	3.1	3.6	2	3.1	3.9	4.5

Following with the previous example (page 23):

$$DER_{lactation} = MER \times 3.5$$

$$DER_{lactation} = (132 \times 32^{0.75}) \times 3.5$$

$$DER_{lactation} = 6{,}215.91 \text{ kcal ME/day}$$

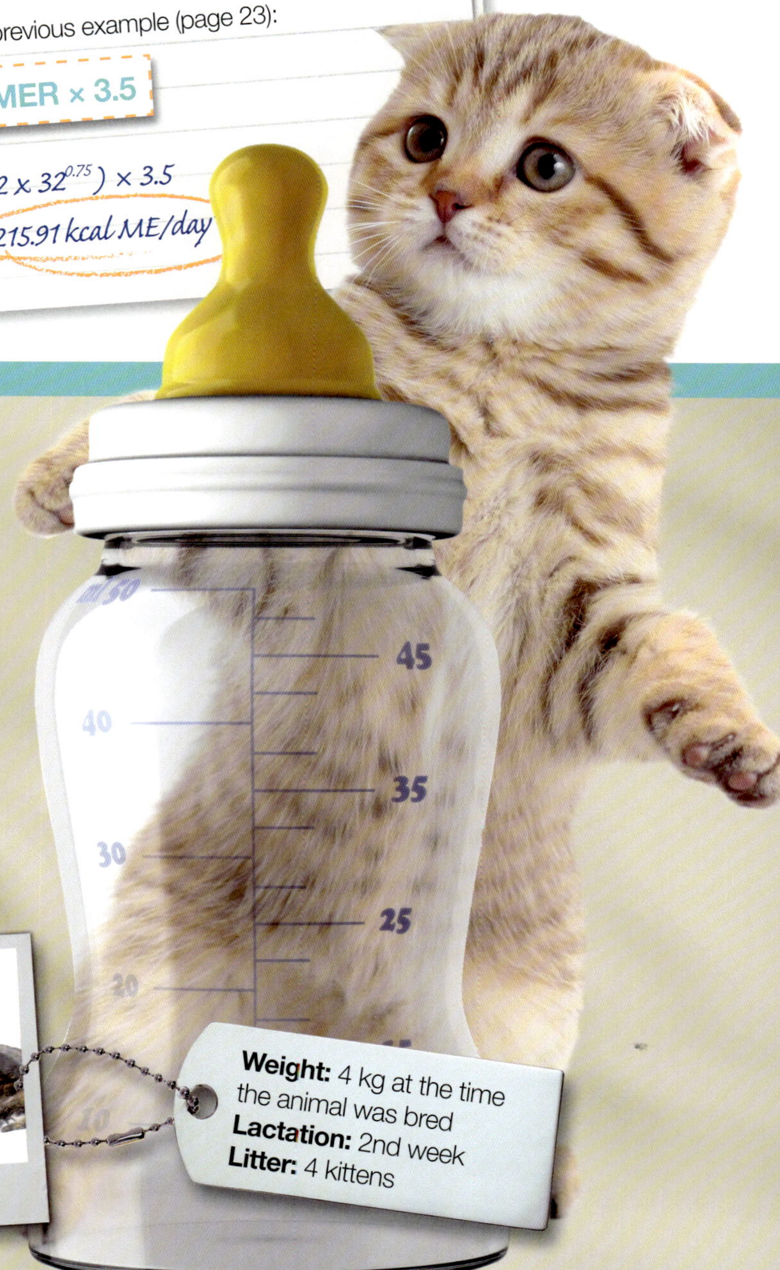

Simplifying the previous equation, we can approximate the requirements during lactation from the MER, depending on the number of puppies or kittens.

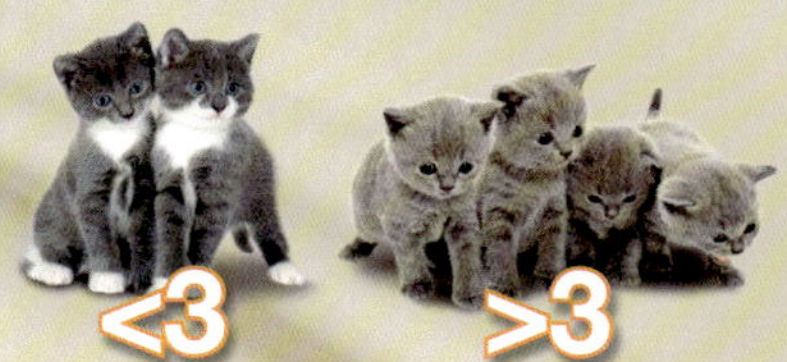

	<3	>3
× MER	1.3	2.1

What are the animal's energy requirements?

$$DER_{lactation}\ (\text{kcal ME/day}) = MER + nK \times BW \times LW$$

$$DER_{lactation} = (100 \times 4^{0.67}) + 60 \times 4 \times 0.9$$

$$DER_{lactation} = 505.15 \text{ kcal ME/day}$$

According to the table:

$$DER_{lactation} = MER \times 2.1 = 531.62 \text{ kcal ME/day}$$

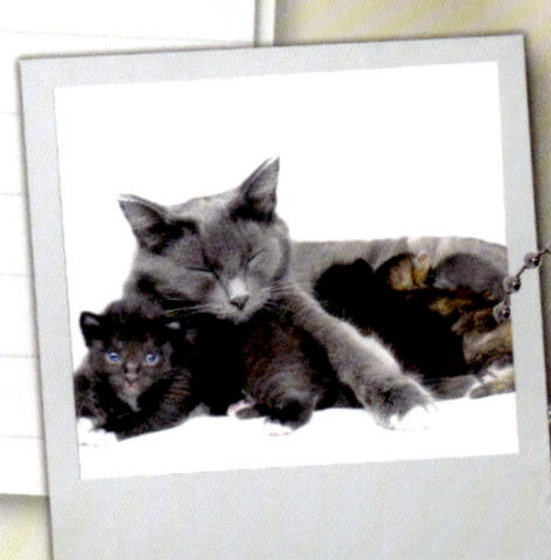

Weight: 4 kg at the time the animal was bred
Lactation: 2nd week
Litter: 4 kittens

4 Weight recovery for the following cycles

- ✔ Female animals should reach their next reproductive cycle with adequate weight and body condition. If the animal has lost large amounts of weight, we must ensure that the characteristics of the food ration and the feeding program during lactation are lengthened for at least 3 weeks after weaning, until the animal once again has adequate nutrient reserves.

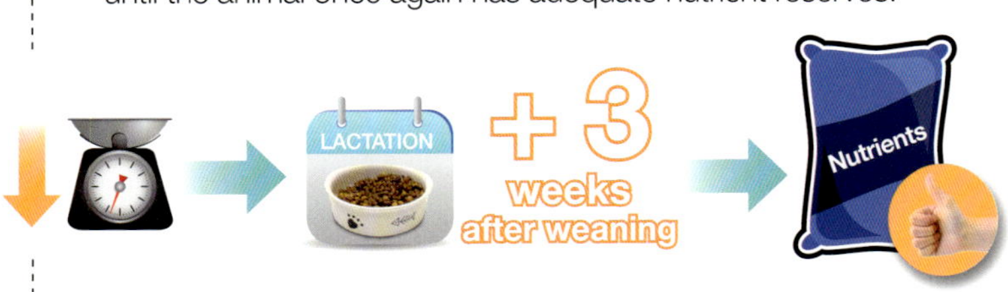

- ✔ During this period, 1.25 to 1.50 × MER is recommended to recover any weight lost. The type of diet should be high in energy (>4.3 Mcal/kg DM) and have a high digestibility of nutrients.

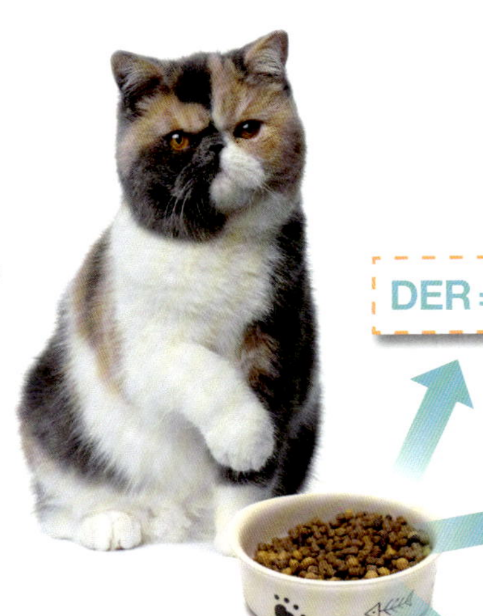

$$DER = MER \times 1.25 \text{ to } 1.50$$

>4.3 Mcal/kg DM

High digestibility

Nutrients and during lactation

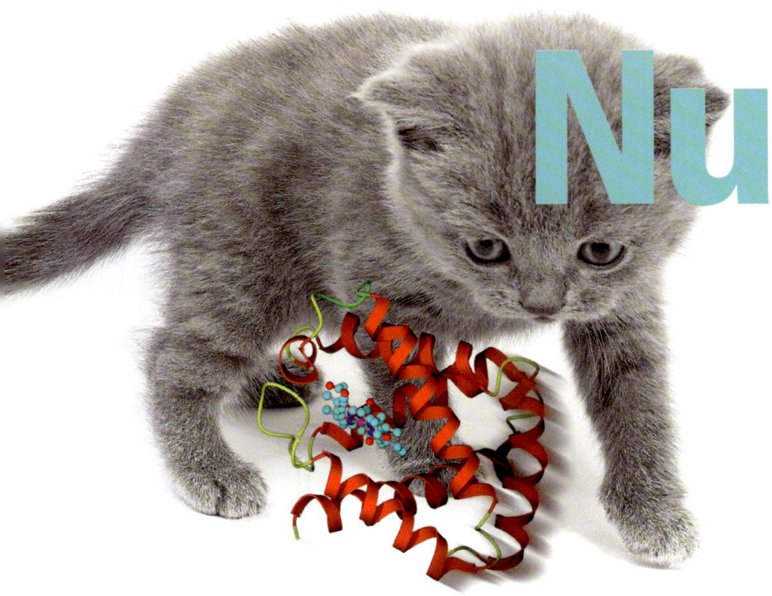

Regarding nutrients, there are no great differences in terms of the requirements for pregnant females. In this section, we will review some of these nutrients.

1 Protein

In cats, recommendations for protein during this phase are increased compared to the requirements for pregnancy and maintenance by 6 % and 50 %, respectively. The recommendations for lactating female cats are 75 g of protein/1,000 kcal ME.

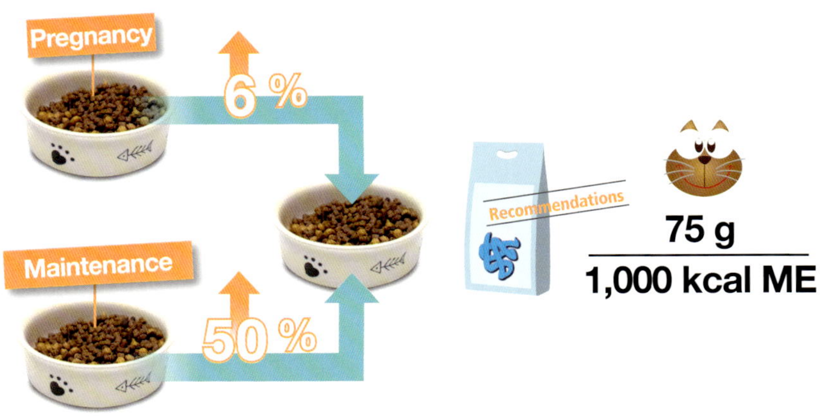

2 Fat and fatty acids

Source of energy for puppies and kittens

Although the NRC recommendations are lower, it is important that the fat levels are high (50 g/1,000 kcal ME) as this increases the concentration of fat in the milk, which benefits newborn puppies and kittens, as they are born with very little fat reserves (<1.5 %). This modification in the energy density of the ration should be accompanied by increasing the rest of the nutrients to ensure a balanced diet.

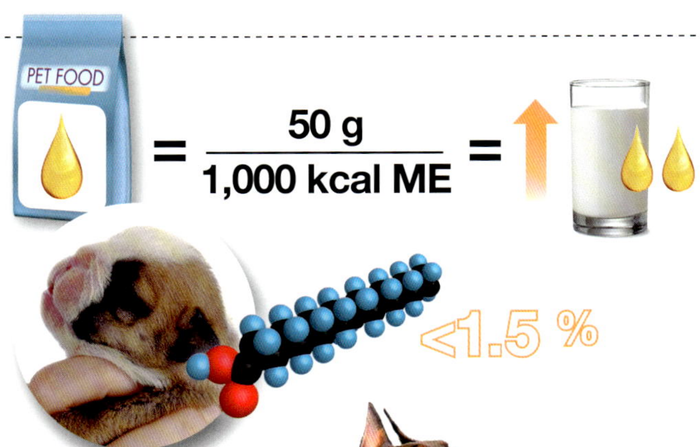

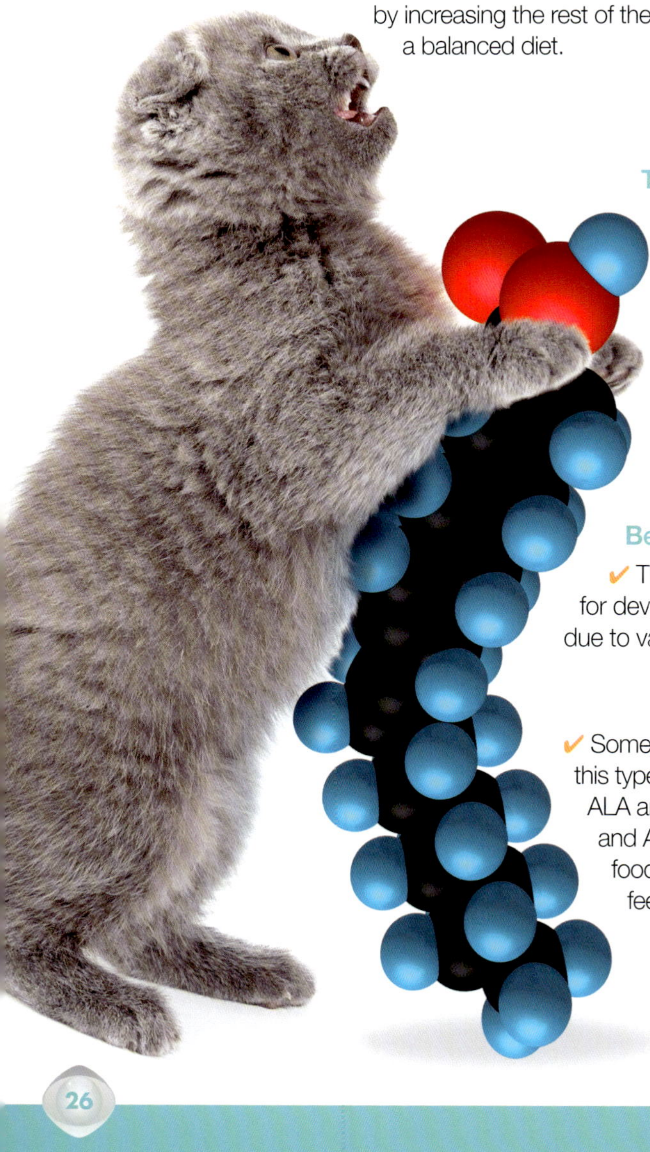

The fat profile of the milk depends on the fat provided in the food ration

Generally, the fat profile of pets is high in PUFAs, especially linoleic acid. When we increase the concentrations of certain FAs of the n-3 and n-6 series (ALA, DHA and AA) in the lactating female dogs' food, an increase in the plasmatic concentrations of these FAs is observed in the puppies.

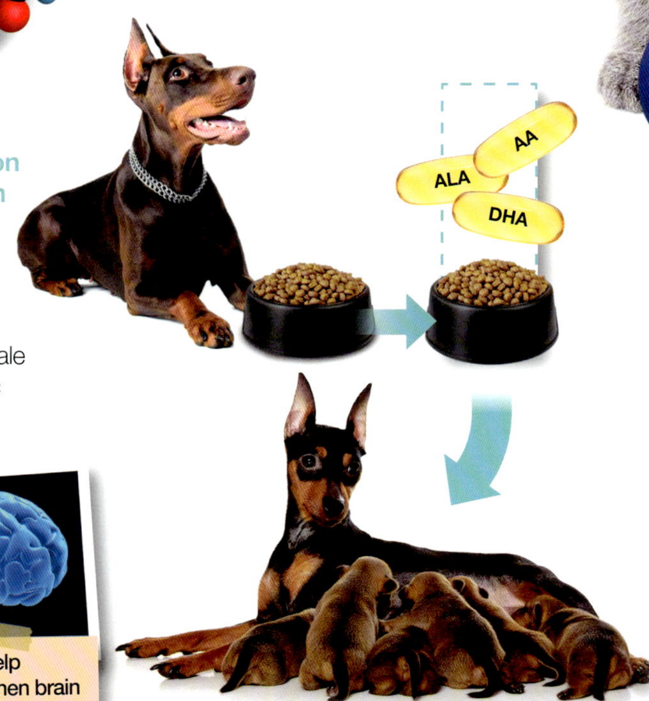

AA
ALA
DHA

Benefits of FAs

✔ They are important for developing animals due to various factors:

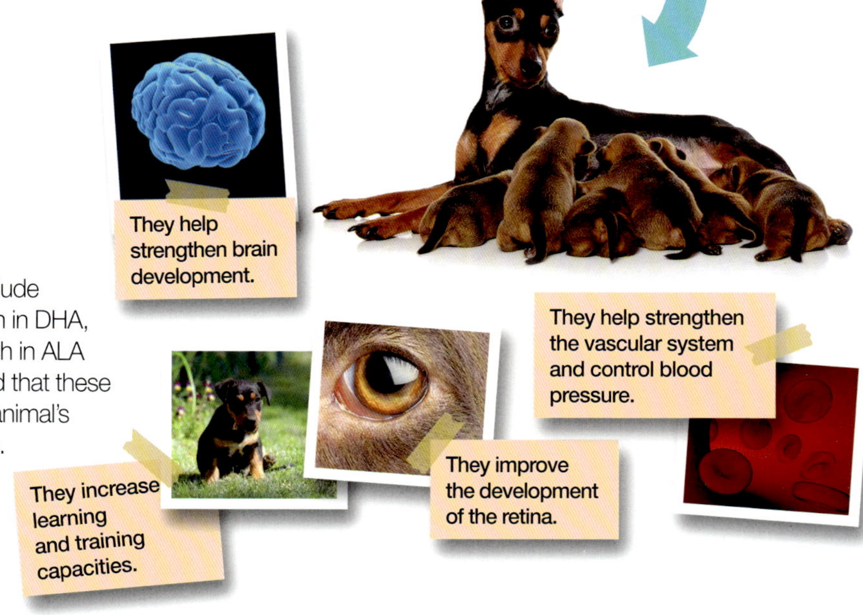

They help strengthen brain development.
They help strengthen the vascular system and control blood pressure.
They improve the development of the retina.
They increase learning and training capacities.

✔ Some raw materials that include this type of FAs are fish oil (rich in DHA, ALA and AA) and fowl fat (rich in ALA and AA). It is recommended that these foods are included in the animal's feeding during this stage.

management

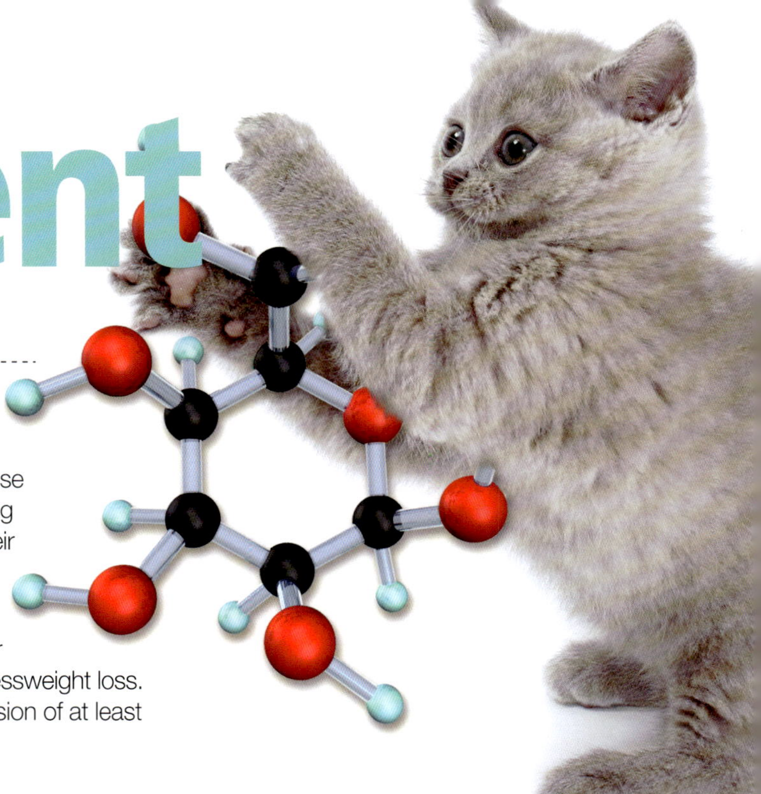

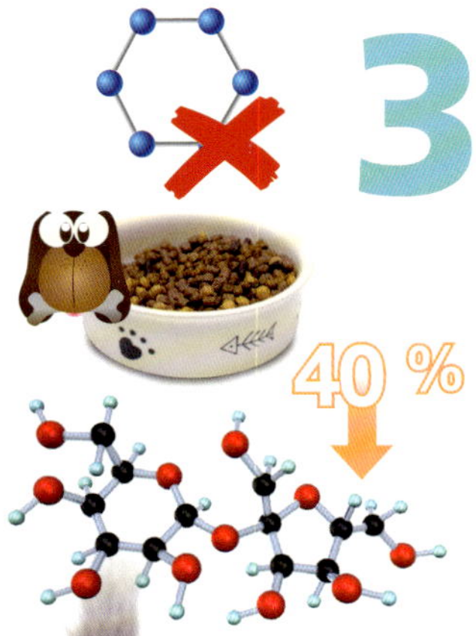

Lactose

3 Carbohydrates

- Feeding female dogs with food rations that lack carbohydrates determines that the concentration in lactose will be reduced by 40 %. To avoid this, a minimum of 60 g of digestible CH/1,000 kcal ME should be included in their food rations, or the protein levels of the rations themselves should be modified.
- Although carbohydrates are not necessary for cats, their inclusion in lactating female cats' rations avoids any excessweight loss. While more complete studies are not available, the inclusion of at least 25 g/1,000 kcal ME is recommended for this species.

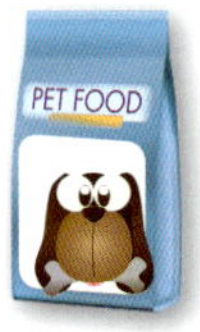

$$= \frac{60 \text{ g CH}}{1{,}000 \text{ kcal ME}}$$

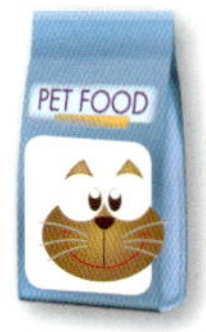

$$= \frac{25 \text{ g CH}}{1{,}000 \text{ kcal ME}}$$

4 Minerals

Depending on the number of puppies or kittens, the requirements for calcium and phosphorus are increased up to 5 times compared to maintenance. If we follow the recommendations for gestation, we ensure that the ingestion of all minerals is adequate.

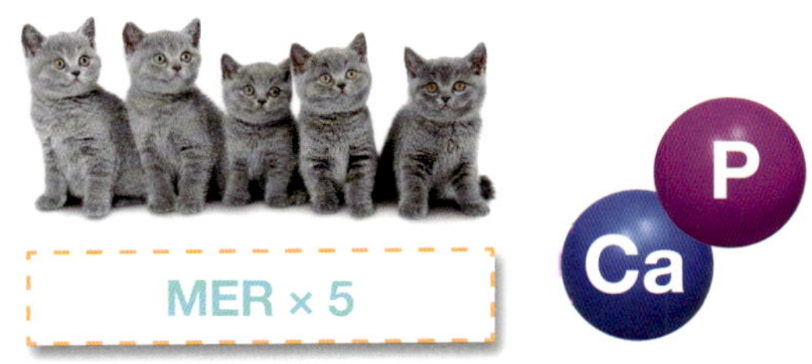

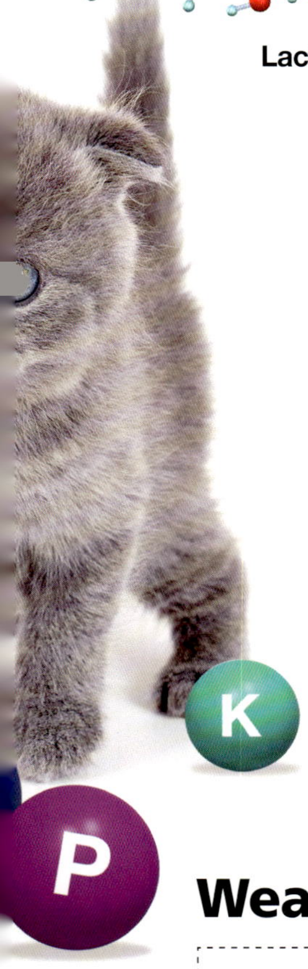

5 Water

Water is a very important nutrient as almost 80 % of milk is water. The correct ingestion of water (the female's requirements plus the daily production of milk) is essential to synthesize the correct volume of milk.

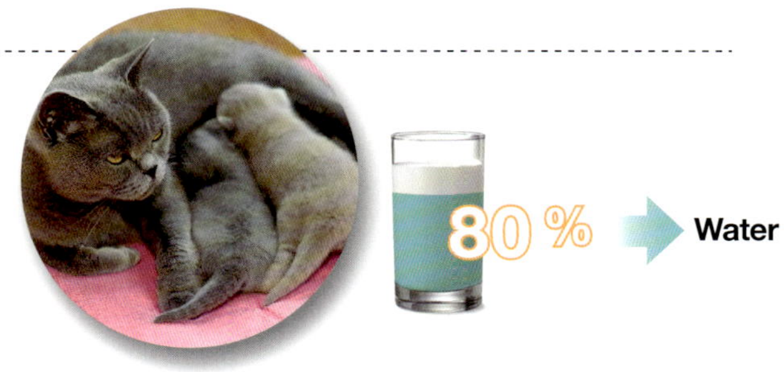

Weaning

5 weeks after birth

Weaning naturally begins 5 weeks after birth, which is when milk production begins to decline. Puppies and kittens usually ingest solid food on a regular basis at 6 weeks of age, although many breeders force early weaning around 4-5 weeks of age.

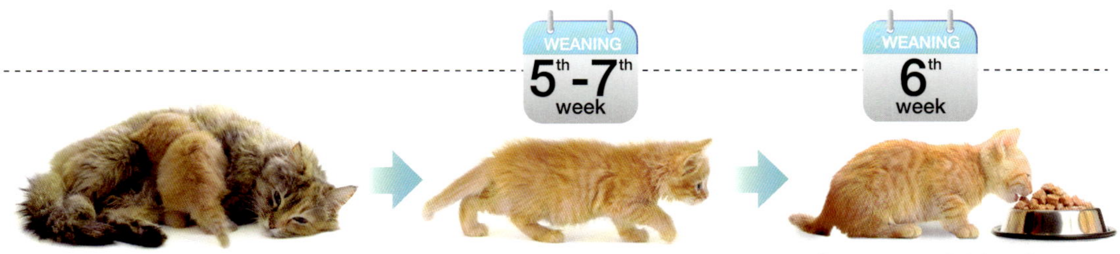

Beneficial for the female

For the mother, weaning has two purposes: it reduces the nutritional load impcsed on her, and it avoids mammary congestion and possible mastitis.

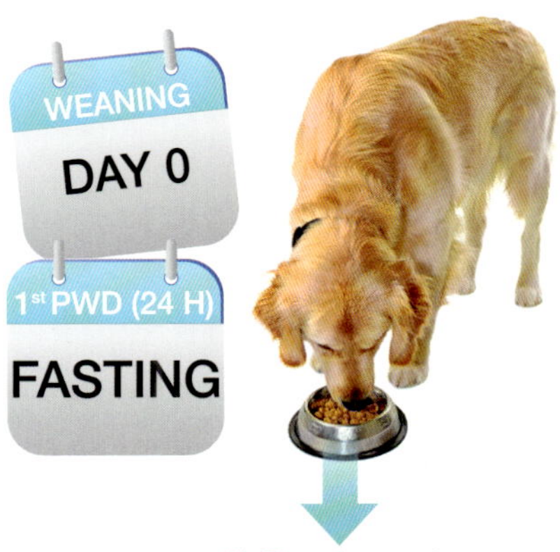

% Requirements post-weaning days (PWD)

Removing all of the offspring and fasting

To achieve the complete elimination of the production of milk, all offspring must be taken away from the mother. Also, on the day that weaning begins, we should keep the mother fasting for 24 hours, as long as her body condition is adequate (4-5/9). From this time, we will begin to increase the daily ration.

Post-weaning days				
1st	2nd and 3rd	4th	5th	6th
Fasting	25% MER	50% MER	75% MER	MER

To be taken into account

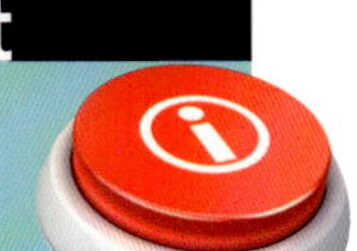

Weight control

During this phase, mothers usually lose some body weight. Their body condition should be reviewed at this time, making sure that they don't lose more than 10-15 % of their weight. For values over this amount, their diet will have to be reevaluated.

Puppy and kitten

1

Growth stages

The adult size, weight, body conformation and behavior of a dog varies greatly from one breed to another, while the differences in the adult weight and body conformation of cats are not as obvious. However, their growth is similar in all cases.

Three periods can be distinguished:

- ✔ Intrauterine growth and development.
- ✔ From birth until weaning.
- ✔ Actual growth (until adult age).

2

A diet for each stage

Diet at this stage of life is very varied as a result of development: animals start with their mother's milk or with milk replacers, they are then fed post-weaning diets and finally growth diets.

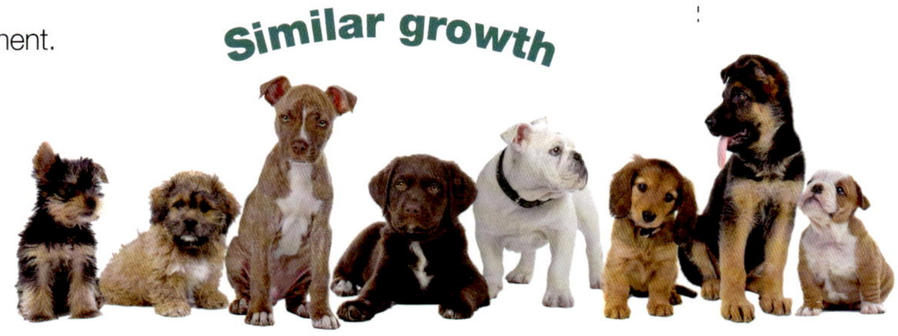

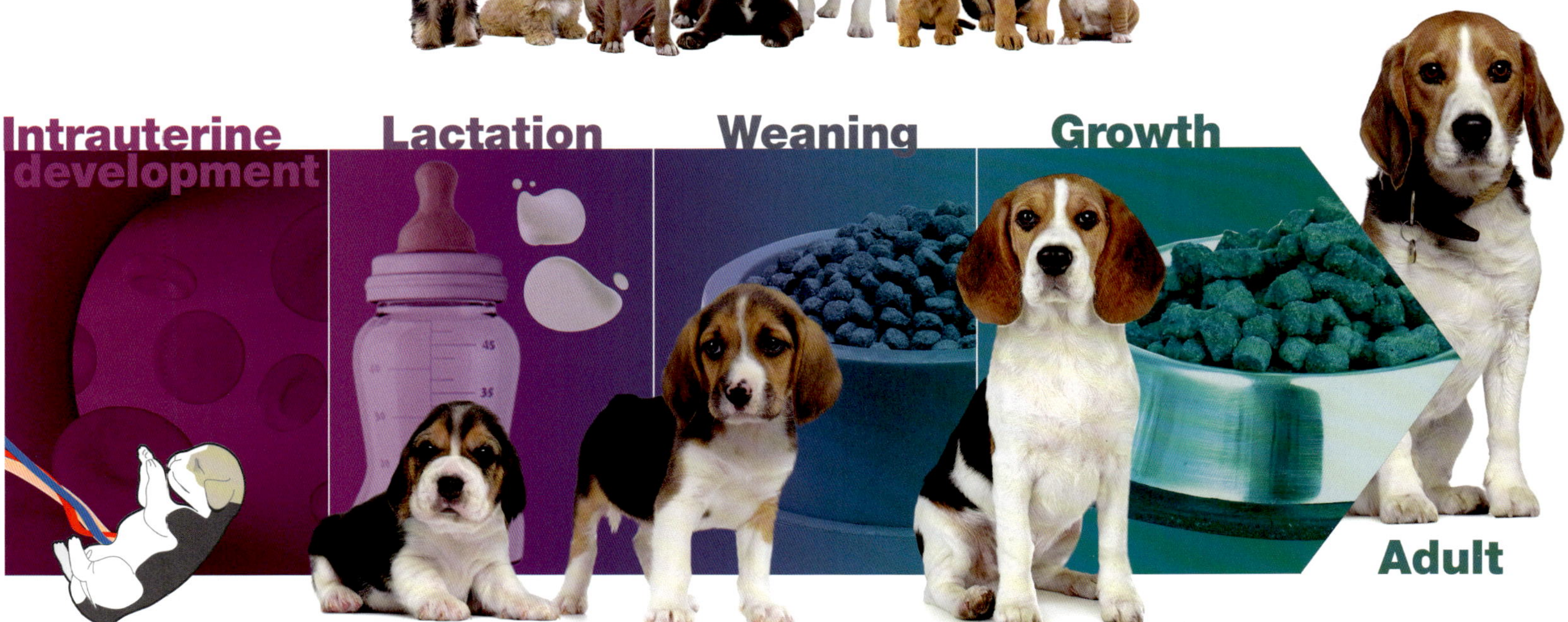

3

Neonatal survival

- ✔ There is a series of very important parameters at the neonatal stage that need to be considered, since neonatal survival depends on them (mortality reaches 20 % in the first two weeks): body temperature (related to the ambient temperature), hydration status and nutrient delivery (related to the quantity and quality of the milk).
- ✔ In their first stage of life, puppies and kittens have very little body fat (1.5 %) in comparison with adults (20 %) and they have not developed the shivering reflex yet, which makes them very sensitive to cold. This can actually lead to their death. The lower critical temperature of puppies and kittens is 32–34 °C; at this temperature, digestive enzymes do not function correctly.

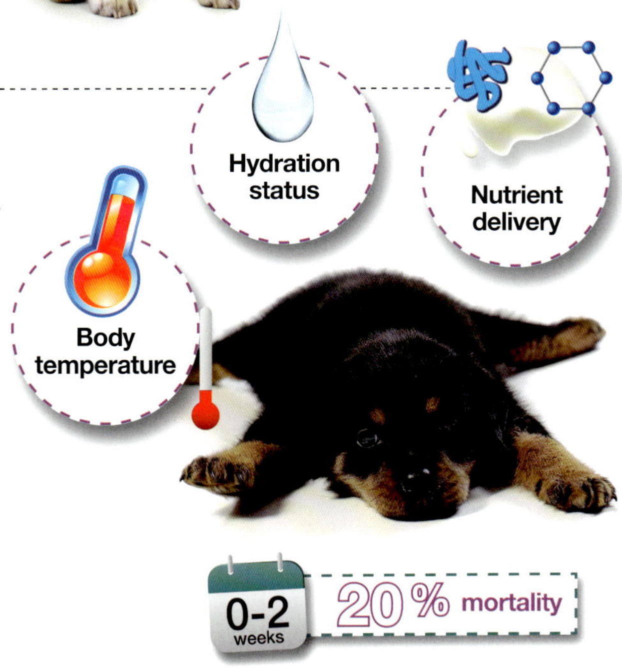

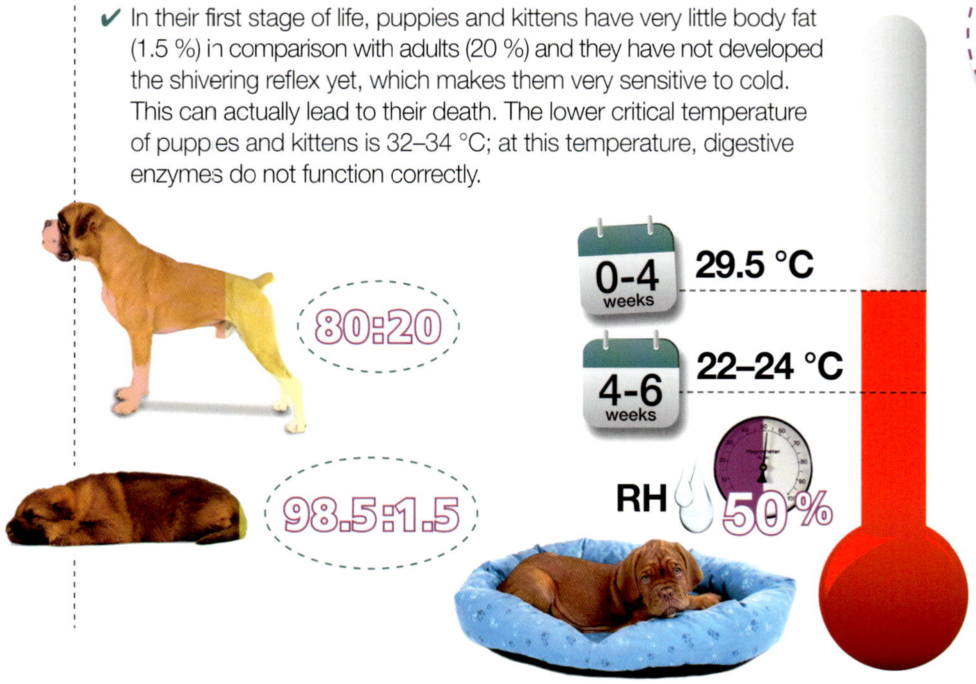

- ✔ A 50 % relative humidity and an average temperature of 29.5 °C are recommended in the room where they are kept during the first few weeks of life and 22–24 °C until 6 weeks of life.

growth

0–3 months

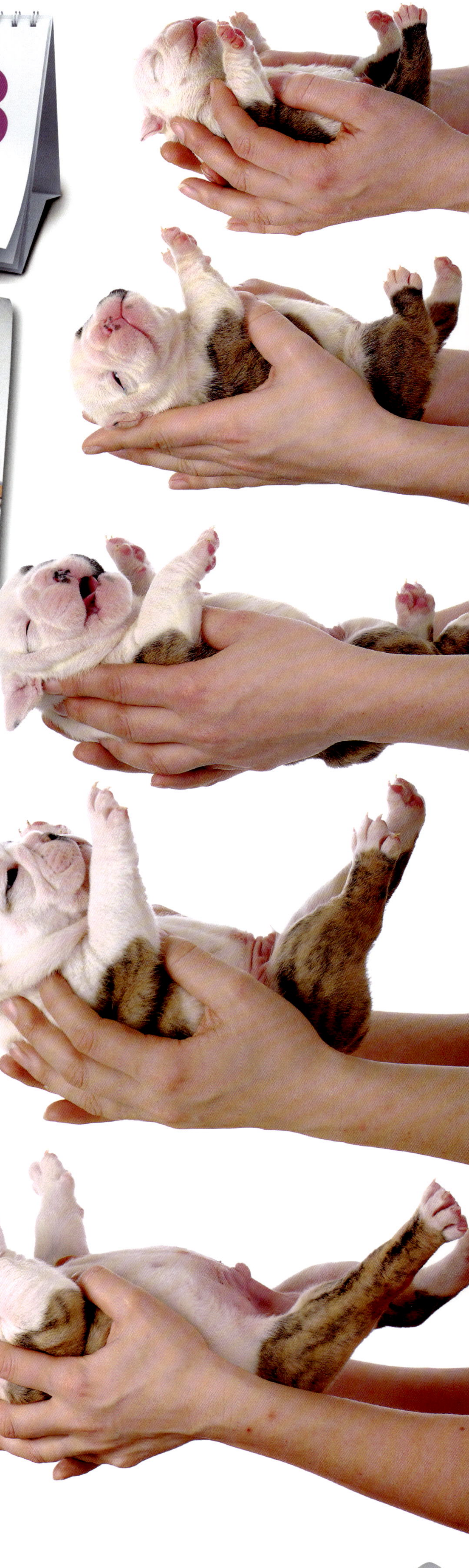

4 Puppy and kitten behavior

Knowing their behavior during the first three months of life helps us to care for them, especially in the case of orphaned animals. Three periods can be distinguished:

1 Neonatal period
First stage of growth

- ✔ Puppies and kittens spend most of their time sleeping (80 %) and suckling.
- ✔ Their sleep is not deep, with involuntary movements and irregular breathing.
- ✔ They usually suckle strongly.
- ✔ They cry when they are hungry.
- ✔ The basis of their diet is their mother's milk.
- ✔ The perianal area must be stimulated for urination and defecation.
- ✔ They start walking at about 10 days old.

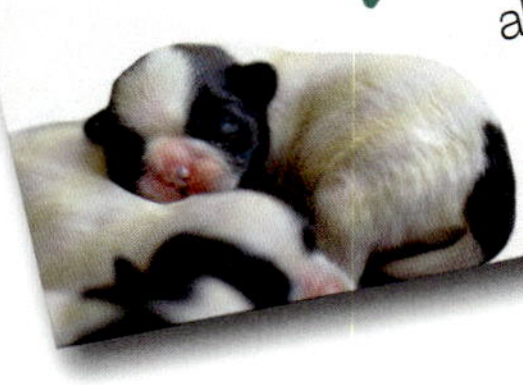

2 Transition

- ✔ This stage is marked by the opening of the eyes (15–18 days) and dental eruption (day 21).
- ✔ They start to explore the environment and to eat part of their mother's food.
- ✔ Urination and defecation is voluntary.
- ✔ They gain their sight and hearing and respond to external stimuli.
- ✔ They start playing with each other.

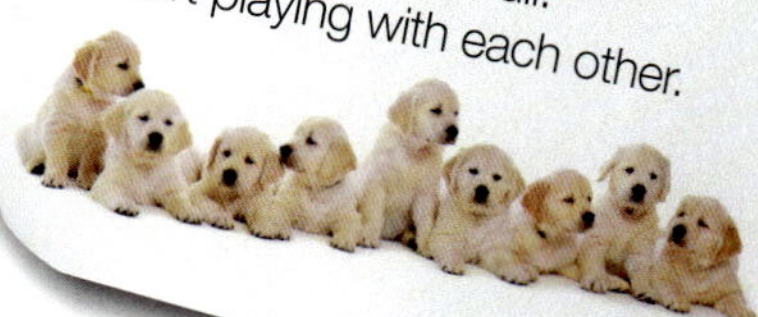

3 Socialization
(until 8 weeks of age)

- ✔ They interact with their mother, siblings and owners.
- ✔ The group hierarchy is gradually established.
- ✔ Natural weaning takes place.

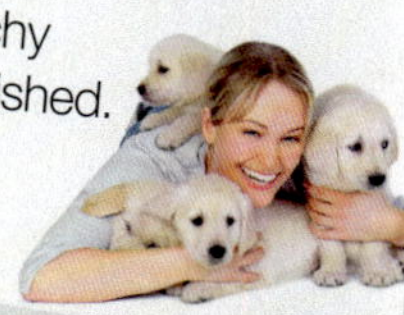

5 Objectives for optimal growth

- ✔ The objectives are very clear: healthy growth, maximum training and minimum diseases associated with growth (obesity and orthopedic diseases).

Healthy growth | **Maximum training** | **Minimum diseases associated with growth**

- ✔ The growth of these animals depends on the diet's energy density and on the amount provided. The needs of puppies and kittens must be calculated to ensure optimal growth for bone development rather than to achieve maximum weight gain.
- ✔ Feeding to achieve maximum growth could cause skeletal abnormalities as well as a lower life expectancy.
- ✔ Puppy and kitten growth can be assessed twice a month based on the evolution of their weight and BCS. They should be weighed every 24–48 hours in the first two weeks of life, especially when their weight at birth is lower than expected.

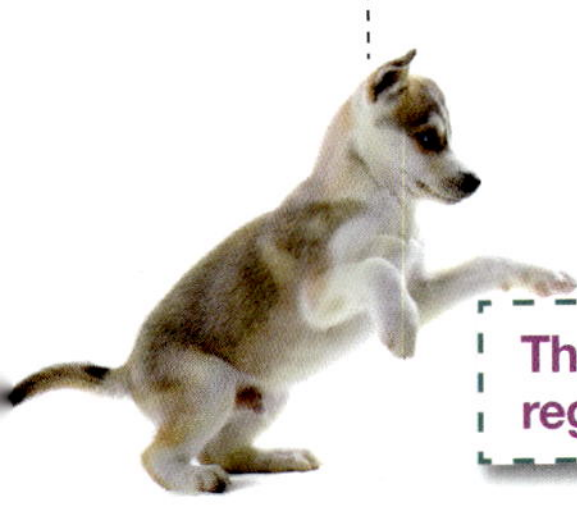

The animal's adult size will be the same regardless of the growth rate.

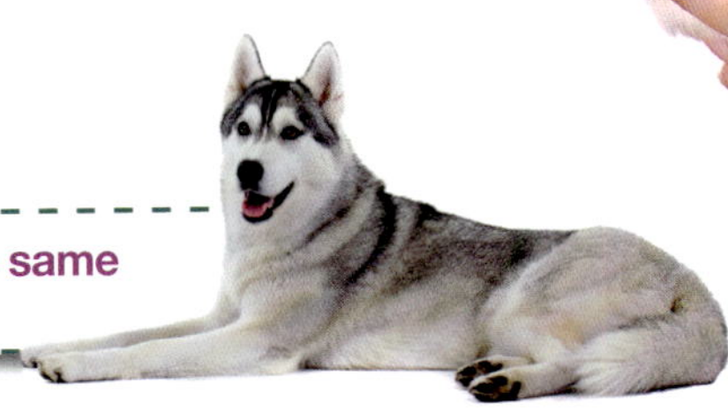

Weight gain in puppies

1 Growth prediction in puppies and kittens

There are two ways to predict growth in puppies and kittens. Weight gain in puppies and kittens is the most important criterion to evaluate their feeding and serves as a reflection of survival during the first stages of life.

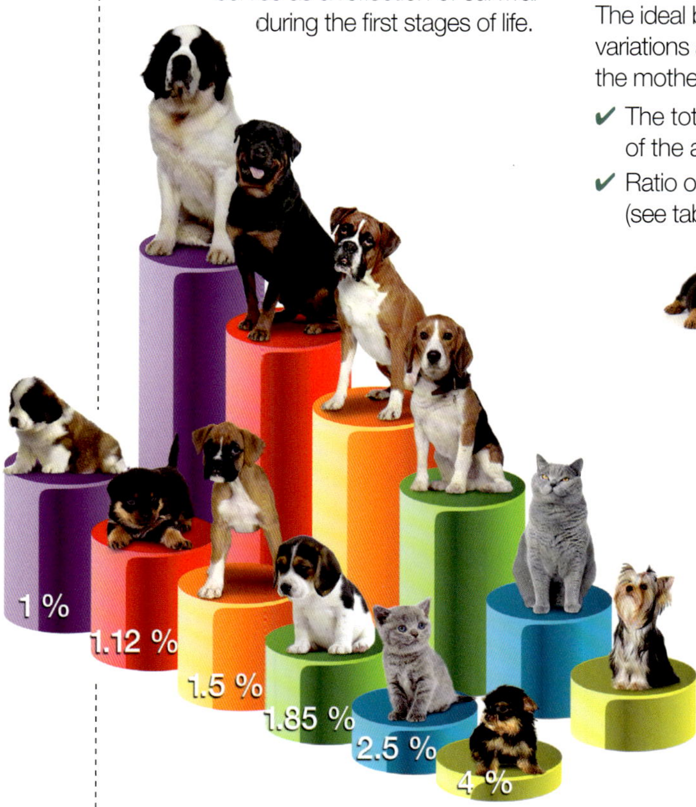

For example, kittens that are born weighing less than 80 g have a high mortality rate and require intensive care.
The prediction methods are as follows:

Birth weight

The ideal birth weight is not easy to determine, as there are different variations among breeds. In spite of this, there is a correlation between the mother's weight and the birth weight of the offspring:

- ✔ The total weight of the litter represents 12-14 % of the adult's weight.
- ✔ Ratio of mother's weight:newborn's weight (%) (see table).

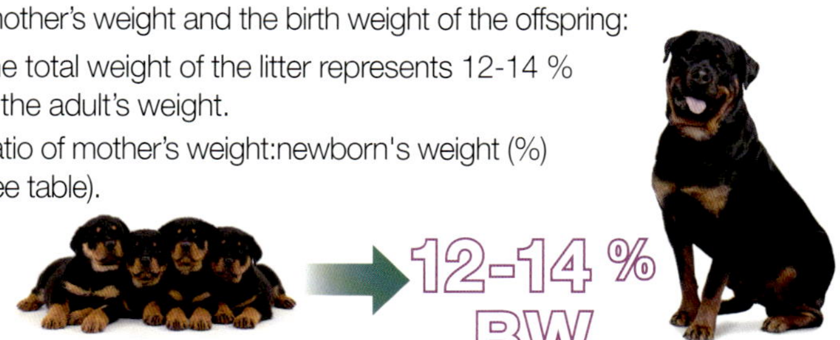

Breed	Female's weight (kg)	% over FW	Newborn's weight (g)
Yorkshire	2.5	4	100
Cats	4	2.5	100
Beagle	13	1.85	240
Boxer	28	1.5	410
Rottweiler	40	1.12	450
Saint Bernard	65	1	650

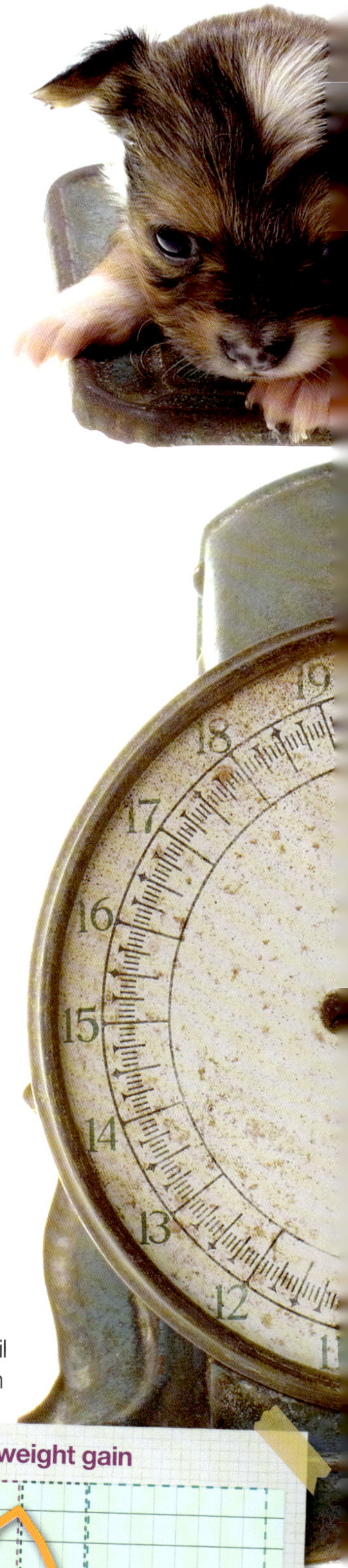

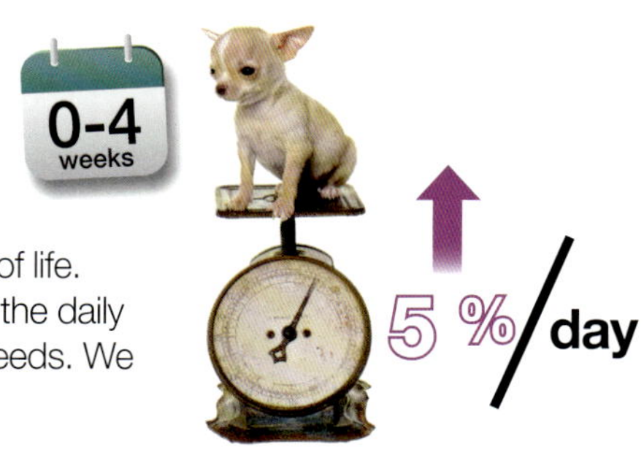

Weight gain

Puppies and kittens gain an average of 5 % daily during the first 4 weeks of life. This primarily corresponds with the accumulation of nutrient stores. Later, the daily weight gain (DWG) varies following a sigmoid curve that is similar for all breeds. We can distinguish three well-differentiated stages in this curve:

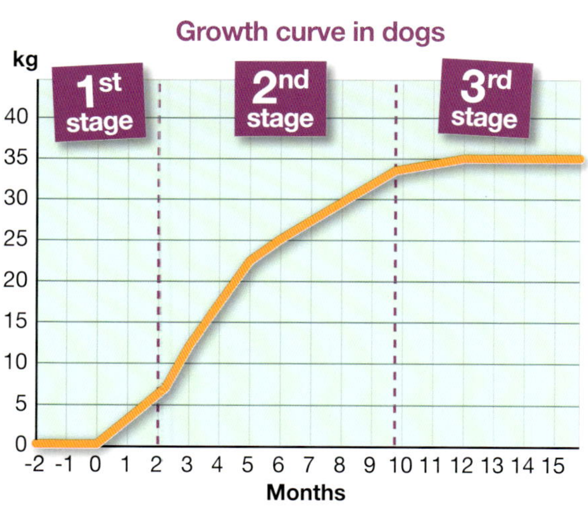

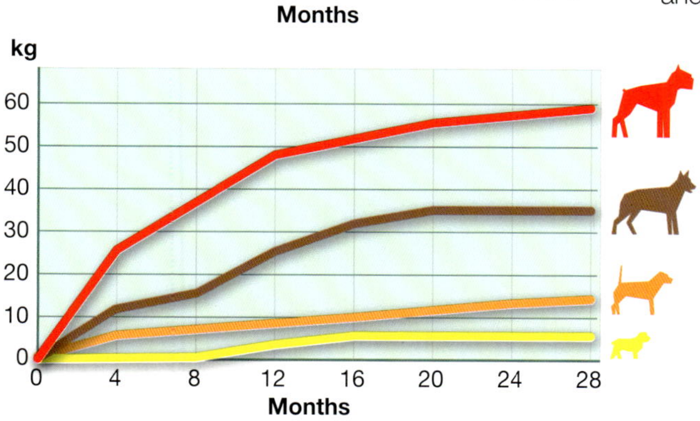

First stage: growth is slow. The energy requirements correspond with the accumulation of nutrient stores and maintenance while at rest (MAR). The puppies and kittens spend most of the day asleep.

Second stage: this stage starts with weaning and goes until the animal reaches 80 % of its adult weight. Here the growth is exponential, with different periods in the daily increases of weight (g/day) that will influence the daily energy requirements (DER). In this case, the energy is divided approximately as follows: 50 % maintenance and 50 % growth.

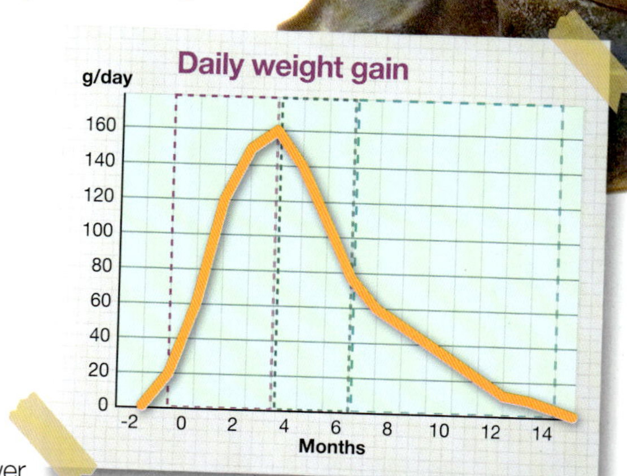

Third stage: the third stage corresponds with the plateau. Growth is slower and most of the energy used is for maintenance (90 %). Although ossification has been completed, a portion of the energy will be used for muscle development (maturation).

and kittens

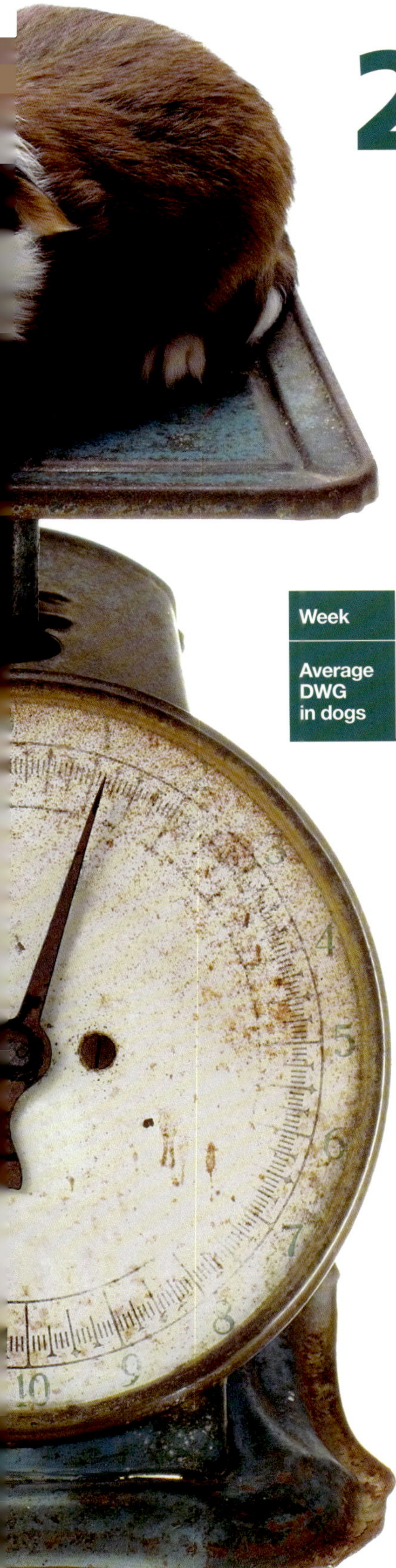

2 Progression to adult weight

All dog breeds reach approximately 50 % of their adult weight between the age of 4-5 months. After this point, and until they finish growing (adults), is where the greatest differences take place:

- ✔ **Small and medium breeds** reach 80 % of their adult weight at 9-10 months of age, reaching their full size at 12 months.

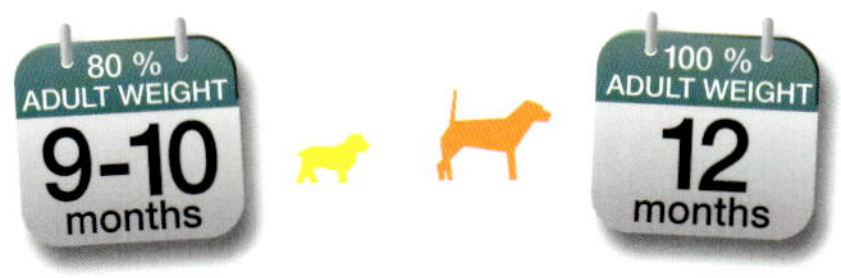

- ✔ **Large and giant breeds** take twice as long to reach maturity. They reach 80 % of their adult weight at 11-15 months of age, reaching their full size between 18-24 months.

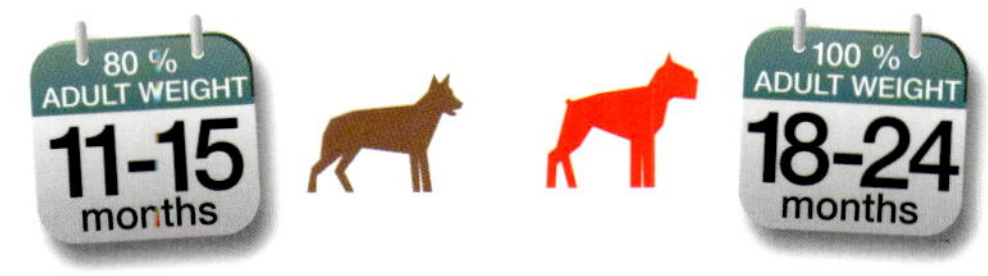

Average curve of weight gain

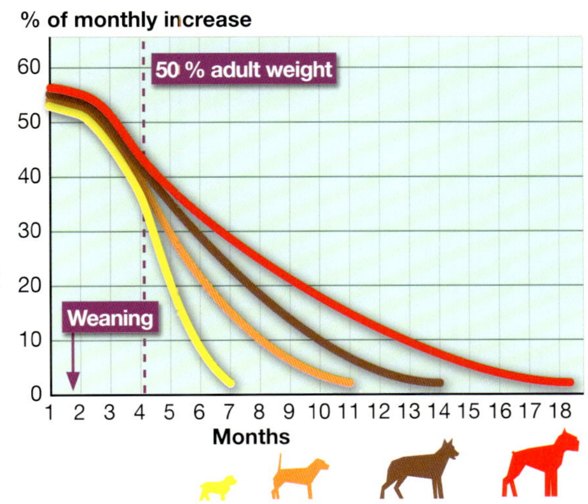

Week	1	2	3	4	4 to 8	Greater than 8	16	20	32	Greater than 40	40 to 60	48 to 96
Average DWG in dogs	8 % current weight	6 % current weight	4 % current weight	3.5 % current weight	3 g/kg adult weight	2-4 g/kg adult weight	50 % adult weight (dogs <25 kg)	50 % adult weight (dogs >25 kg)	65 % adult weight	80 % adult weight	100 % adult weight (according to breeds)	complete development (according to breeds)

3 Weight in kittens

- ✔ For cats, the average weight gain is 100 g per week for the first 6 months of life.
- ✔ From this point on, growth is slower: males gain an average of 20 g/day, while females gain approximately half of that. At 10 months of age, the growth plates are closed and growth has completed, although after they reach one year old, they will gain a small amount of weight as a result of the maturation stage.
  Cats are sterilized during this stage: growth is not affected by the surgery; however, the energy recommendations are affected.

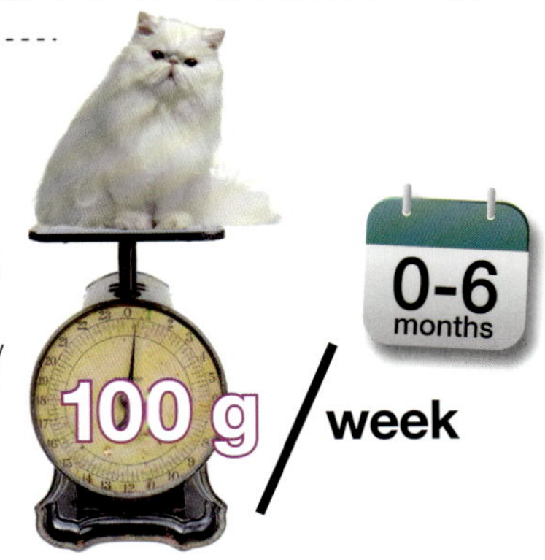

Growth curve in cats

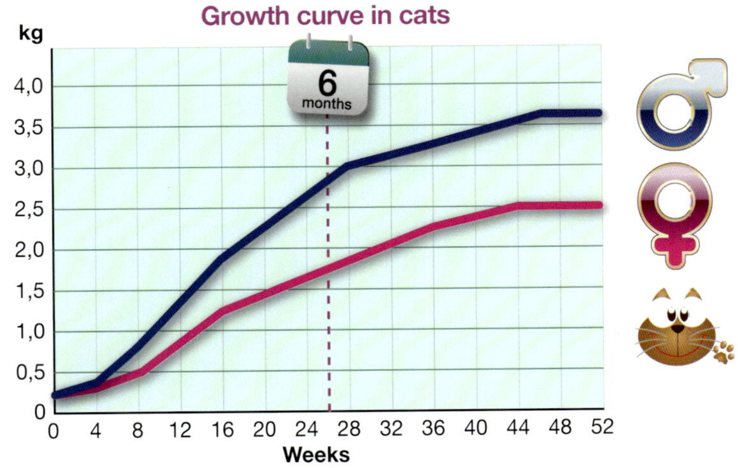

- ✔ The differences of growth according to sex are very obvious after 4 weeks of age: females grow slower and weigh less than males.

4 Growth according to genotype

- ✔ On the other hand, growth and development in dogs will be different depending on the genotype of each specific breed: Greyhounds, for example, will develop long limbs and a broad thorax, while Rottweilers will develop more muscle mass.
- ✔ These differences in conformation will also affect the animals' feeding, which is why there are different food products available on the market. Most studies have been focused on giant and miniature breeds given the existing differences.

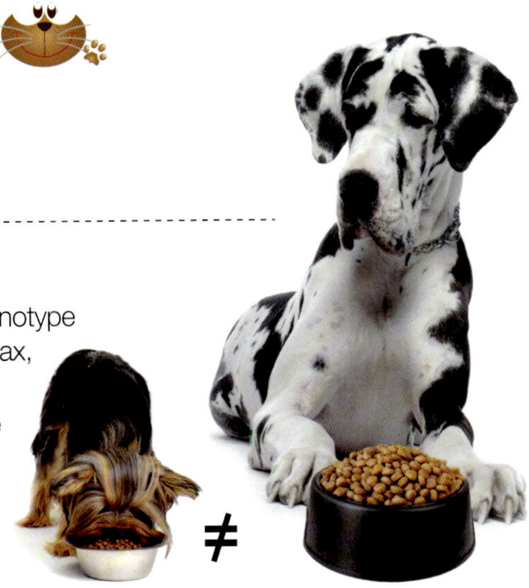

It is widely accepted that milk is a complete and unique food for newborns. However, as animals grow, the nutrients it provides become limited, and solid food must be introduced by the 4th week of life.

Lactation and

Mother's milk

1 Different proportion of nutrients between species

- ✔ The milk of different mammals has the same components but with different proportions. Extrapolating values from one species to another is thus useless. For example, as a consequence of a greater fat content, the milk of female dogs is more calorie-dense than that of female cats (34 % more).
- ✔ On the other hand, milk from dogs and cats is rich in long-chain FAs, especially linoleic and arachydonic acids, as well as in taurine, arginine, iron, calcium, and phosphorus, when compared with other species (for example, cows and humans).

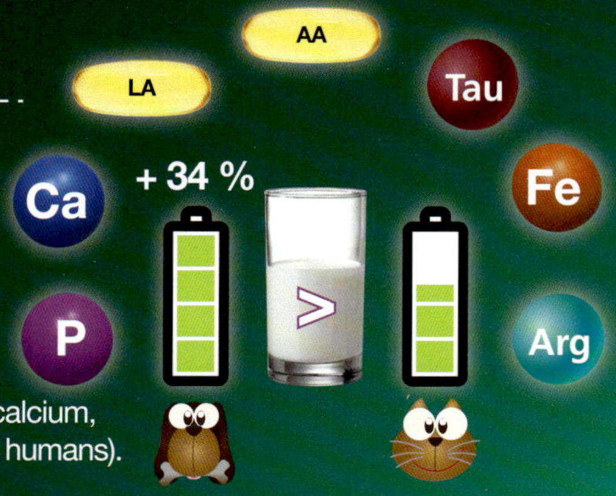

2 Different proportions of nutrients depending on the lactation period

The milk's composition is modified along a curve:

- ✔ **Protein:** protein levels are high during the first days (10 %) and decrease until the third week (8 %) where there is a small upturn until weaning.

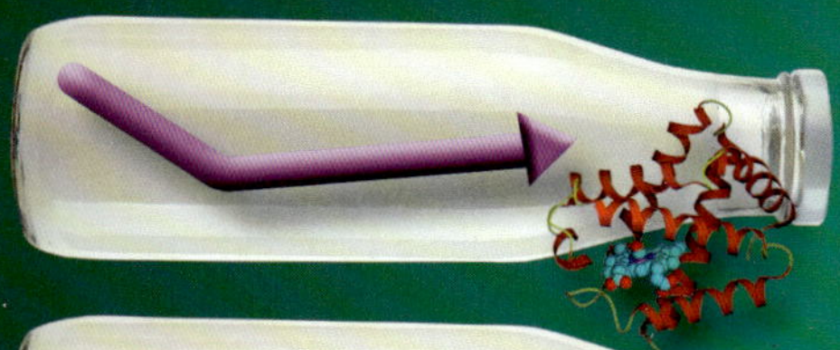

- ✔ **Fat:** fat levels start out very high but decrease drastically on the third day. They subsequently increase again until reaching maximum levels in the second week until weaning.

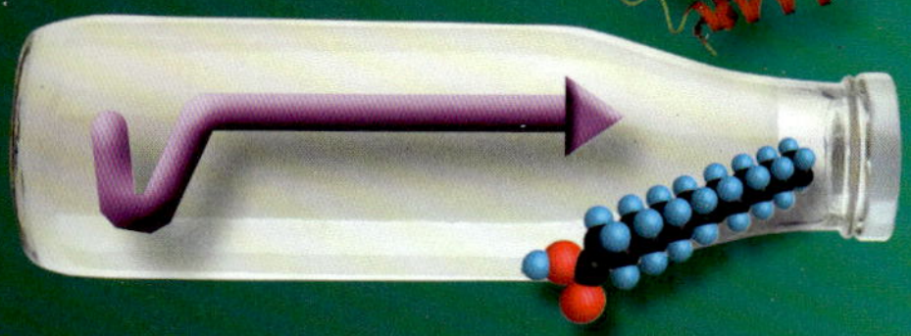

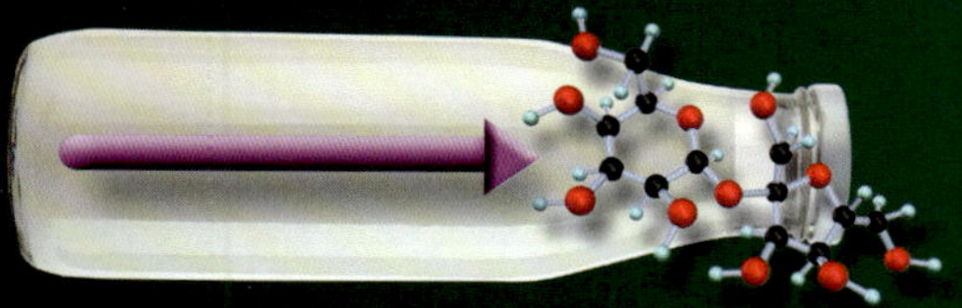

- ✔ **Lactose:** there are no variations throughout the cycle and lactose levels remain constant.

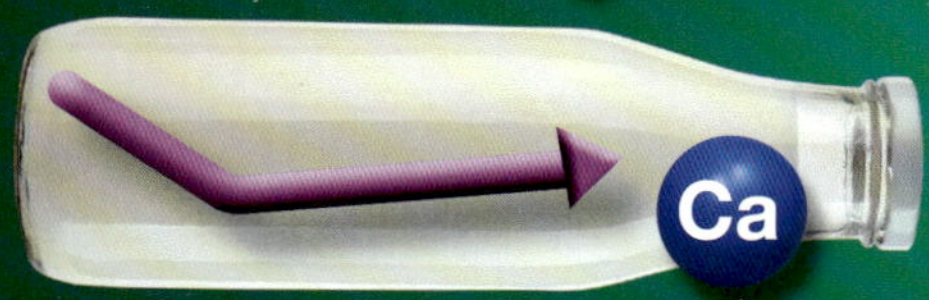

- ✔ **Calcium:** the calcium level changes are proportional to the protein content.

3 Milk proteins with biological activity

There is a multitude of proteins with biological activities related to the following:

Defense system:
Lysozyme, lactoferrin, lactoperoxidase.

Provision of nutrients:
- ✔ Bile salt-stimulated lipase, which favors the secretion of bile and the absorption of fats in newborns.
- ✔ α-amylase.
- ✔ Vitamin-transporting proteins:
  - β-lactoglobulin for vitamin A.
  - Vitamin B_{12} and folic acid transport proteins.
- ✔ Phosphopeptidases that solubilize calcium and favor its absorption.

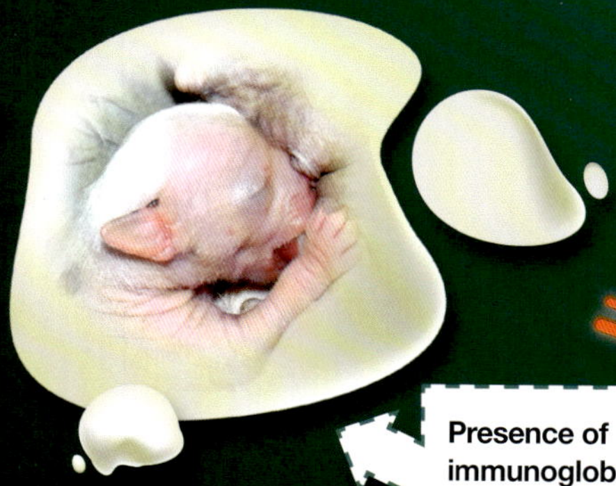

Growth factors of the IGF-1 and IGF-2 type.

Presence of immunoglobulins:
Specific IgA present in milk and other secretions that impede the adherence of antigens to the surface of the intestine.

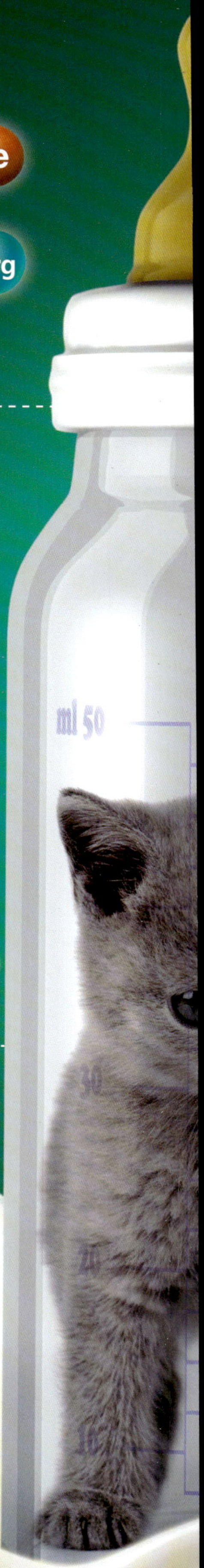

milk replacements

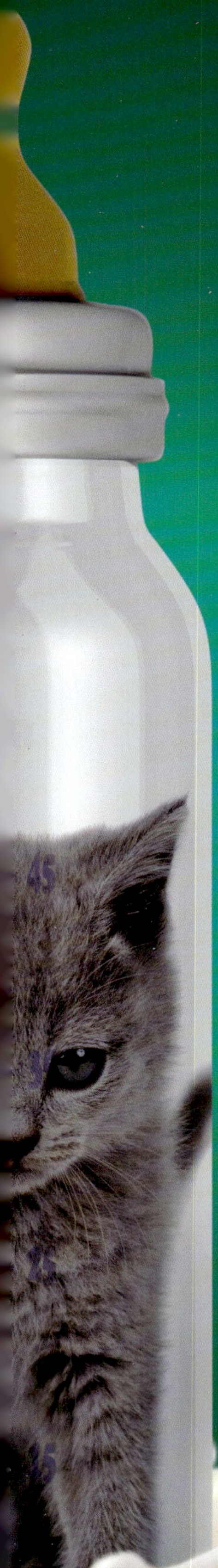

Artificial milk

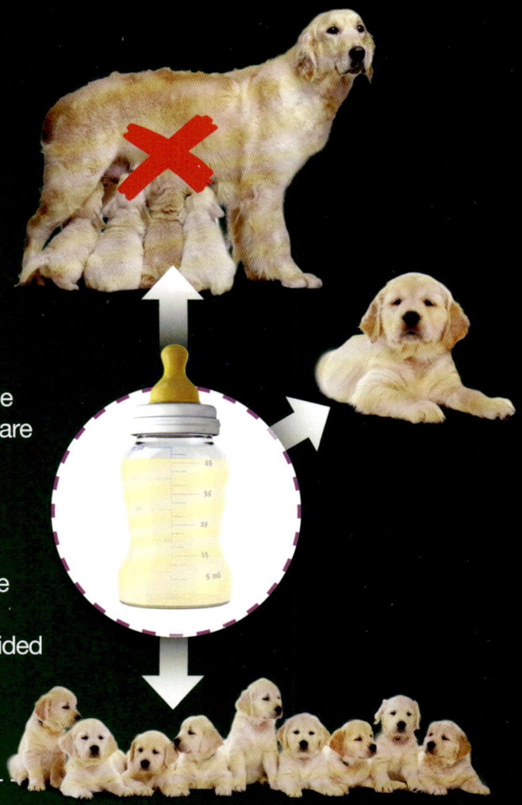

- ✔ Milk substitutes represent a good alternative in dog and cat nutrition when litters are large and the mother's milk does not fulfill the requirements of all of the offspring, or when we are rearing orphaned puppies or kittens.
- ✔ Designing adequate artificial milk is not simple given the characteristics of the milk from our pets. The formula should be as similar as possible to natural milk.
- ✔ The mixtures of fats or of different types of carbohydrates (for example, substituting lactose for other glucose polymers) contribute to the creation of a good product, occasionally with health benefits for the puppy or kitten: high levels of lactose cause diarrhea that can be avoided with maltodextrin, for example.

1 How is a good milk replacement designed?

✔ The challenge lies in the quality of the milk proteins. They are highly digestible proteins (90 %), which belong to three classes:

Casein: it is the predominant protein and is synthesized in the mammary gland.

Serum proteins: albumin passes directly from the circulation to the gland.

Lipoproteins from the fat globules: this fraction is of little significance to us.

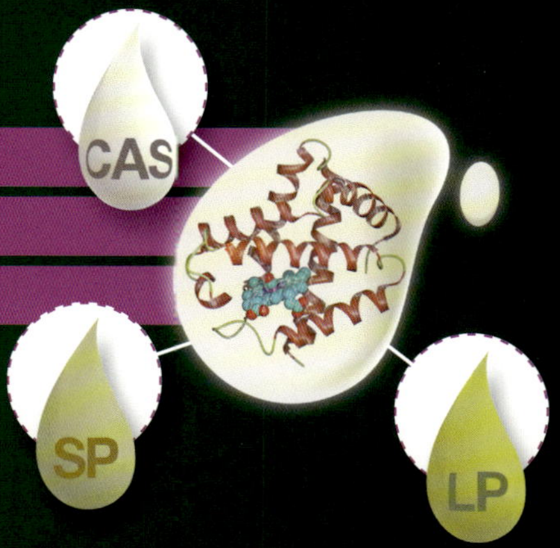

✔ Also, the amino acid profile is different among them.

Protein type	Amino acid profile
Casein	↓ Cys
Serum proteins	↑ Thr Ile Leu Trp

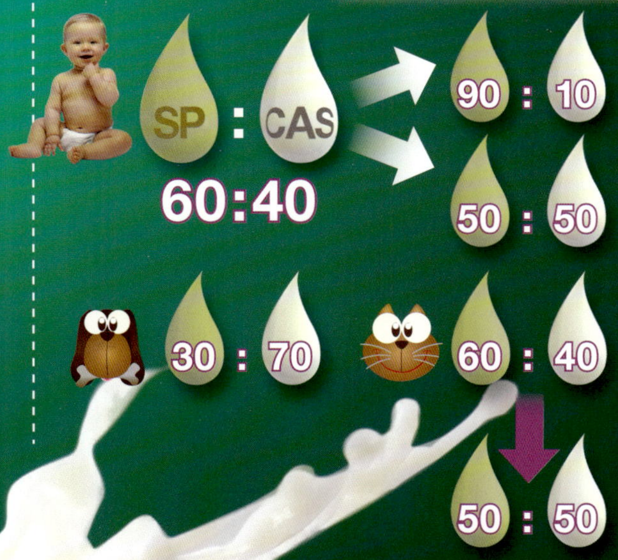

- ✔ As a result, the serum protein:casein ratio determines the quality of the milk replacement depending on the requirements and conditions their manufacturing. For example, formulas for children are predominantly 60:40, but throughout the lactation cycle, these proportions vary (90:10 to 50:50). That said, few substitutes for dogs and cats have been formulated taking into account these premises.
- ✔ In dogs, the serum protein:casein ratio is 30:70 and remains constant throughout the entire lactation cycle, while in cats, the ratio is 60:40 and decreases to 50:50 throughout the cycle.
- ✔ As we can see, casein is the predominant protein in dog's milk (similar to cow's milk), while in female cats, there is an equal division between both categories (similar to the case with mares). The predominance of casein affects the digestion of protein, amino acids and minerals.

2 Composition of milk substitutes

Base composition	Powdered nonfat milk and whey.	**Animal and plant-based fats** (fish fats are of special interest due to their richness in DHA).	**Vitamins and minerals** and enriched with certain amino acids (for example, arginine and taurine).

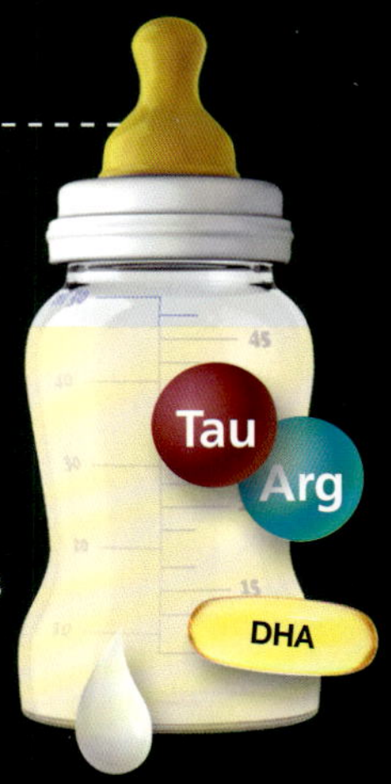

Plant-based proteins have been used in certain recipes; however, this is not ideal due to their richness in anti-nutritional factors, low digestibility, and the development of food allergies (for example, gluten).

Enzymatic

1 Enzymatic activity during growth

- ✔ During the growth of puppies and kittens, not only does their size and weight vary, but changes also take place with their digestive enzymes and the hydrolyzing capacity of these enzymes, which will affect the use of nutrients.
- ✔ Generally, the development of the digestive system, in size and absorption capacity, from the moment of birth until maturity is greater in cats than dogs. In both species, and for all enzymes, the activity is minimal on the first day of life.

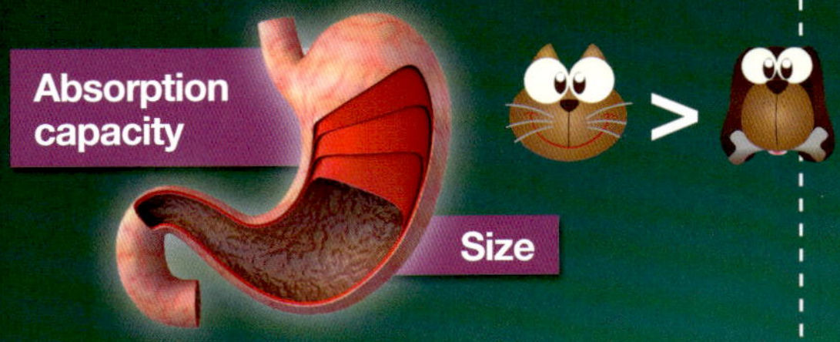

2 How do enzymes vary in the first stages of life?

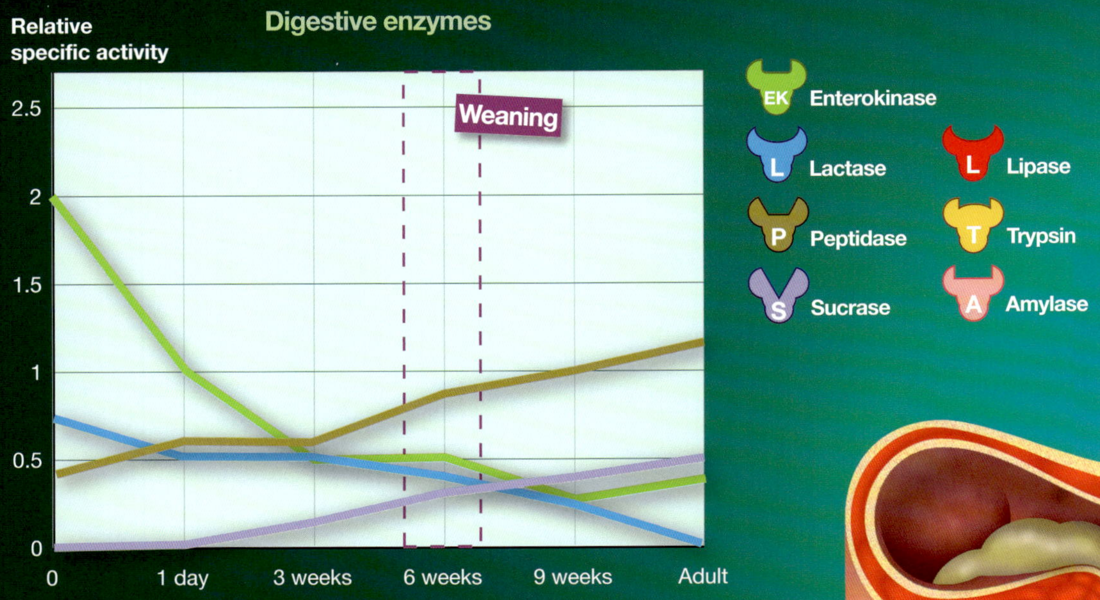

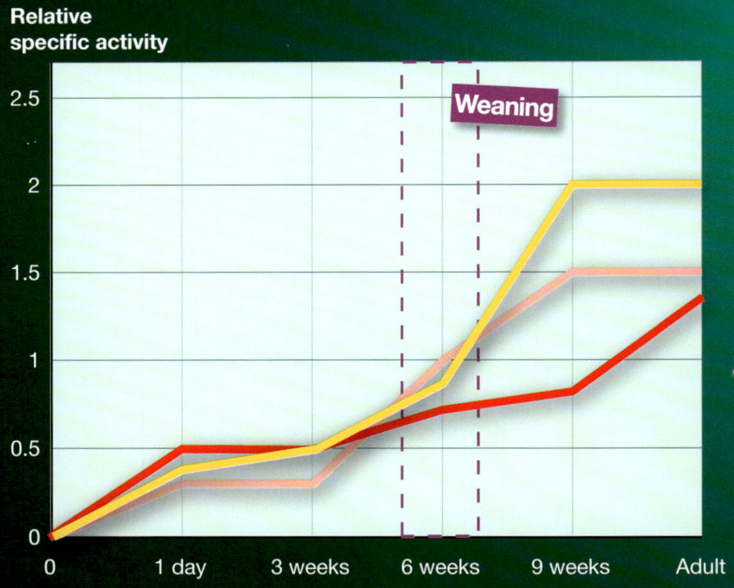

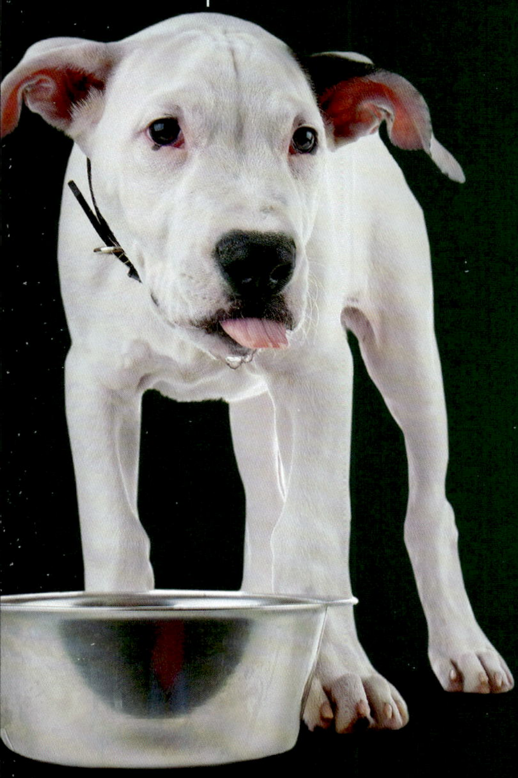

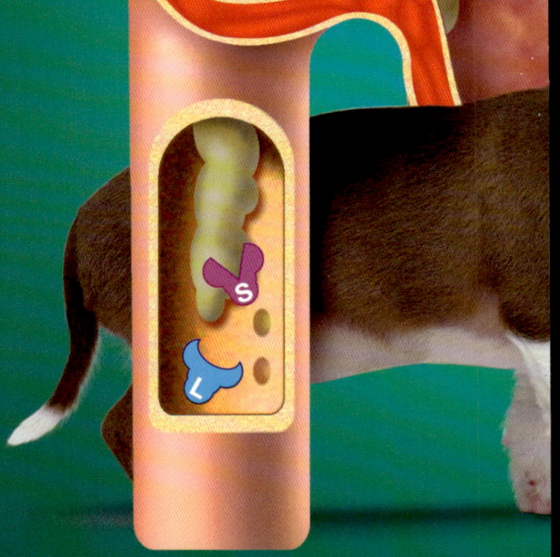

3 Digestive efficiency in puppies and kittens

- ✔ As we see, the digestive system of puppies and kittens has an elevated efficiency to utilize nutrients fully when the food offered is of high quality. For this reason, residues are usually not found undigested in their stool, except when pathologies are present.
- ✔ The different nutrient transporters (glucose, amino acids, dipeptides) present an elevated functional capacity up to 6 weeks, when the values are stabilized at levels similar to those of adults.

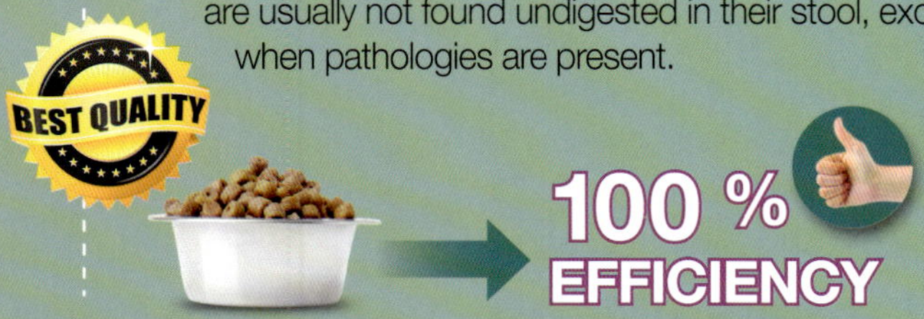

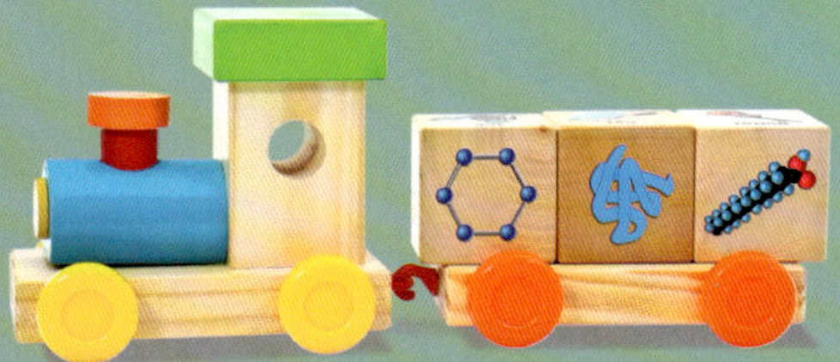

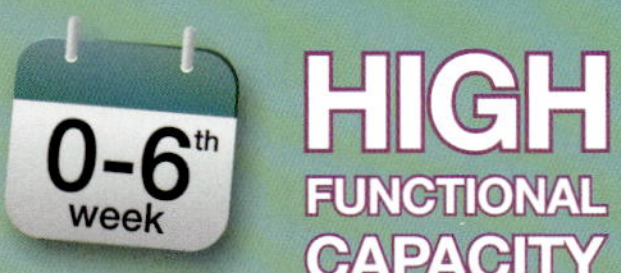

development
of the digestive system

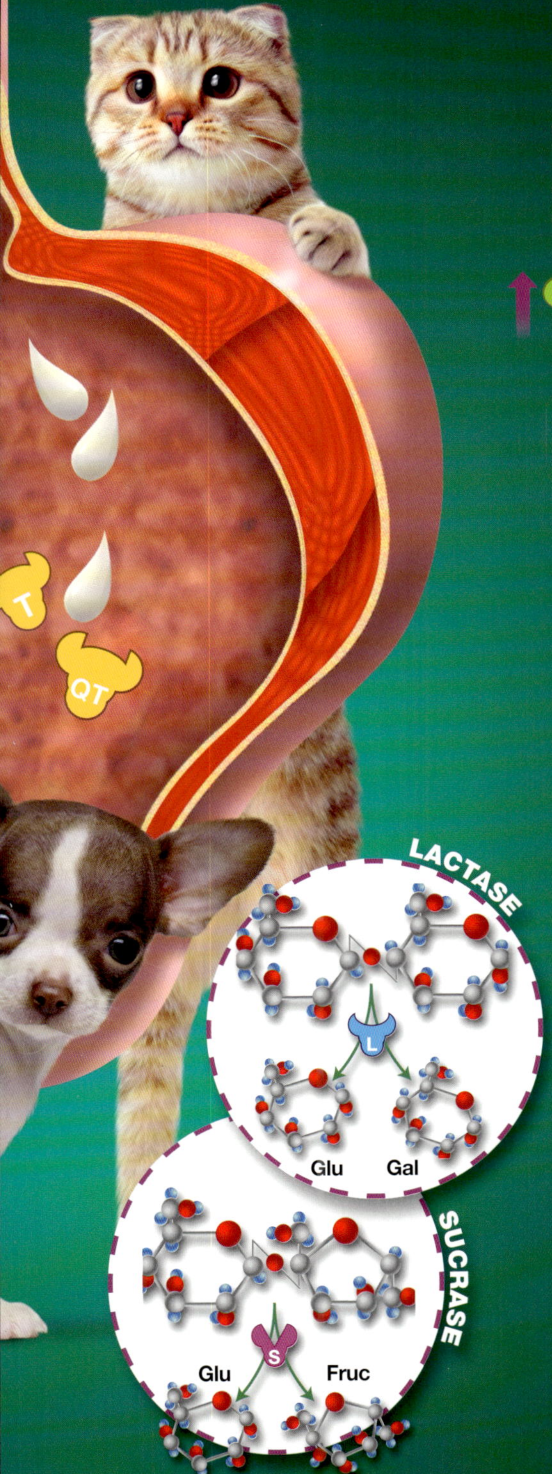

PERIODS of maximun enzymatic activity

Enterokinase (activates trypsinogen to trypsin)

Presents elevated activity since birth and decreases until 6 weeks of life, when it reaches the same levels as those found in adults. Its high levels, together with low levels of trypsin and the presence of trypsin inhibitors in colostrum represent a paradoxical fact: the possibility of absorbing unaltered macromolecules during a brief period of time.

EK + T + T → **Absorption of macromolecules**

Trypsin, chymotrypsin and lipase

Trypsin, chymotrypsin (this represents only 2 % of trypsin) and lipase reach their maximum activity between the 3rd and 9th week in dogs, while in cats, growth takes place throughout their entire lives.

Other peptidases

For example: aminopeptidases A and N, leucine aminopeptidase and γ-glutamyl transpeptidase present variable activities from the moment of birth, increasing their levels from the 6th to 9th weeks.

Lactase

- ✔ It splits the sugars found in milk (lactose) in glucose and galactose, and is present during the first 3 weeks of life. After the 6th week (weaning), its activity is no longer detected.
- ✔ The levels of lactase in cats is lower than in dogs (possibly due to a lower lactose content) and also, a certain amount of activity persists in adults.

Sucrase

- ✔ It splits common sugar (sucrose) in glucose and fructose; it is undetectable at birth, but appears at 3 weeks of life, reaching its maximum level at 9 weeks, doubling its activity until reaching the adult age.
- ✔ In cats, sucrase reaches constant, very low levels from birth until reaching adult age.
- ✔ For this reason, giving sugar to puppies or kittens can be harmful.

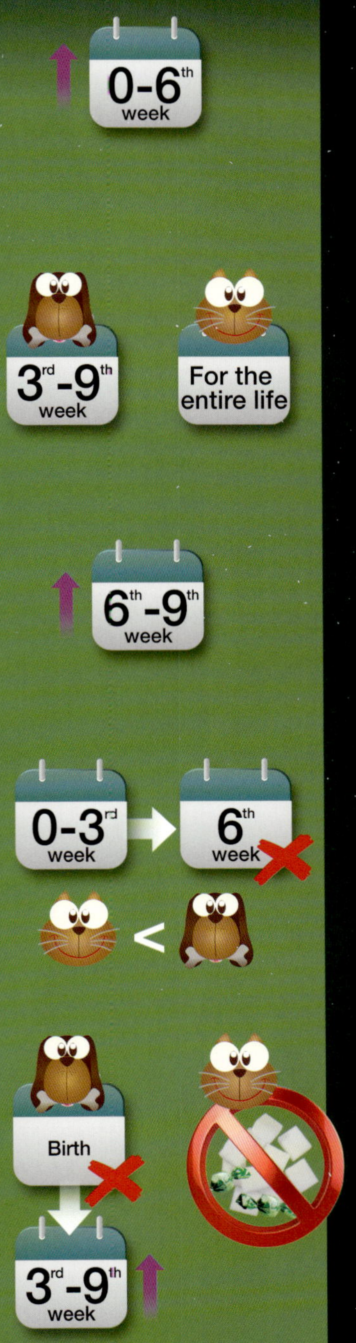

4 The right time to wean

From the previous reading, we know that puppies and kittens have a limited capacity to modify the absorption of nutrients of the apical cells, or brush-border cells, depending on the diet composition and any changes made to the diet. Correct comprehension of the processes hereby explained will help us understand when is the best moment to wean the offspring from the mother, and what the composition of the blended foods for weaning should be, without causing any digestive problems.

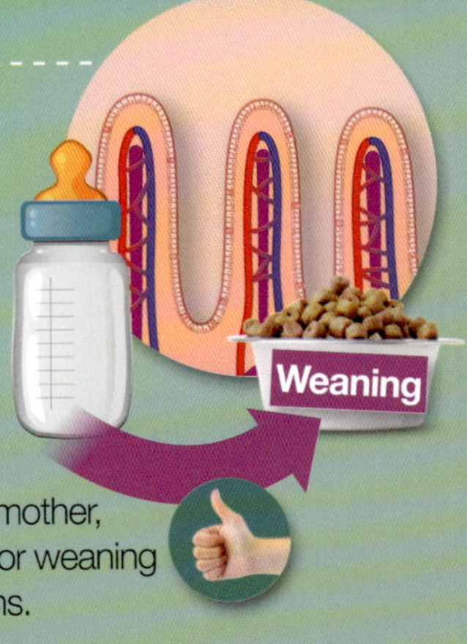

To be taken into account

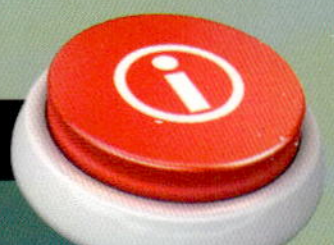

We must not forget, therefore, that weaning is a physiological period of adaptation where the gastrointestinal system is highly involved. The interpretation of the dental age in puppies and kittens can help us to decide which is the best nutritional strategy at each moment of their lives.

Requirements

1 Energy

✔ We have already seen what the growth curve looks like and learned about daily weight gain. According to that information, the daily energy requirements (DER) for growth will be multiples of the MER, and they include the requirements for growth and maintenance.

$$DER = \times\ MER\ (ER_{growth} + ER_{maintenance})$$

0-2 weeks DER = MER **PAUSE**

✔ We only consider that the metabolism is at rest during the first 2 weeks given that at this age, baby animals sleep all day.

✔ The energy requirements are different for cats, small and medium dogs, than for large and giant dogs (see graph).

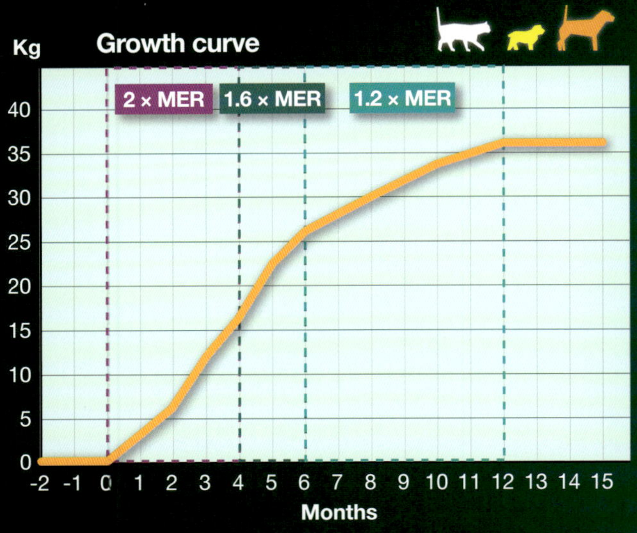

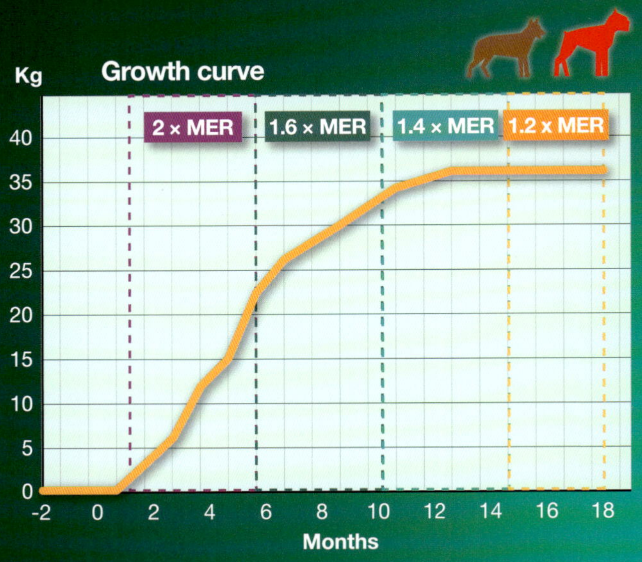

As we have seen in the graphs, the DER_{growth} are conditioned by the growth rate.

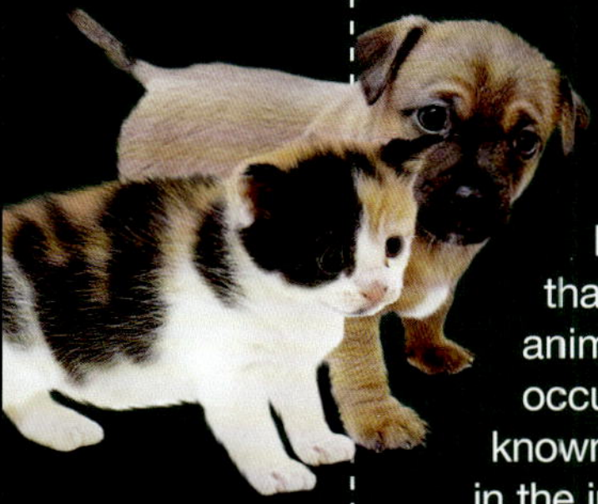

Be careful with obesity!

In small and medium dog breeds and in cats, controlling a pet's ingestion prevents obesity. It has been documented in various species that during infancy and adolescence, while the animal is growing, adipocyte hyperplasia occurs, although the precise age is not known in dogs and cats. Any imbalance in the ingestion of energy during growth will favor growth of the fatty tissue and will therefore be a predisposing factor for the animal being overweight as an adult.

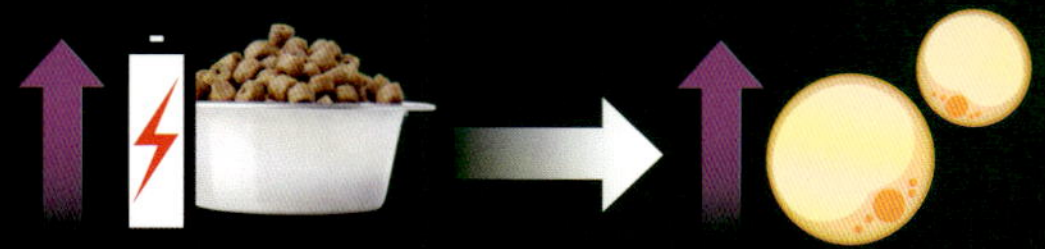

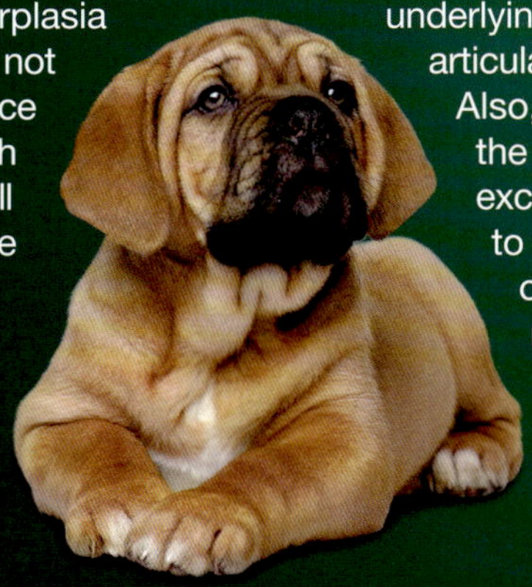

Be careful with excess calories in large breeds!

In large and giant breeds, fast growth is incompatible with a healthy bone structure: the bone becomes thinner and weaker than normal and cannot support the underlying joint. Damage to the cartilage produces articular incongruity (similar to osteochondrosis). Also, all of the aforementioned is favored by the pressure exerted on the joints due to the excess weight. These animals have a capacity to grow very quickly until they are 6 months old. For this reason, energy and protein restrictions in these breeds are more important than in others.

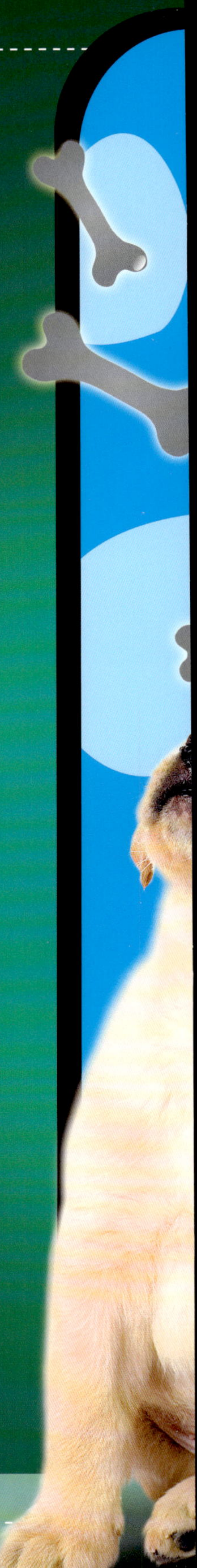

2 Water

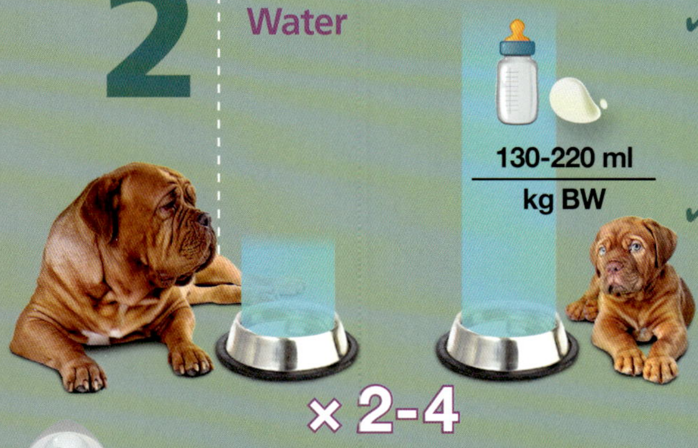

✔ Water is important during the lactation stage. The amount of liquid ingested by the puppies and kittens is much higher than that of weaned animals and adults.

✔ It is estimated that a puppy or kitten needs 130-220 ml of liquid/kg of body weight, between 2 and 4 times more than an adult. This volume of liquid will be provided with the mother's milk or with the corresponding milk substitute.

3 Carbohydrates

There are no specific requirements for this nutrient, except for the carbohydrates provided by the milk. In any case, the age at which the growing animals are capable of using these nutrients should be taken into account.

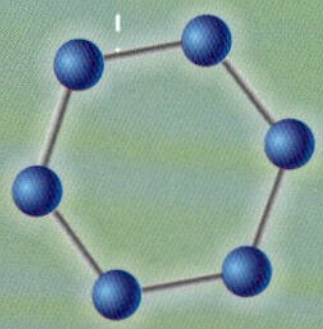

during growth (I)

The nutrient requirements during this stage are greatly increased, only surpassed by those needed during lactation. In general, they are twice as much as the needs of adults of the same weight.

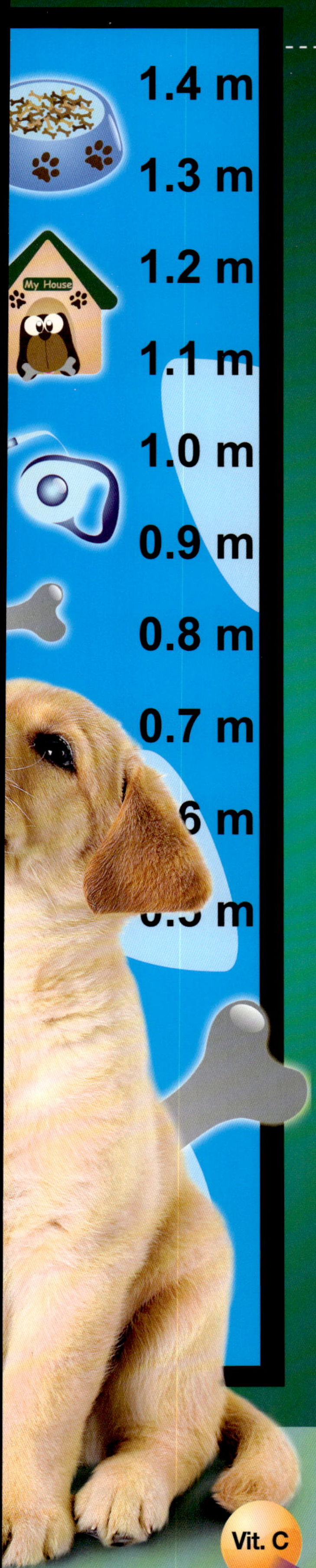

Calculation of the daily energy requirements

We can calculate the DER using the following formulas:

$$DER_{growth} = MER \times 3.2 \times [e^{(-0.87w)} - 0.1]$$

$$DER_{growth} = MER \times 6.7 \times [e^{(-0.189p)} - 0.66]$$

Where:

w = current weight (kg)/expected adult weight (kg)

e = 2.718

As an approximation of the previous equations, and for easy clinical use, the following table can be used. In large and giant breeds, it has been considered that a restriction of 30 % in the requirements leads to slower growth but decreases musculoskeletal problems.

	Energy requirements during growth						
	DER_{growth} = × MER						
Age (months)	Birth-2nd week	2nd week-weaning	Weaning-4	4-6	6-10	10-12	
Small and medium	0.55	1.9	2	1.6	1.2	1	
Large and giant	0.55	2.3	Weaning-4	4-8	9-12	12-18	18-24
			2	1.6	1.4	1.2	1
	Birth-2nd week	2nd week-weaning	Weaning-5	5-6	7-8.5	9-11	12
Cats	1.6	2-2.5	2.5	1.7	1.4	1.2	1

Example

What are the requirements of a male Beagle puppy that is 5 months old, with a current weight of 8 kg?

Standard male Beagle weight: 14 kg.

$$DER_{growth} = MER \times 3.2 \times [e^{(-0.87w)} - 0.1]$$

$$MER = 132 \times BW^{0.75}$$

$$DER_{growth} = [132 \times 8^{0.75}] \times 3.2 \times [e^{(-0.87 \times 8/14)} - 0.1]$$

$$DER_{growth} = \text{1,005.8 kcal ME/day}$$

Or by using the values in the table:

$$DER_{growth} = MER \times 1.6 = [132 \times 8^{0.75}] \times 1.6$$

$$DER_{growth} = \text{1,004.6 kcal ME/day}$$

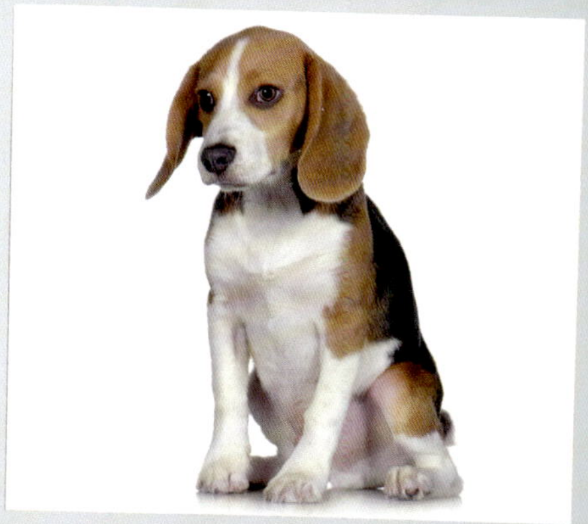

Beagle **Age:** 5 months **Weight:** 8 kg

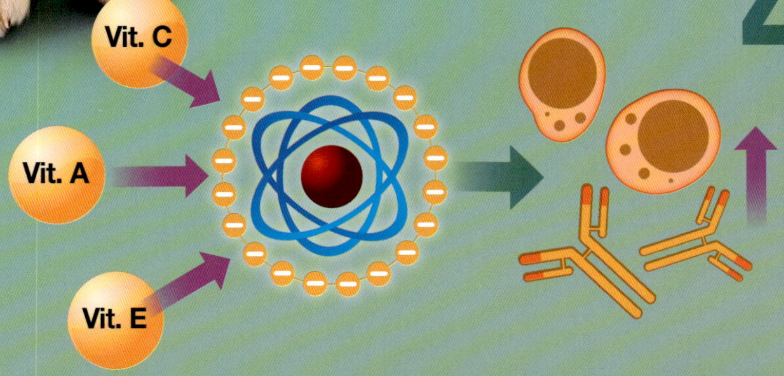

4 Vitamins

Vaccination programs are also implemented during the growth period of our pets. Although there are few studies that connect nutrition with the immune response in puppies and kittens, it seems that the incorporation of certain vitamins with antioxidant effects (vitamins A, C, and E) in foods offers certain benefits in periods of immunological activity: a proliferation of lymphocytes, high levels of IgM and an increased vaccine antibody titer have been described. More conclusive studies are needed.

Requirements

1 Protein

- ✔ Protein needs are higher in young animals than in adult animals: this is due to the growth and development of the body.
- ✔ On the other hand, the quality and digestibility of the protein must be high given that it needs to provide the animal with essential amino acids. In this sense, it is of great importance that the minimum amount of animal-based protein in food rations for growing dogs and cats be at least 19 %.
- ✔ As always, it is important that the proportions of proteins correspond with the calories of ME ingested. The requirements are maximum during weaning and from that point on, they decrease.

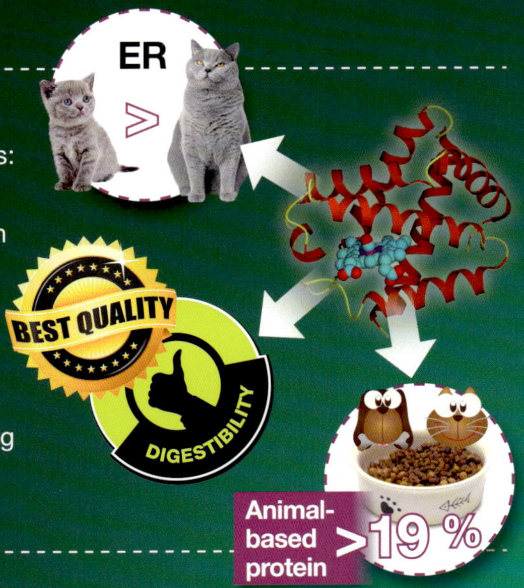

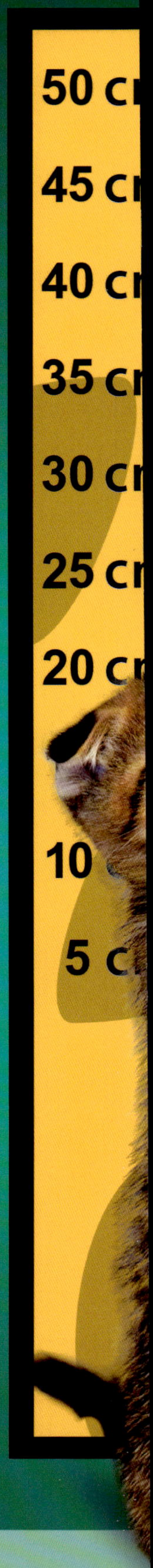

2 Important amino acids during growth

Arginine

Arginine is necessary as ornitine cannot support the urea cycle alone during the growth stage. It absence causes a decrease in the ingestion of food and nervous conditions caused by hyperammonemia. A deficiency causes cataracts in large breed puppies: the explanation is not clear, but it could be due to an increase in the secretion of insulin.

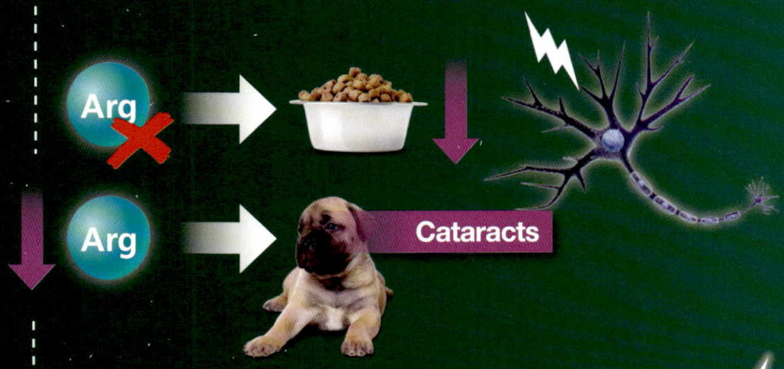

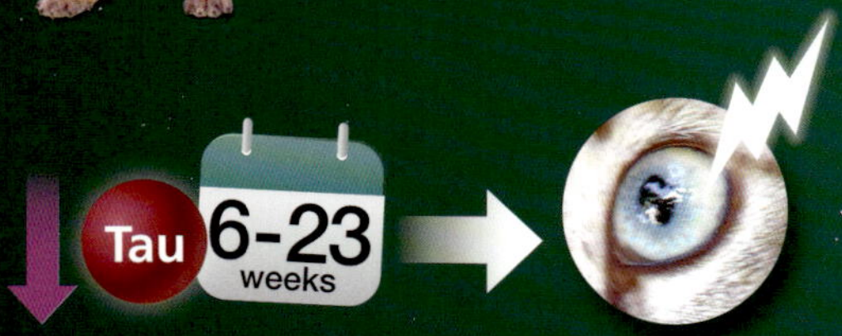

Taurine

Taurine is important for the development of eyes and vision during growth. A deficiency at 6 weeks of age that lasts for longer than 4 months will cause degeneration of the photoreceptors of the retina and will lead to blindness. The condition is similar to the central retinal degeneration syndrome in cats.

Tryptophan

Tryptophan is involved in the ingestion of food. A deficiency in kittens determines a decrease in the consumption of food of up to 13 g/day.

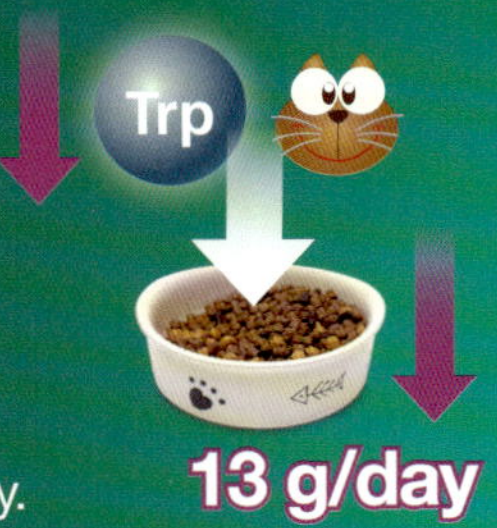

Phenylalanine and tyrosine

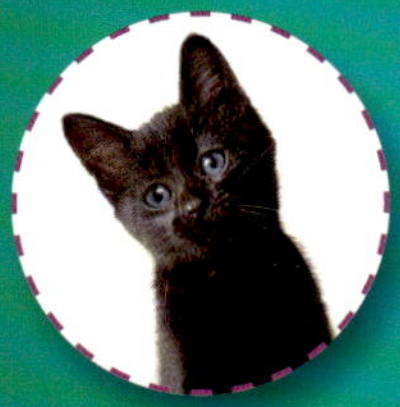

These proteins affect the black color of an animal's fur. Its absence in kittens causes their coat to turn brown. In addition, its deficiency in kittens causes the degeneration of the axons and collapse of myelin; the effect is a nervous condition that manifests as an unstable gait, the tail held bent forward, hyperactivity, vocalization, and excessive salivation.

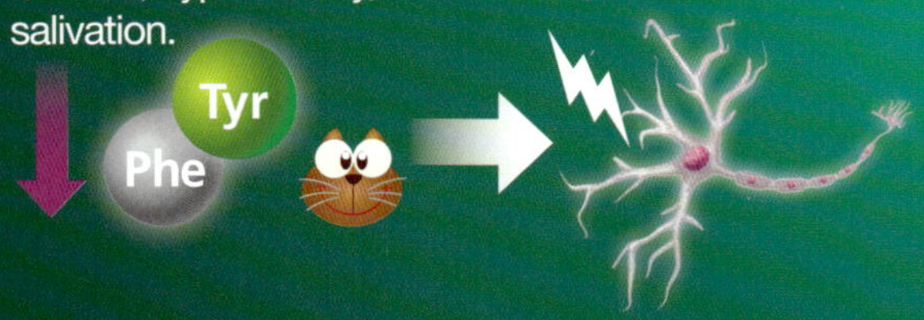

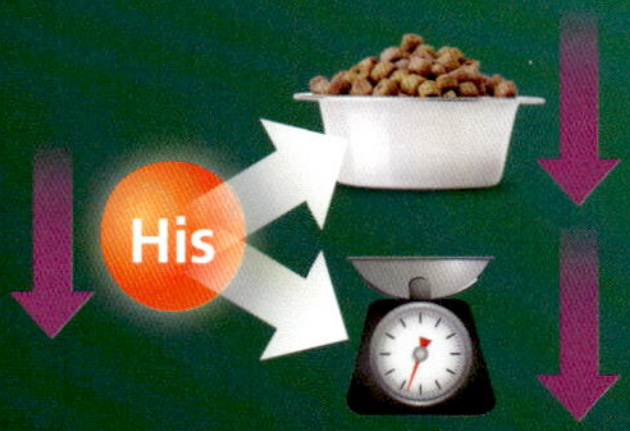

Histidine

Due to its participation in the synthesis of various neuro-active precursors, a deficiency of histidine causes lack of appetite and weight loss.

4 Minerals: calcium and phosphorus

- ✔ Calcium is another important nutrient in the growth and development of puppies and kittens, especially in large or giant breed dogs due to its involvement in bone growth.
- ✔ The requirements for certain vitamins and minerals are shown in the following table.

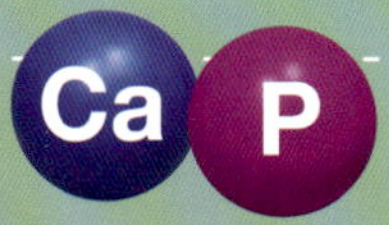

	Nutrient/1,000 kcal ME			
	Calcium (g)	Phosphorus (g)	Ca:P	Vitamin D (µg)
Small/medium breeds	3	2.5	1:1-1.5:1-1.8:1	3.4
Large/giant breeds	2-2.2	1.5-2	1.2:1	3.4
Cats	2	1.8	1:1	1.4

during growth (II)

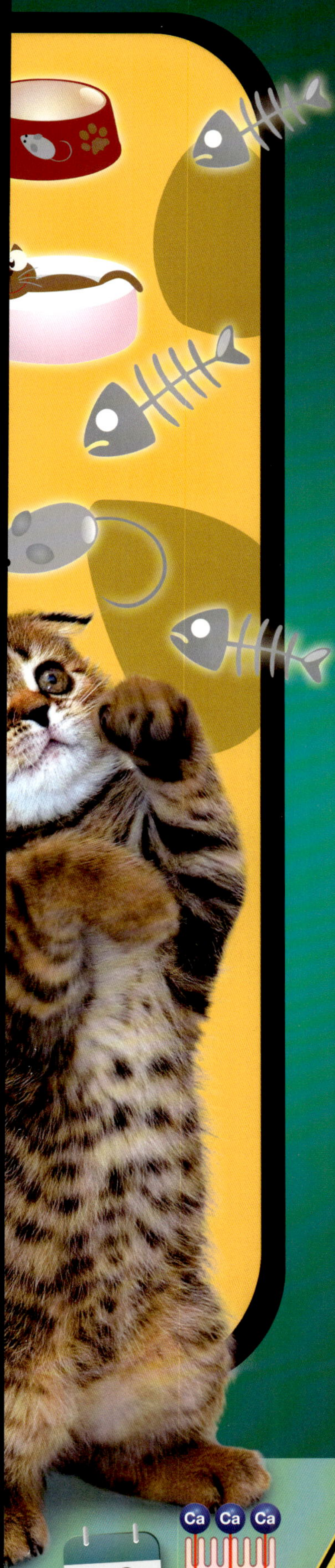

Recommendations regarding amino acids

As there are differences between species and between certain dog breeds, the following table summarizes the recommendations.

	Nutrient (g)/1,000 kcal ME							
	Protein		Arg	Phe-Tyr	Trp	Tau	His
	NRC 2006	AAFCO/FEDIAF	NRC 2006, AAFCO and FEDIAF				
Cats	56.3	65/75 to 90	2.4 (max. 8.75)	4.78	0.4 (max. 4.25)	0.25-0.6	0.83
Dogs 4-14 weeks	56.3	56.25/72.5 to 80	1.98	3.25	0.58	No	0.98
Dogs >14 weeks	43.8	55 to 62.5	1.65 to 1.78	2.50	0.45	No	0.63
Great Dane	-	65	-	-	-	-	-

3 Fat and fatty acids

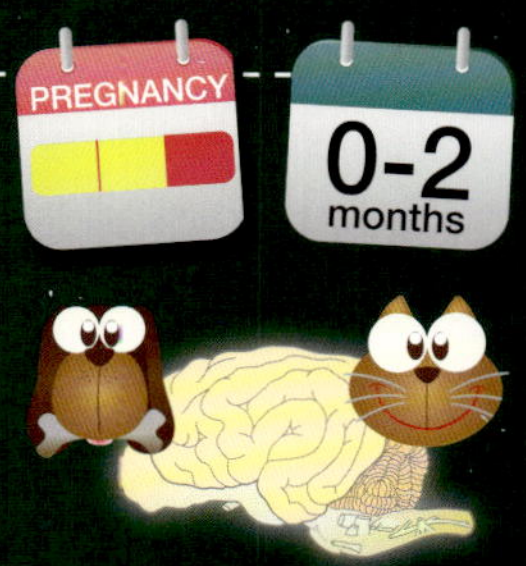

Nervous system development

Fat and fatty acids play an important role in the development of the nervous system, the retina, sense of hearing, learning, and memory in growing cats and dogs. The development of the nervous system of our puppies and kittens has two phases: in the last third of gestation and in the first 2 months of life.

High content in mothers' milk

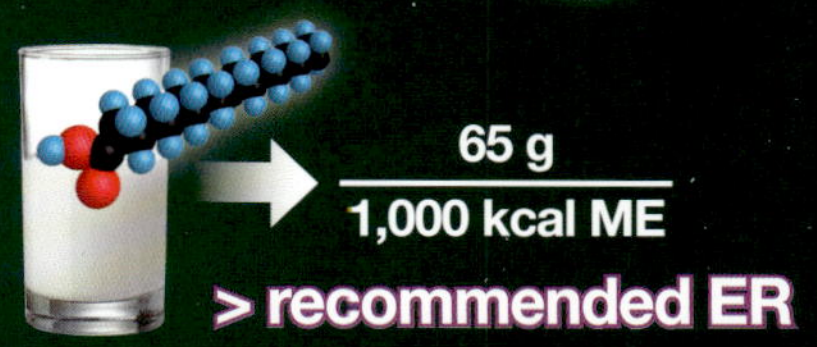

The concentration in fat (65 g/1,000 kcal ME) and EFAs is much higher in the milk (for example, linolenic acid-7.6 g/1,000 kcal ME-) than the recommendations; this could explain why the growth of lactating puppies and kittens is so fast during this period.

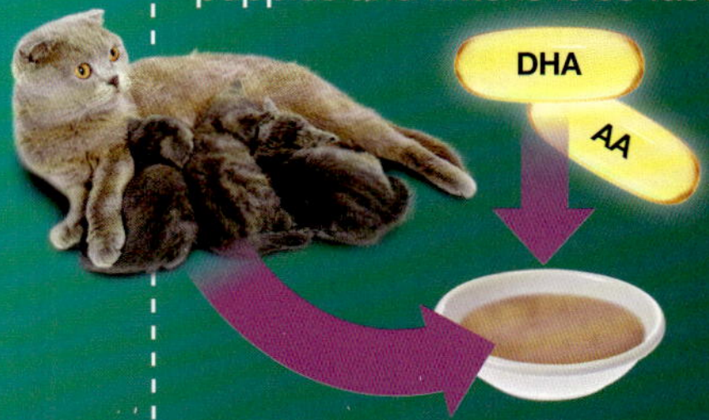

Incorporation of long-chain FAs in an animal's diet

On the other hand, puppies and kittens are inefficient in the elongation or obtention of long-chain FAs, such as DHA and AA, and therefore these must be added to their food rations in the peri-natal period, although they are capable of converting the α-linolenic acid into DHA, with poor efficiency, from the mother's milk.

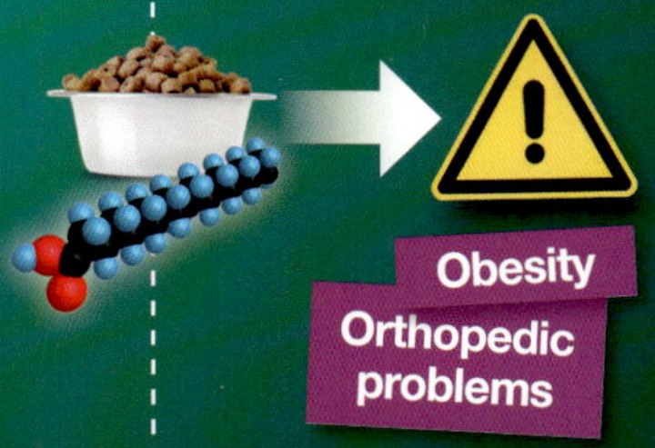

Monitoring to prevent fast growth

Providing fat in the food rations of growing animals must be monitored to avoid orthopedic problems due to excessively fast growth, as well as to prevent obesity. The table summarizes the recommendations for weaned puppies and kittens.

	Nutrient (g)/1,000 kcal ME				
	Fat	Linoleic acid	α-linolenic acid	Arachydonic acid	EPA + DHA
	21.3	3.3	0.2	0.08	0.13
	22.5	1.4	0.05	0.05	0.025

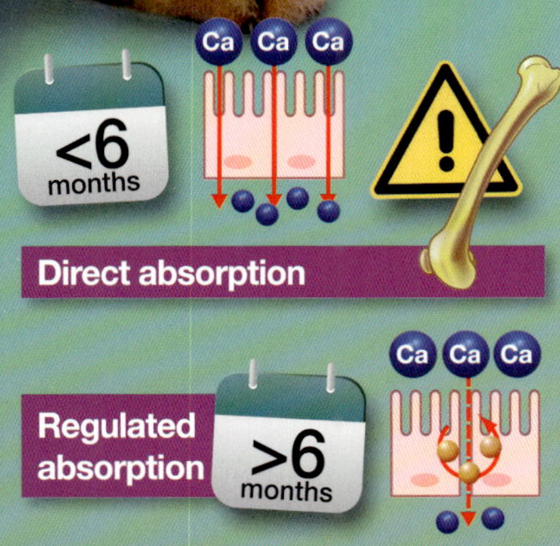

Calcium and growth

The capacity to regulate the metabolism of calcium is not achieved until 6 months of age. Until this age, most of the calcium is directly absorbed in the intestines in a passive manner and depends, therefore, on the concentration of the food ration. Puppies and kittens lack the autoregulation mechanisms (vitamin D, calcitonin, GH and PTH) that control and protect them from this massive ingestion of the mineral. All of this coincides with the maximum growth phase between 3 and 5 months. The result could be the presentation of orthopedic abnormalities. However, this possibility has only been observed in large and giant breeds, especially in Great Danes, and not in small/medium breeds or in cats. This suggests the possible existence of genetic differences between the different dog breeds. This explanation could be supported by the variations in metabolizing vitamin D that exist between different breeds and their relationship with the growth hormone. More research is needed to confirm this effect.

Food management in

1 Milk substitutes

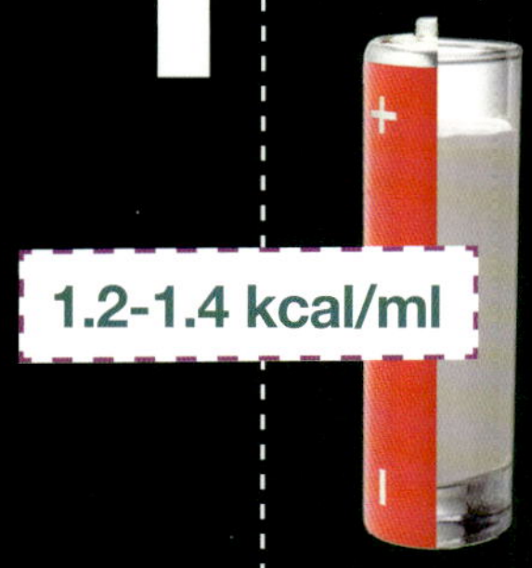

✔ The energy concentration of milk varies between 1.2 and 1.4 kcal/ml; we can thus use this value to adjust the volume of milk to the requirements of unweaned animals. Depending on the digestive capacity at these ages, during the 1st week, 8 to 12 doses per day are recommended, and 4 to 6 after the 2nd week of life.

✔ When administrating milk substitutes as reinforcement in large litters or for ophaned animals, all of the animals in the litter are always taken into account. Certain guidelines should be followed when preparing the milk substitute.

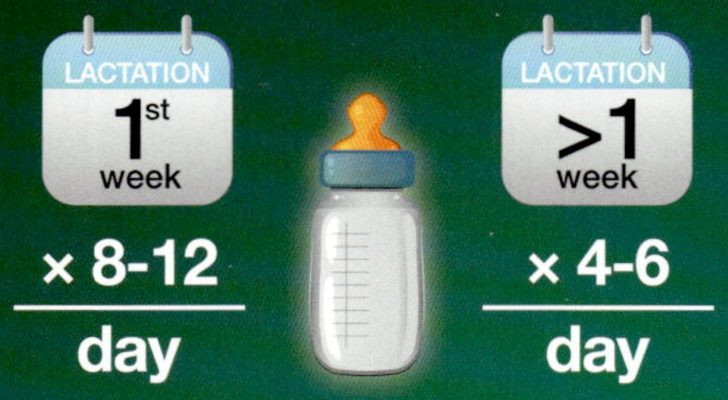

Guidelines for preparing milk replacements

✔ Make sure that the powder:liquid ratio is correct. This way we will avoid diarrhea and vomiting (primarily due to the content in DM, lactose, and minerals).

✔ Maximum cleanliness of the materials.

✔ We can prepare the daily volume and store it at 4 °C, to later administer the needed quantity for each dose. If any product is left over, it should be discarded.

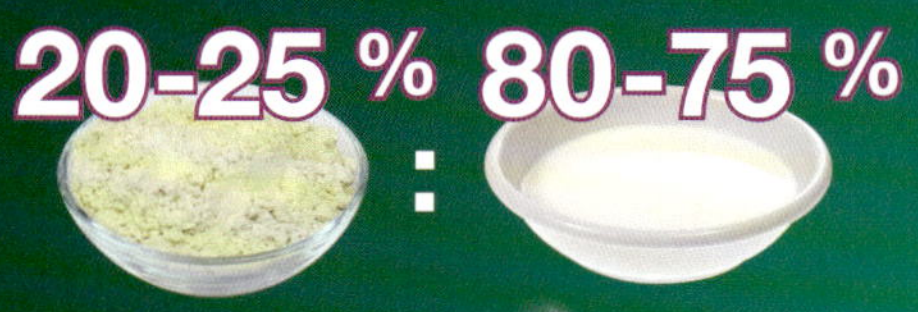

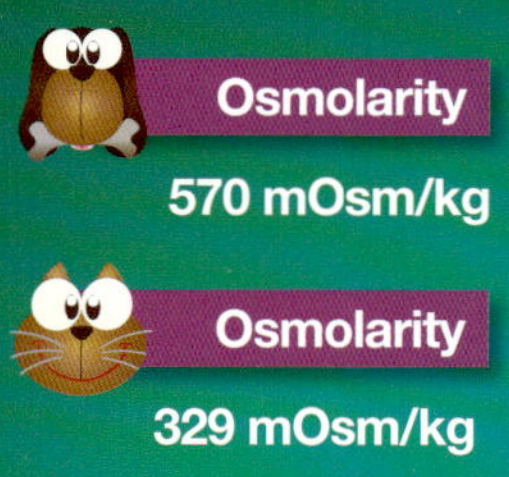

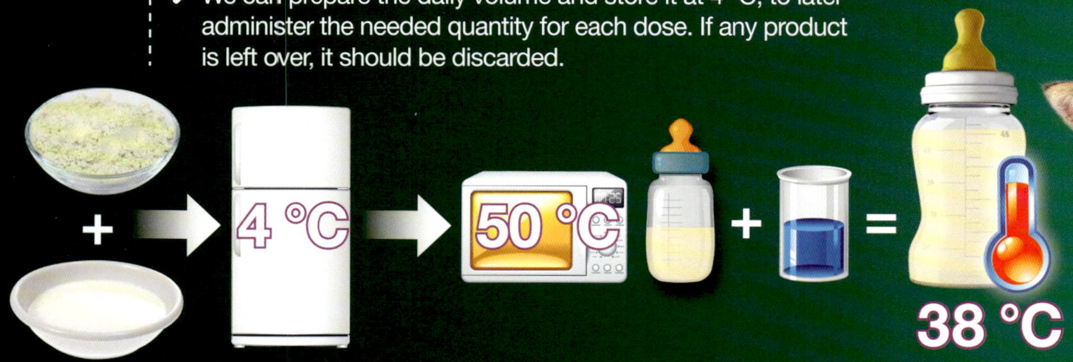

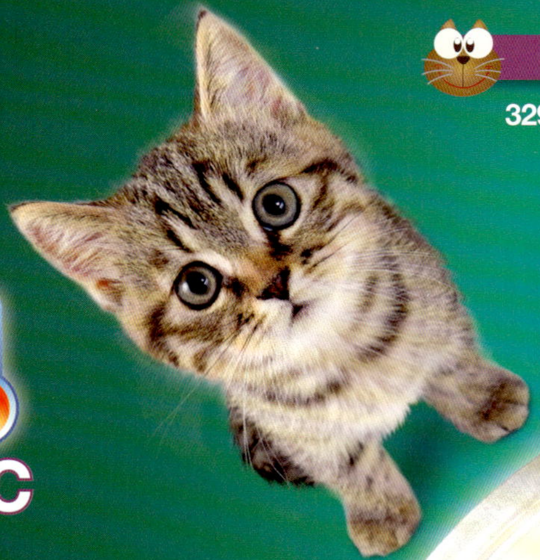

✔ To prepare the formula, we will heat half of the estimated dose to 50 °C until a homogeneous mixture is obtained. Then we will add lukewarm water until reaching the total volume, making sure that the temperature is 38 °C.

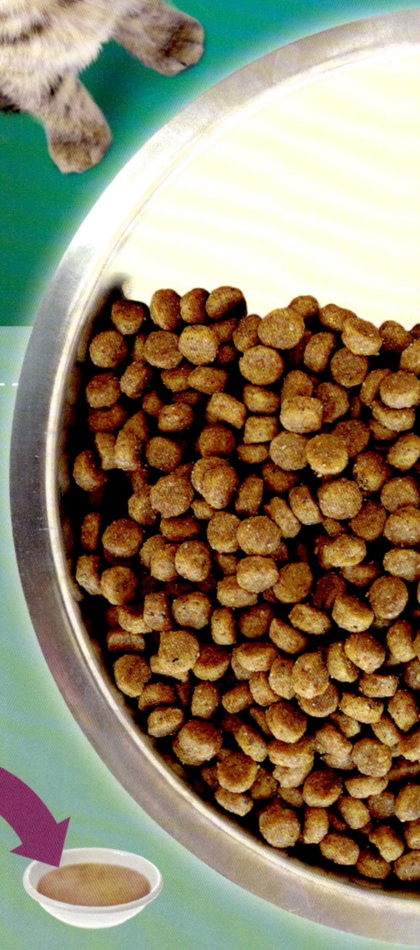

2 Weaning

✔ Weaning should start in a natural manner when the puppies or kittens are 4 weeks old, and end when they are around 7-8 weeks old (although in reality this is different, closer to 3-4 weeks) with foods created especially for this purpose, with characteristics similar to the following example:

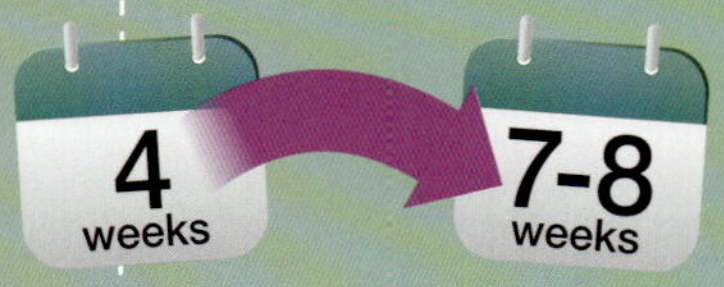

Nutrient (g)/1,000 kcal ME									ME Mcal/kg DM
Protein	Arg	Tau	Carbohydrates	Fat	Fiber	EPA-DHA	Ca	P	
>65	4	0.47	60	50	14	0.7	2.7	2.1	>4

✔ An alternative to stimulate the consumption of solids is to mix commercial wet or dry foods for growing animals with warm water, in different proportions (30 to 50 %). It is recommended that the dilution be mixed and homogenized correctly.

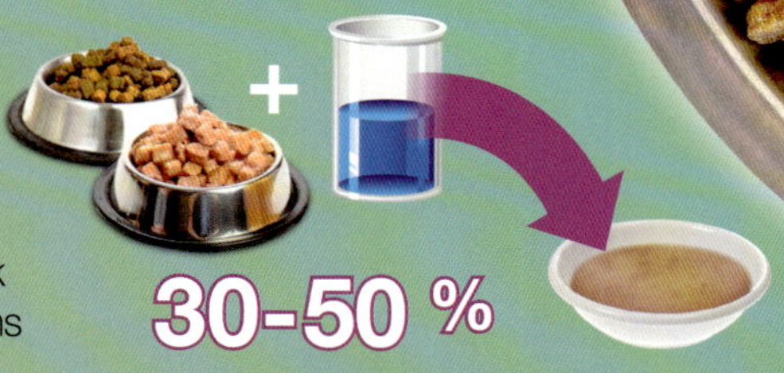

✔ To ensure that the food recommendations are correct, it is important to check the weight and BCS weekly or bi-weekly, to determine whether our predictions were right or whether any adjustments to the food ration are needed.

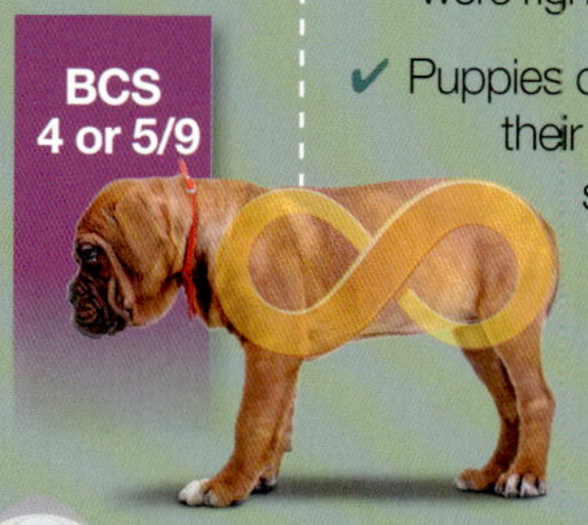

✔ Puppies or kittens should grow with a BCS of 4 or 5/9 and their silhouette should look like an infinite mathematical sign (∞), where the baby animal's waist is visible and the bone prominences and the ribs should be easily palpable.

✔ During the growth period, the use of supplements, extra food, or treats is not recommended (for example, a hot-dog sausage has nearly 200 kcal). The family and any other people that may be in contact with the puppy or kitten (trainers) should be informed of this. These attitudes have a double effect; they modify the acceptability of foods and predispose the animal to obesity (although it is not rare to see overweight puppies and kittens at 6-7 months of age).

puppies and kittens

Administration

The administration will be performed with a bottle or a gastric tube, depending on the newborn's strength.

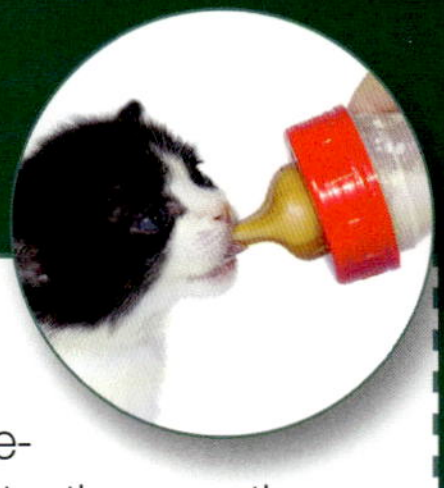

Bottles are reserved for strong animals with a good sucking reflex. It is important that only one drop comes out of the bottle's nipple when the bottle is turned upside-down. Making a cut in the tip of the bottle's nipple is better than creating a hole, allowing control of the suction and avoiding aspiration pneumonia.

The gastric tube is used in very weak animals. It is very easy to use: it needs to be lubricated and slowly introduced in the oral cavity toward the esophagus. Any coughing indicates that we are in the trachea. The first volumes will be administered very slowly to verify the correct position of the tube.

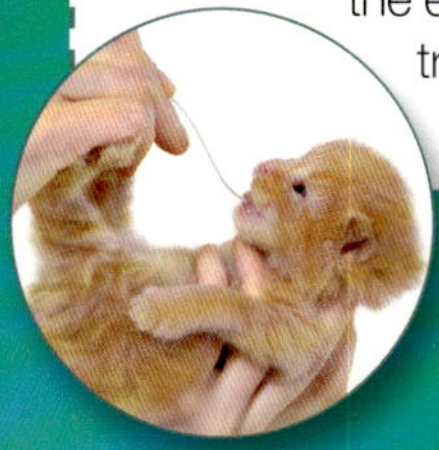

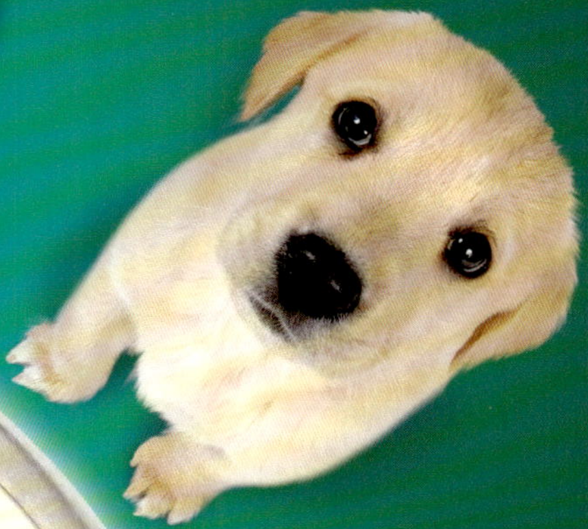

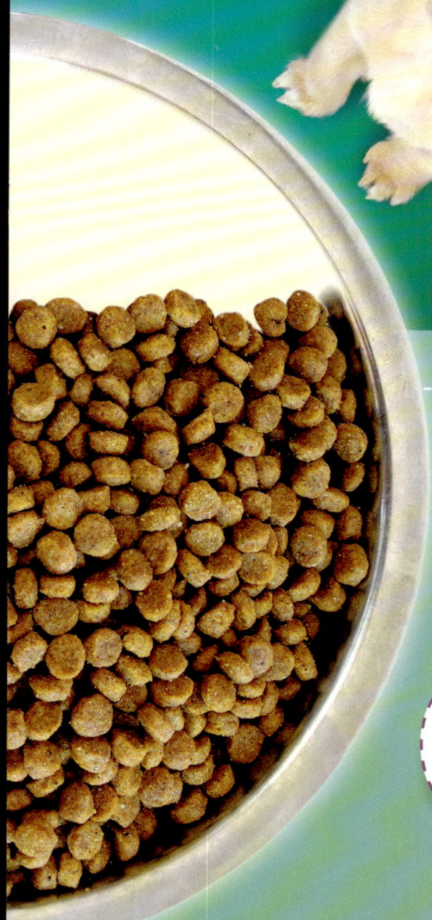

The approximate volume of the substitute recommended is shown in the table.

Volume/unit of weight/day		
Age	0-3 weeks	>4 weeks
	100 ml/kg	150 ml/kg
	20 ml/100 g	25-35 ml/100 g

Example

What would the volume of a milk substitute be for a kitten that is brought to our clinic with its eyes open, with deciduous incisors and slight eruption of the deciduous canine teeth, which weighs 375 g?

✔ Considering the opening of the eyes and the dentition, this animal is about 3 weeks old. At this age, the estimated weight is 400 g. This is a well-fed kitten.

✔ The daily volume should be:

DV = (375 g/100 g) × 20 ml = 75 ml (≈ 100 kcal ME/day)

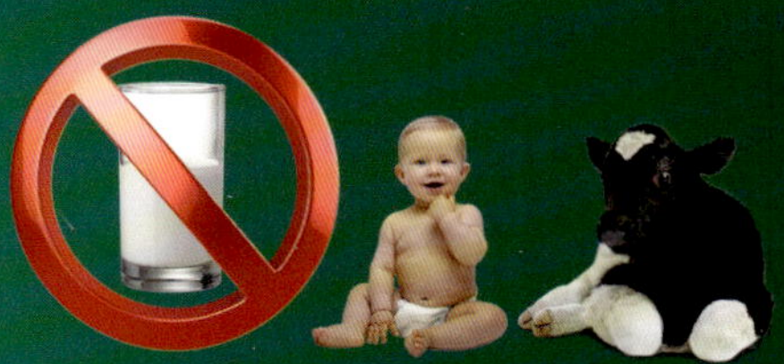

Human infant formulas and cow's milk as milk substitutes are not recommended, due to their low concentration in energy and certain nutrients (for example, protein, arginine, taurine and fat) as well as their high lactose concentration (which causes diarrhea).

The volume is adjusted to the energy recommendations.

$DER_{growth} = MER \times 2$

$MER = 100 \times 0.375^{0.67}$

$DER_{growth} = (100 \times 0.375^{0.67}) \times 2$

$DER_{growth} = 103.7 \text{ kcal ME/day}$

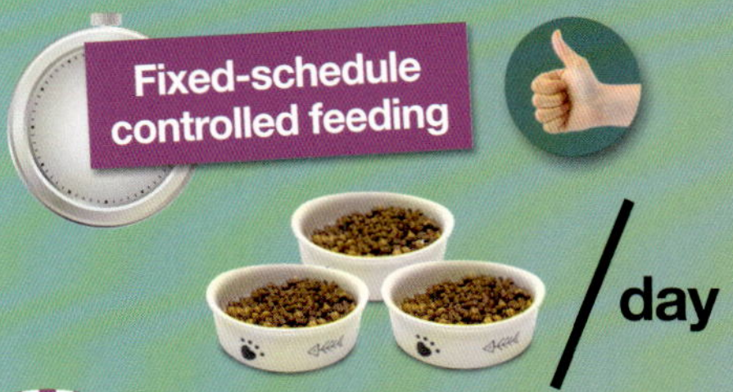

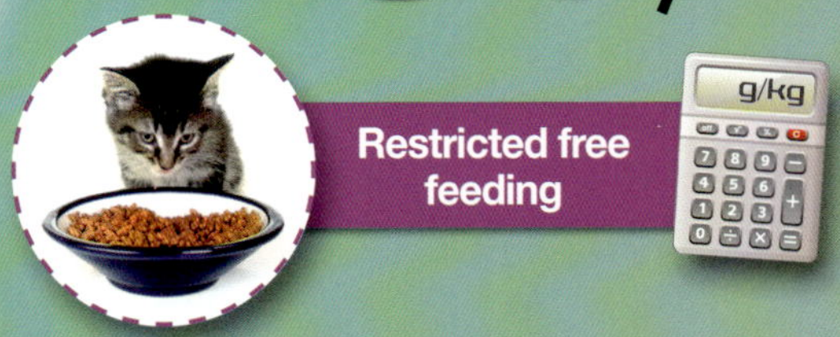

Feeding schedule

✔ The fixed-schedule controlled feeding method is recommended, with 2 or 3 meals per day. If this is not possible, the second-best option is restricted free feeding, especially for cats. Free feeding leads to digestive overloading with the possibility of developing episodes of gastric dilatation-volvulus in dogs.

✔ As a result of development, especially of the volume of the digestive system, of the capacity to utilize the nutrients ingested, and the dentition, the food rations for growing animals should be highly digestible and with an energy content that varies from 3.5-4 or 4-5 Mcal/kg DM in dogs and cats, respectively.

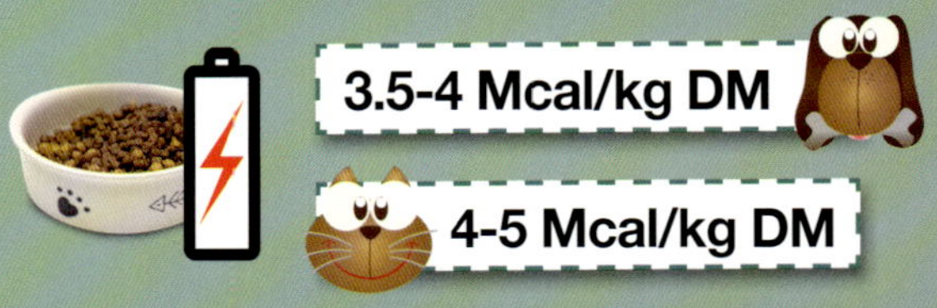

To be taken into account

Much has been speculated about exercise during the growth stage. Moderate exercise allows for there to be a balance between ingestion and energy expenditure and favors the pet's proper muscle conformation. However, in large and giant breed dogs, excessive and continuous exercise during the growth stage, without veterinary monitoring, leads to certain osteo-articular problems, such as osteochondritis dissecans.

✔ In addition, the changes in the type of food given to our pets should be done gradually (see "Diet changes: How should I do it?" in Volume I of the Atlas). This situation is typical at the time a puppy or kitten is purchased or adopted and arrives to its new home.

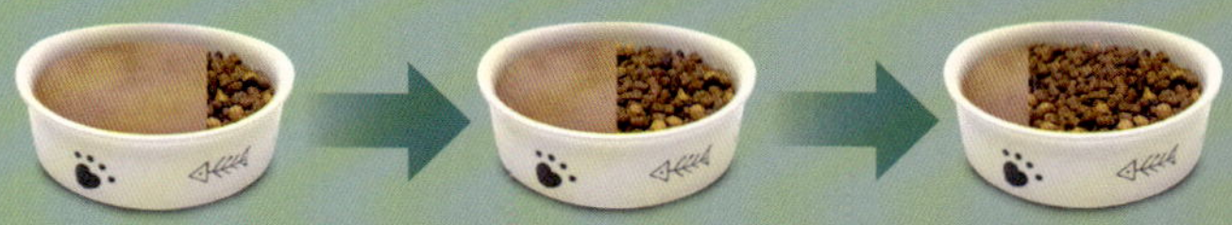

The aging

1 Aging mechanisms

- ✔ Aging is a progressive process that includes physiological, metabolic, and behavioral changes, characterized by decreased functions.
- ✔ It is not a pathological process, but it affects the presentation of certain diseases, particularly cancer, chronic renal failure, and heart disease.
- ✔ The beginning of this stage of life takes place when the animals reach the halfway point of their life expectancy: between 5 and 7 years of age.

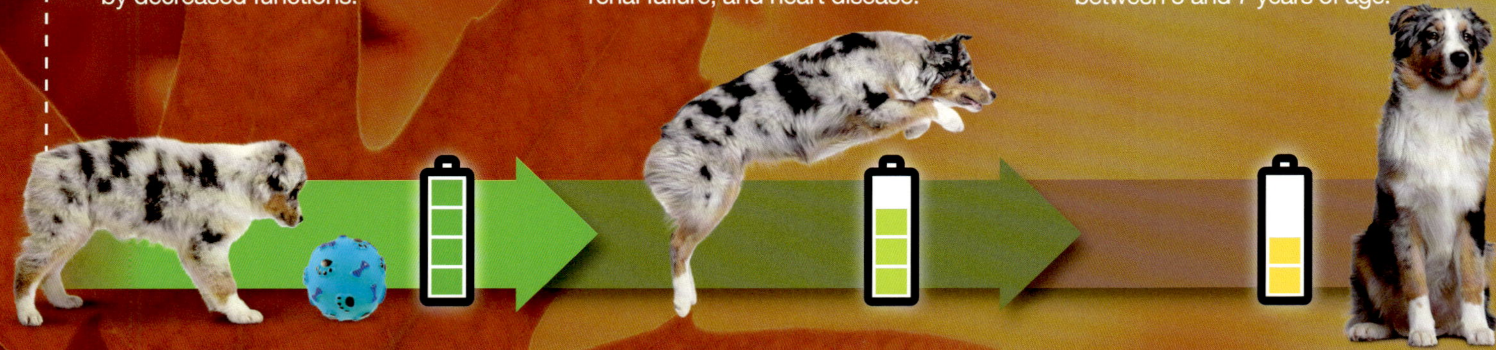

2 Life expectancy

The life expectancy of our domestic dogs and cats represents an exception in the animal kingdom.
In the wild, senile animals, due to natural selection, represent a target for other predators, diseases and accidents.
Pets enjoy old age accompanied with social well-being, in spite of diseases that are a natural part of the degenerative aging process.

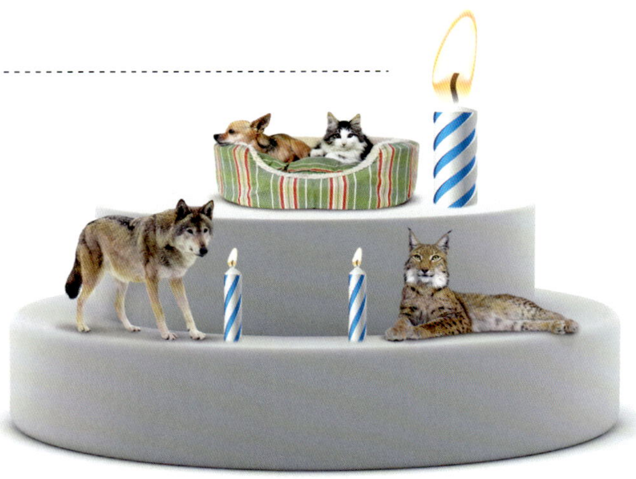

Life expectancy varies with each species

There are records of dogs and cats dying at ages near 30 years old, but this is rare.

- ✔ Cats, on average, live longer: this could be due to a slower aging process. Their life expectancy is similar to small and medium dog breeds.
- ✔ In dogs, there are differences depending on body weight. The weight and the life expectancy are inversely correlated: small dogs live 45 % longer than giant dogs.

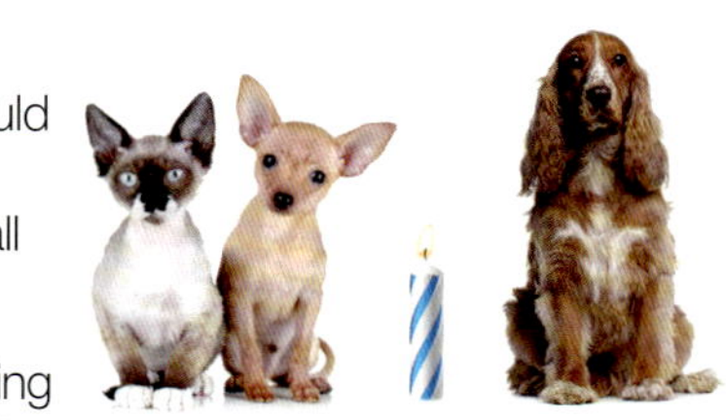

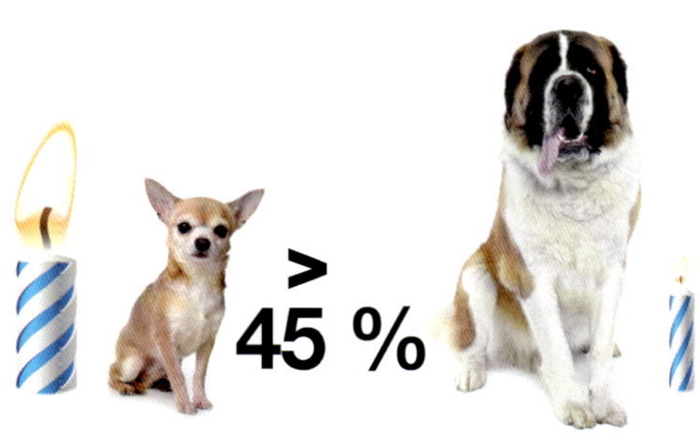

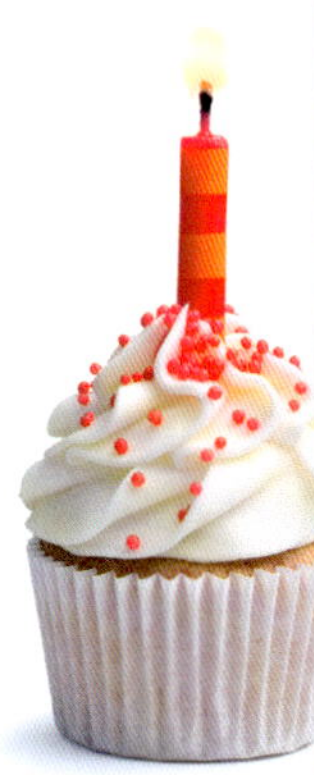

Species and size		Beginning of old age (years)
Small dogs (<10 kg) and cats	<10	11.5-12
Medium-sized dogs (10-25 kg)	10-25	10
Large dogs (25-45 kg)	25-45	9
Giant dogs (>45 kg)	>45	7.5

The breed affects life expectancy

The life expectancy in some breeds is influenced by certain hereditary traits (for example: English Bulldog) or by certain orthopedic conditions caused by high growth rates. A large quantity of hereditary diseases have been reported in purebred dogs that could contribute to the reduction of their life expectancy.

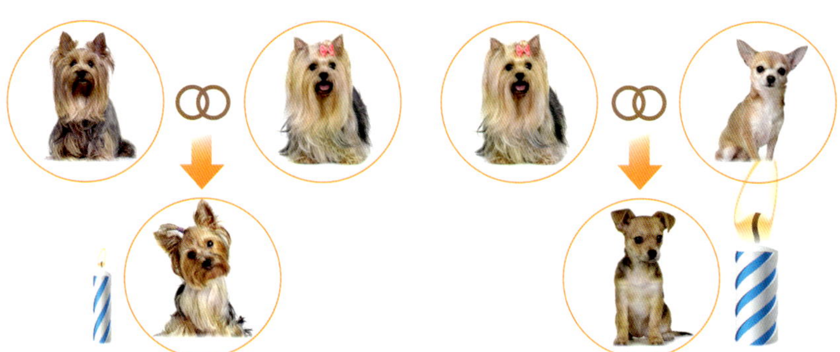

Purebred Mixed breed

process

The mechanisms of aging include:

- Deterioration of the DNA with instability of the genome
- Changes in genetic expression
- Shortening of telomeres
- Non-enzymatic glycosylation of structural proteins
- Oxidative stress

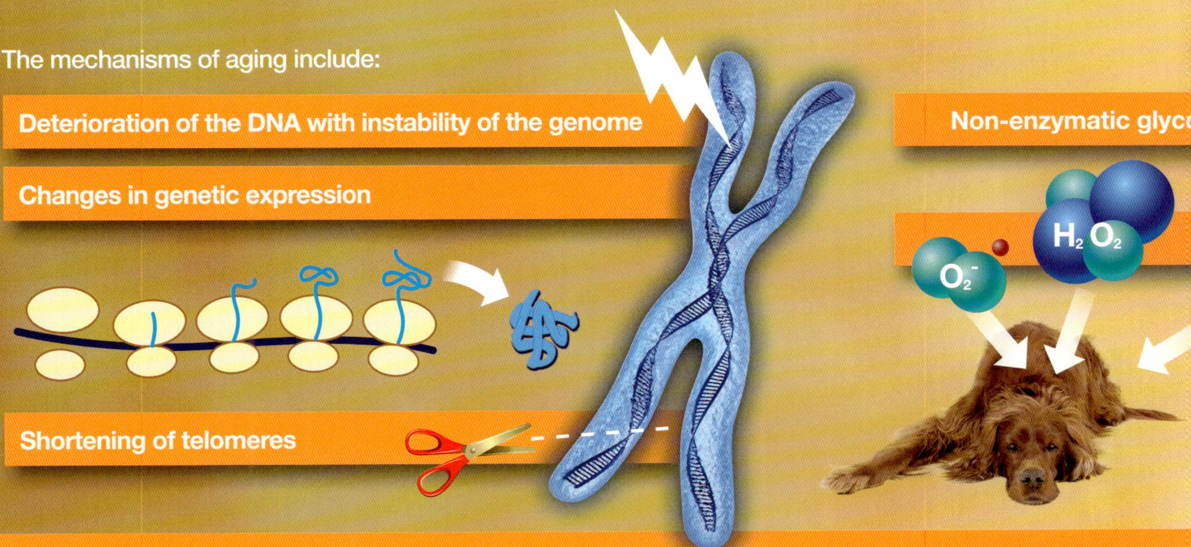

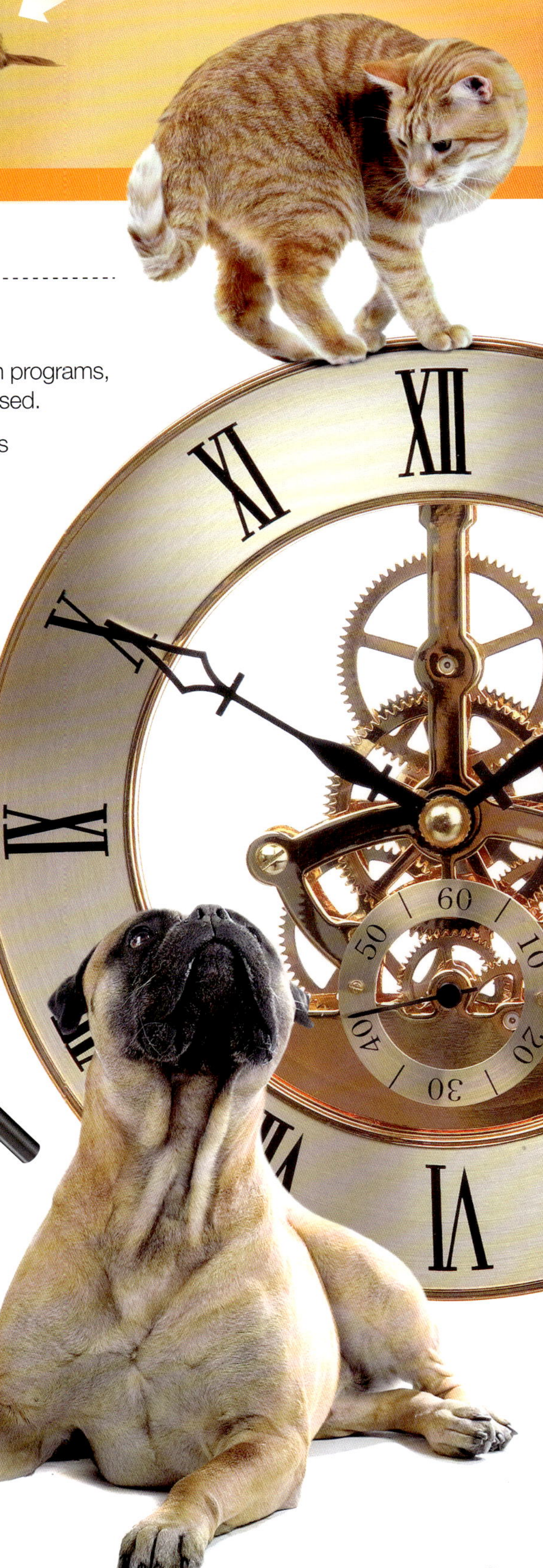

3 Dogs and cats live longer

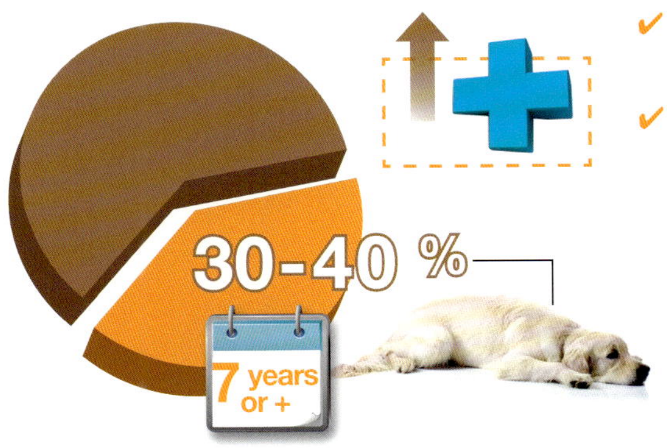

- ✔ Currently, and as a result of the best health programs, the number of geriatric patients has increased.
- ✔ Approximately 30-40 % of pets are 7 years of age or older.

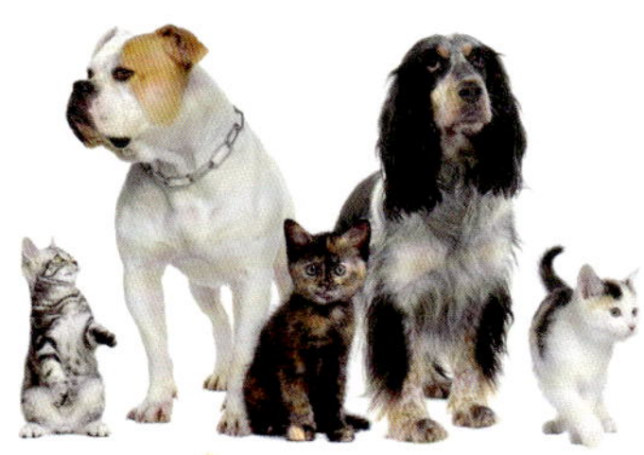

- ✔ Unlike other previous stages where the requirements of the group are considered, in this stage, great individual variations are seen in the animals' state of health. Each patient should be observed individually, evaluating the functional changes more than their chronological age, to establish the nutritional requirements in accordance with their particular status.

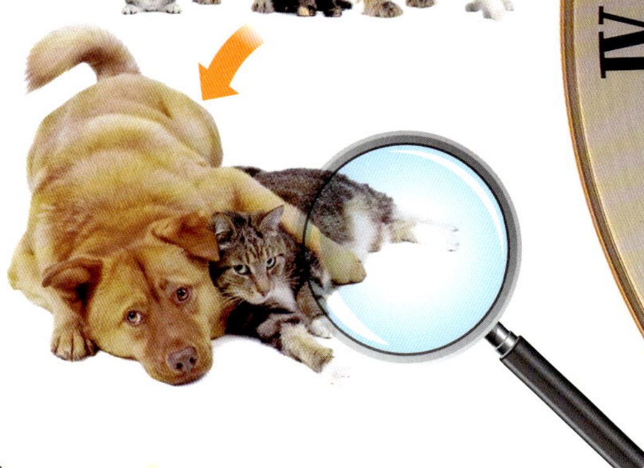

- ✔ The only scientifically proven nutritional factor that prolongs life expectancy and reduces the risk of other pathologies is the decrease in calorie consumption throughout the entire life of the pet.

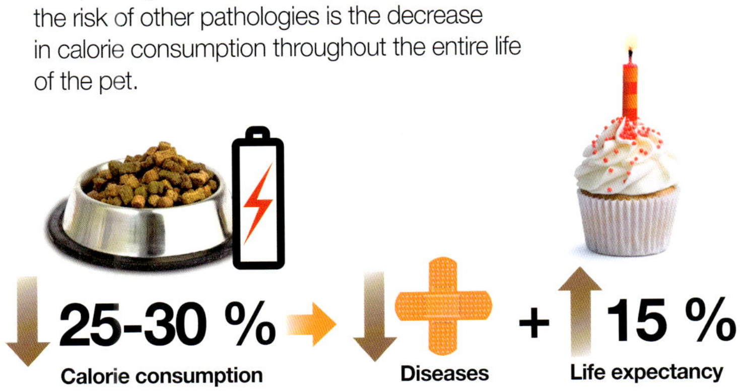

How does

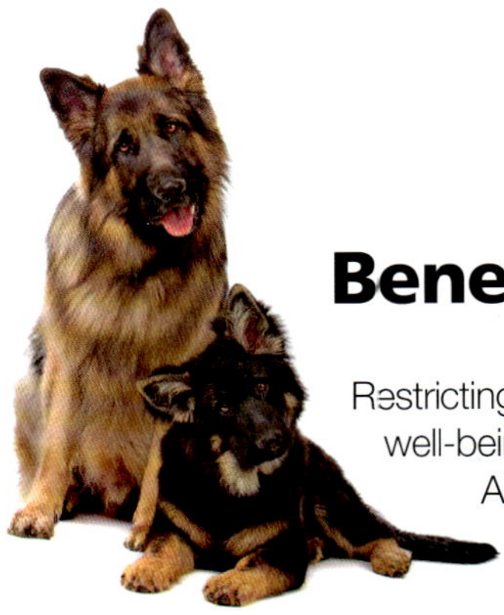

Benefits of calorie restriction

Restricting the daily energy requirements by 25 % in dogs throughout their life offers greater well-being and life expectancy.

Although the intrinsic mechanisms of these processes are not clear, the different observations have revealed certain benefits, generally speaking:

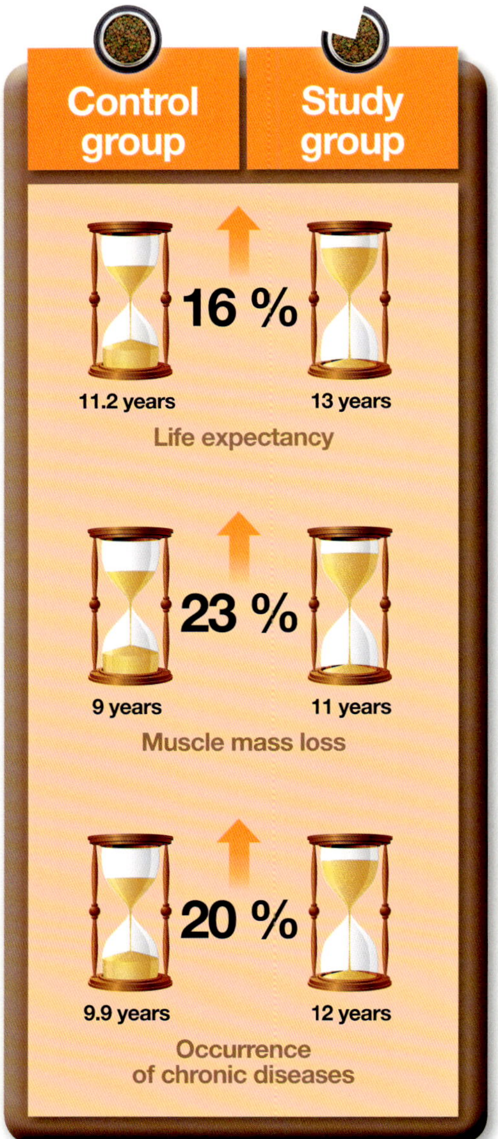

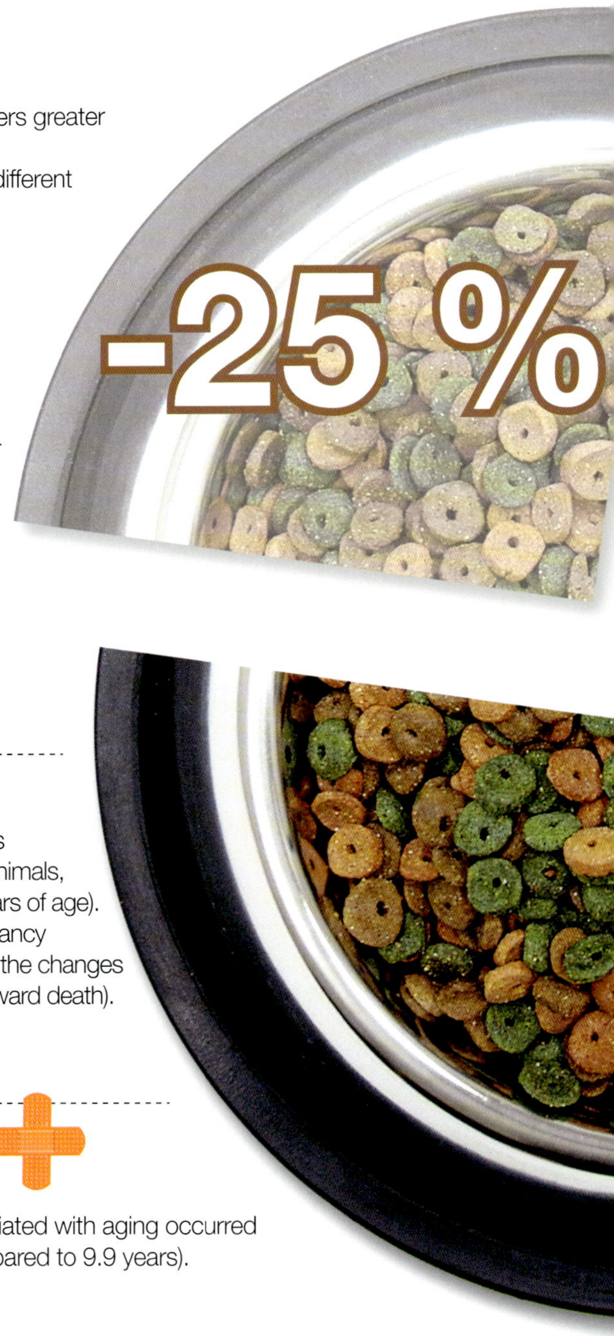

1 Greater life expectancy

The half life is prolonged from 11.2 to 13 years, or, a 16 % increase. At the age by which all of the "control" dogs had died, nearly 40 % of the dogs with diet restriction were still alive.

2 Reduced loss of lean mass

In the control group, the loss of mean mass took place at 9 years of age. In the study animals, this period was nearly 23 % greater (11 years of age). This allows for an increase in the life expectancy (the loss of muscle mass is related with the changes that take place in the trajectory toward death).

3 Delay in the occurrence of chronic diseases

The age at which chronic diseases associated with aging occurred was approximately 20 % higher (12 compared to 9.9 years).

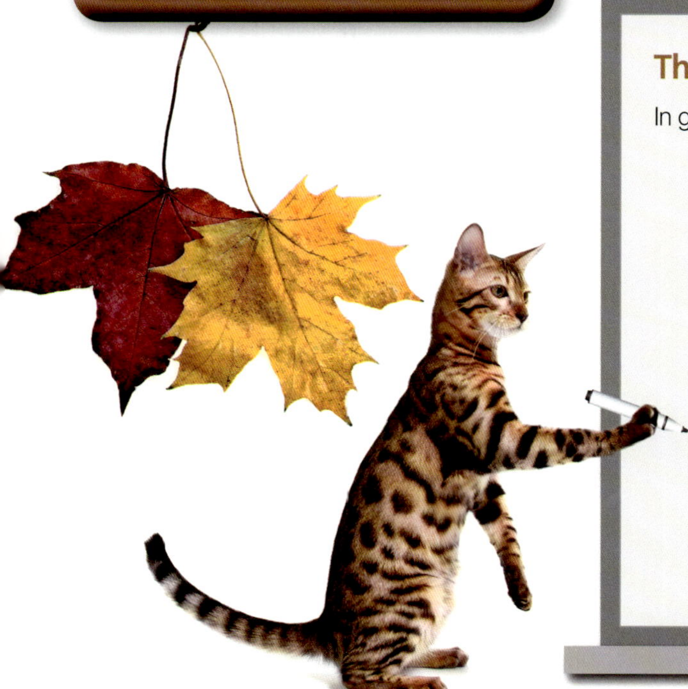

Theories on the effects of calorie restriction

In general, and in different species, the theories about the positive effects are as follows:

- One theory affirms that calorie restriction **reduces the rate of cellular division in many tissues**, which would partially explain its positive effects on cancer.
- Another theory is based on the fact that the **blood glucose level is reduced**, which in turn decreases the rate of accumulation of sugar in the proteins and its destructive effects.
- One interesting hypothesis postulates that it slows down aging given the fact that it **reduces the production of free radicals** due to a lower consumption of oxygen by the mitochondria.
- Recent research shows that calorie restriction leads to a **reduction in triiodothyronine (T_3)**, which is a hormone with an important role in the body's metabolic control.
- The latest studies defend the possible implication of the **PHA-4 gene** as key in the physiological effects of calorie restriction.

food restriction affect aging?

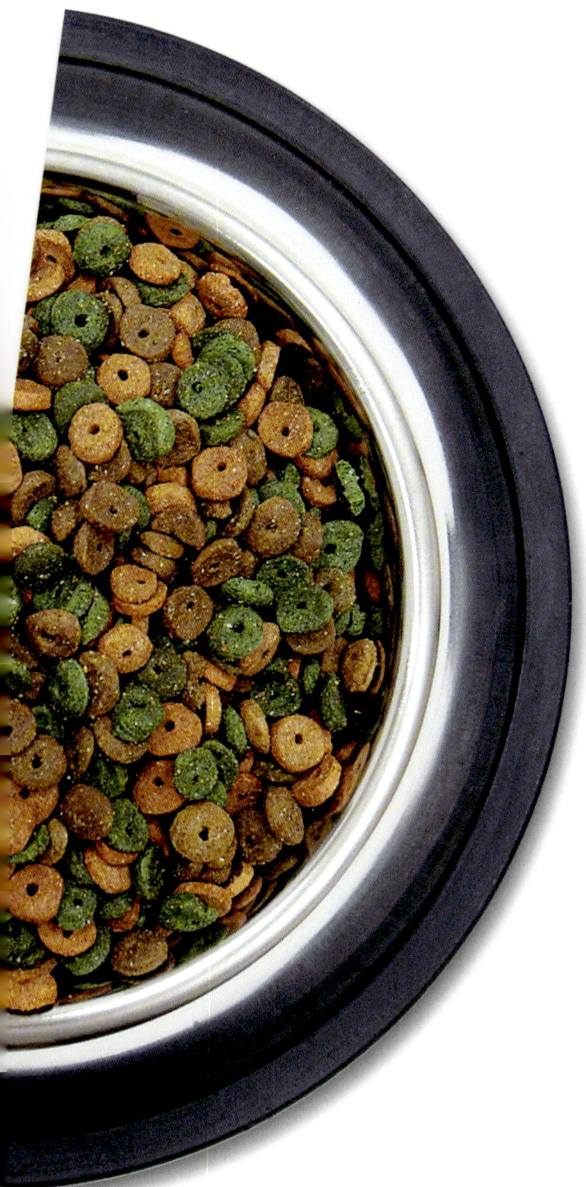

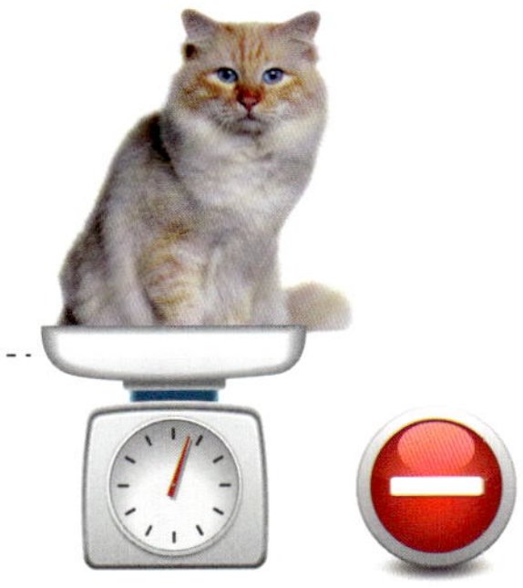

4 Lower weight

The total weight was 25 % lower.

−25 %

5 Better body condition

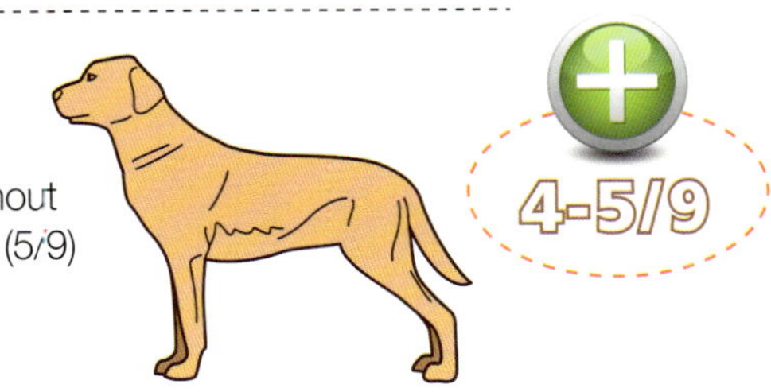

The body condition (based on Laflamme's scale of 9) was kept between 4-5/9 throughout the animals' lives, showing a slight increase (5/9) during the senile phase (10 to 14 years).

6 More muscle mass

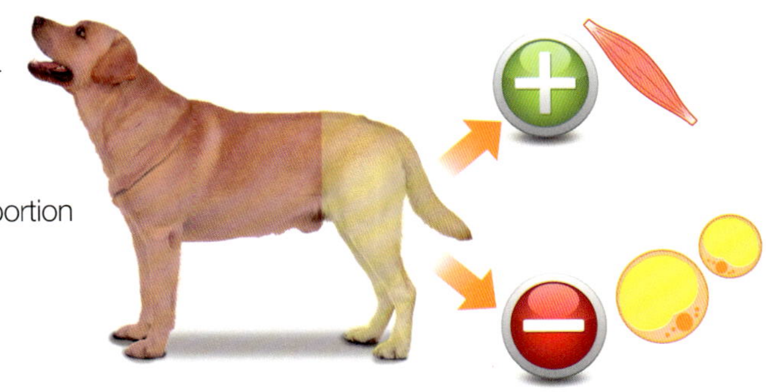

The body fat and lean tissue were lower; however, the proportion of muscle mass was higher.

7 Better bone quality

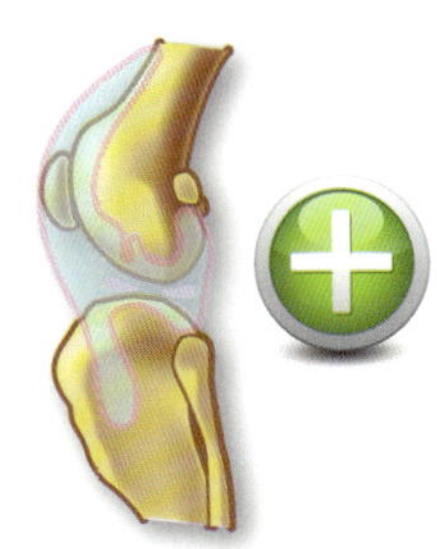

No changes were observed in the maturation, structure, or metabolism of the bone tissue. The density and mineral content of the bones were higher and remained constant between 6-12 years of age. After that age, a decrease in the two parameters occurred, but values higher than those in the control group were maintained.

8 Better immune response

The loss of the immunological response capacity due to aging, measured by the activity of the lymphocyte populations and the lymphoproliferative response to mitogens, was lower and more delayed over time.

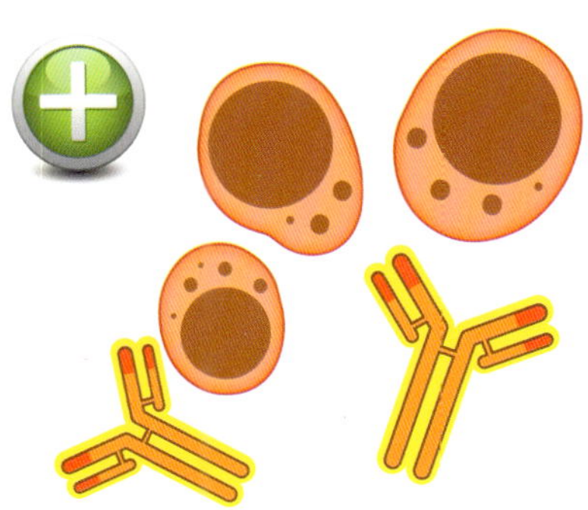

9 Less damage to DNA

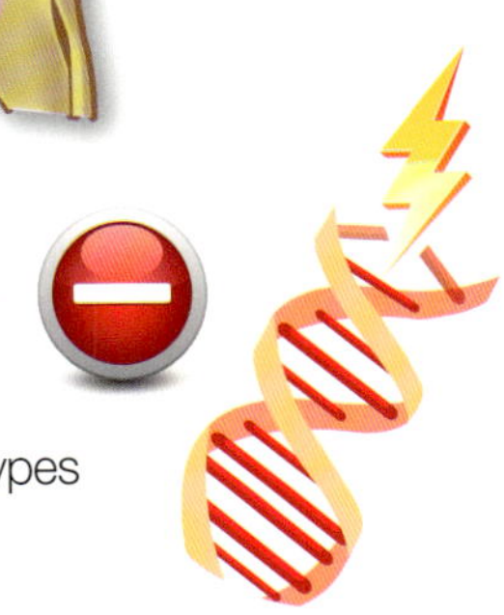

DNA damage was evaluated by the prevalence of the different types of oncological processes and by the rate of mutagenesis.

10 Lower glucose levels

In spite of the fact that baseline glucose levels increase with age, their levels were lower.

Better response to insulin

The sensitivity to insulin was higher. A correlation between insulin resistance and increased body fat has been shown.

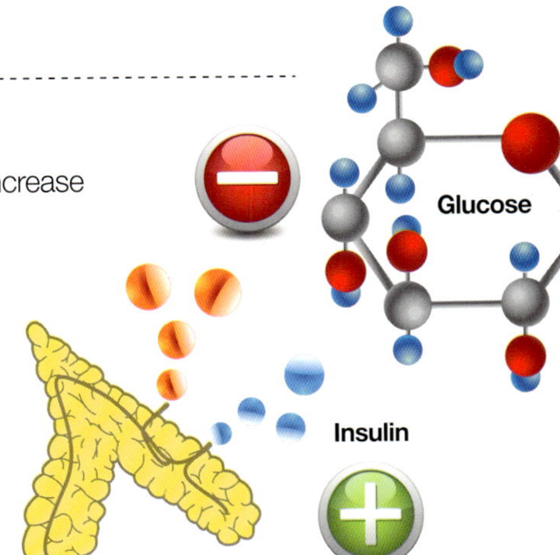

Gastrointestinal

1 Changes in the gastrointestinal tract

There are several hypotheses to explain the changes that take place in the gastrointestinal tract of cats and dogs as a consequence of aging. These include:

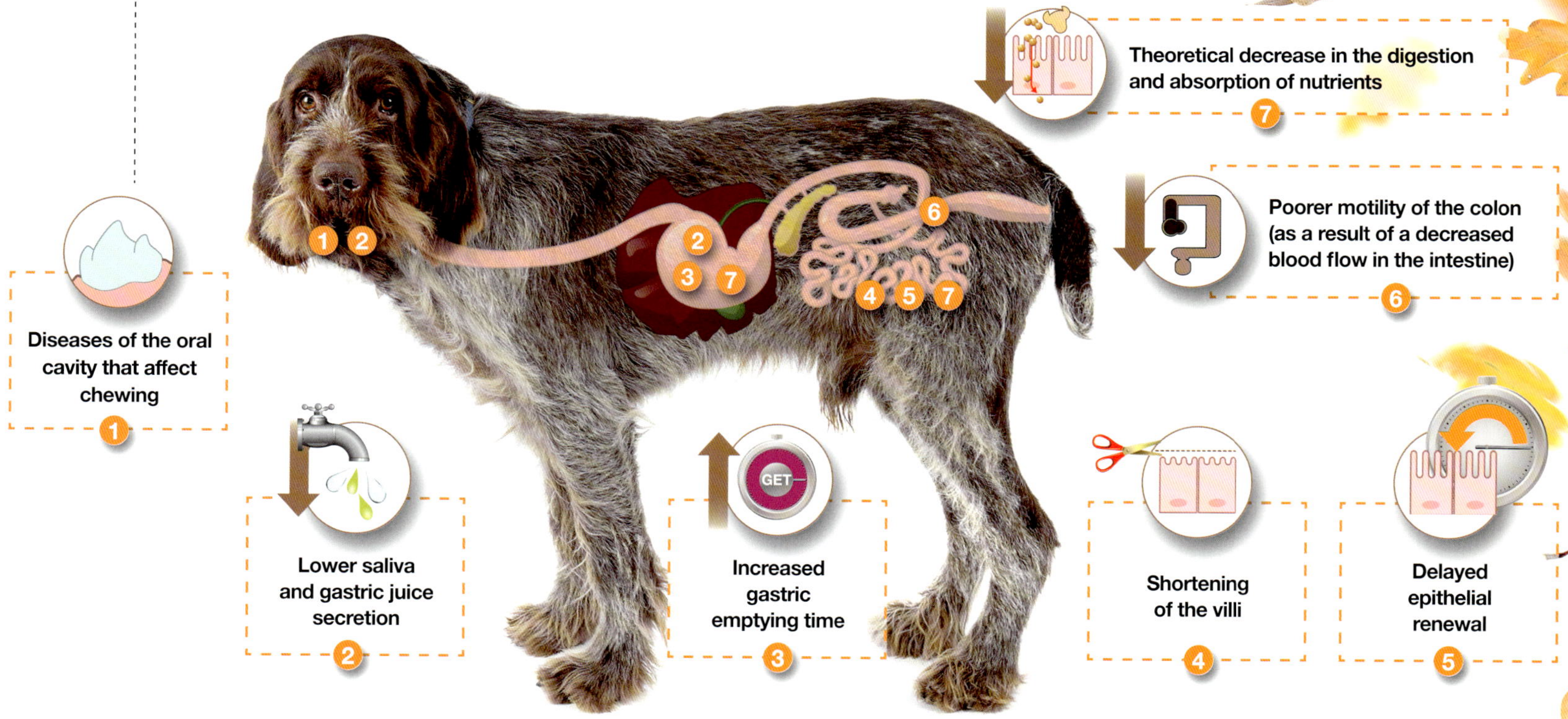

2 Sense deterioration can reduce food intake

- ✔ With age, the number of taste buds and nerve endings in the nasal cavities is reduced, which may be why pets have a decreased interest for food.
- ✔ It is unclear whether this is due to a deterioration of the sense organs or to behavioral changes. The cognitive dysfunction syndrome is a combination of several of these changes.

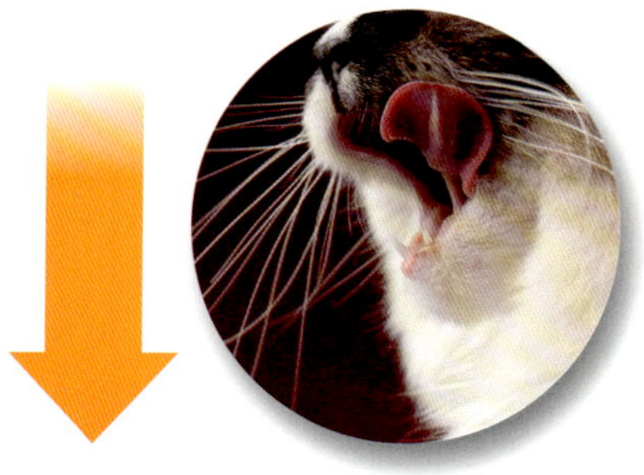

Cognitive dysfunction syndrome

- ✔ It has been reported in cats and dogs. The prevalence of the disease varies with age, with values of 28 % and 50–68 % at 12 and 15 years of age, respectively, in both species. The causes are neurohistopathological and neurochemical; over time, the brain suffers oxidative stress due to its high lipid content.
- ✔ In addition, older animals have acquired routines and are very sensitive to situations of stress (owner's death, a new pet, moving house), which may cause them to display anorexia/hyporexia.
- ✔ In any case, the result of these processes is a progressive loss of weight and muscle mass.

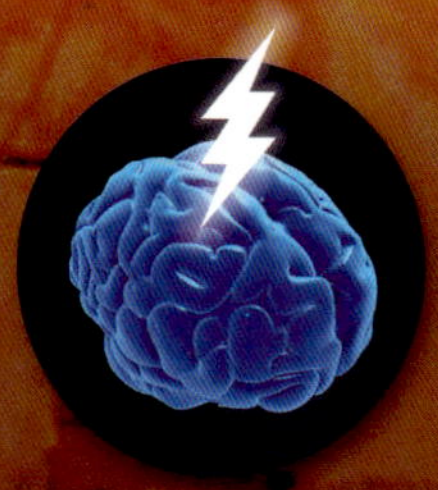

Brain deterioration

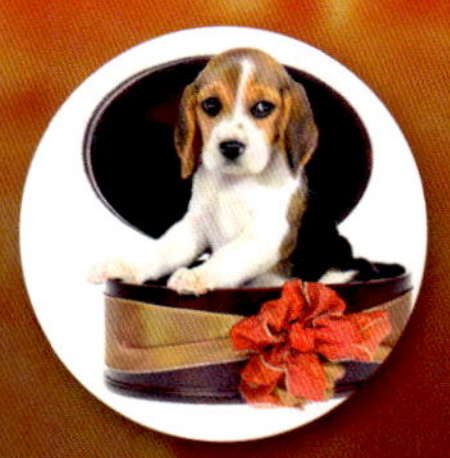

New pets

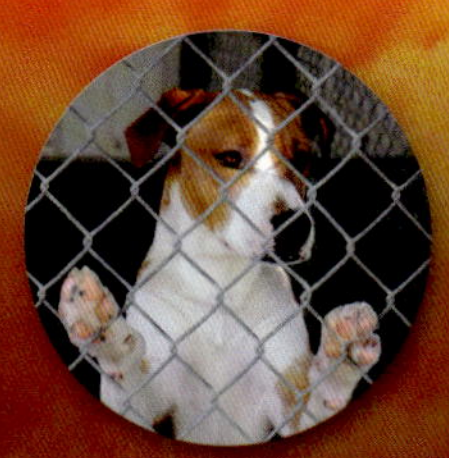

Owner's death

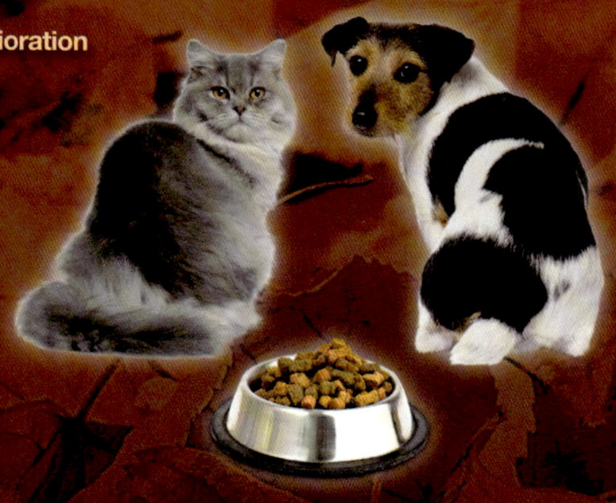

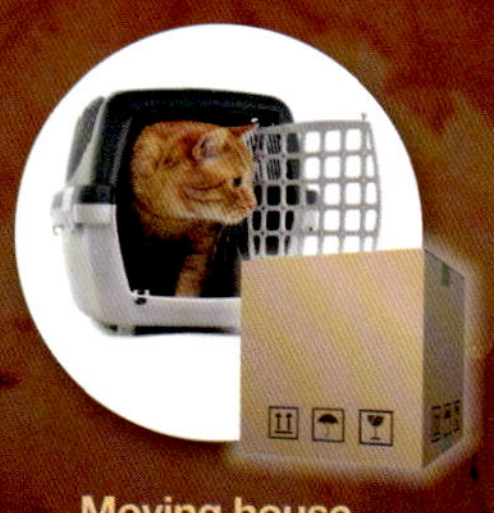

Moving house

changes due to aging

3 Decreased levels of some hormones

- ✔ The levels of some hormones related to food consumption have been reported to decrease with age. This is the case of ghrelin, a hormone synthesized in the gastric mucosa with an orexigenic effect (appetite stimulant), which could contribute to reducing the appetite of senior dogs.

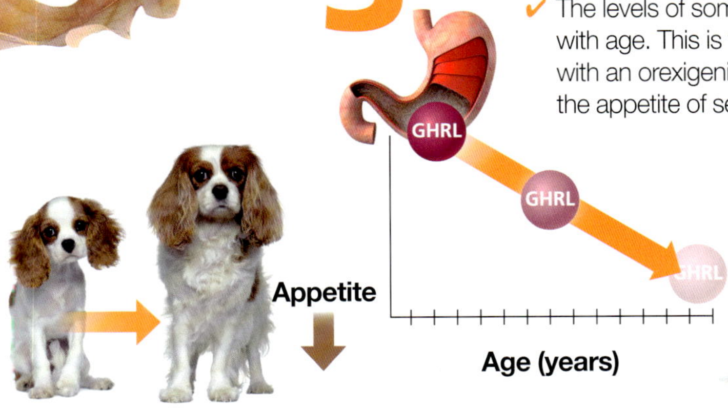

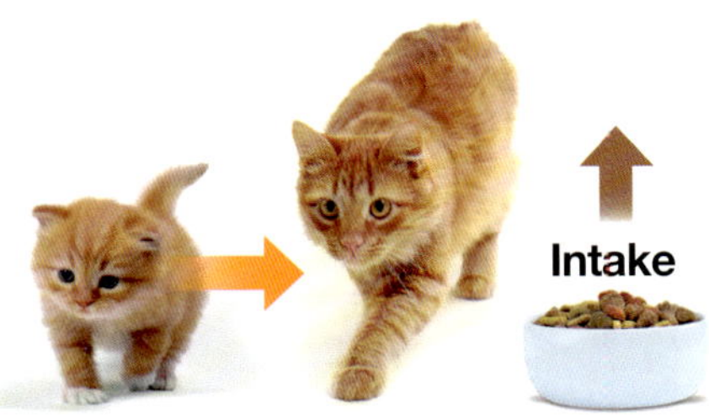

- ✔ Cats are the exception to this weight-loss rule. Healthy old cats increase their food intake to compensate for the deficiencies in their digestive processes.

4 Changes in nutrient digestibility and efficiency

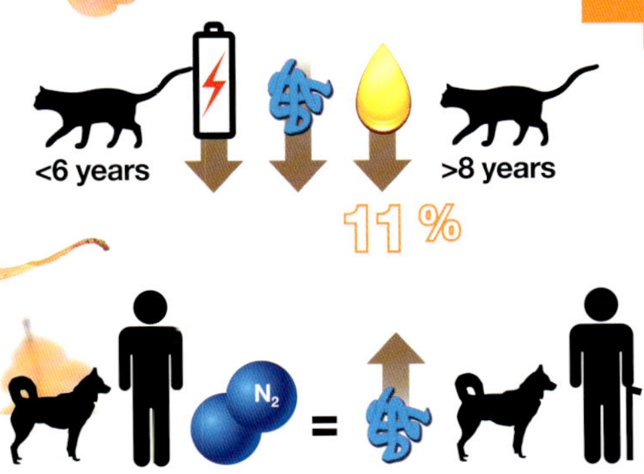

- ✔ There is some controversy on the changes in nutrient digestibility and efficiency of use. No significant results have been obtained, but, when compared with a group of young cats (<6 years), a tendency to a reduced energy and protein digestibility has been observed in older cats (>8 years), as well as significant differences in fat digestibility. The latter value is reduced by approximately **11 %**, although the authors do not consider whether this may be due to a reduction in pancreatic or biliary secretions.
- ✔ In human medicine, the efficiency of protein use has been shown to be reduced in senior patients. Similar studies conducted in dogs reveal similar results: old dogs need approximately **50 % more protein** to maintain and recover their nitrogen reserves.

5 Changes in the intestinal microbiota

- ✔ The digestive tract is sterile at birth, but it is rapidly colonized by the microbiota of the environment, which will suffer changes as a result of diet and age.
- ✔ In general, and although some genera increase their population, the total number of bacteria in the large intestine decreases by approximately 11 % compared with adult animals.
- ✔ In senior dogs, bacteria of the following genera are increased: *Clostridium* spp. (by up to 300 %), *Streptococcus* spp., *E.coli*, *Lactobacillus* spp. and *Bacteroides* spp. when compared with adult dogs. On the other hand, bacteria of the genera *Bifidobacterium* spp. and *Eubacteria* spp. are lower in number.
- ✔ This type of changes in the microbiota, particularly in the amount of clostridia, may affect the physiology of the digestive tract, e.g., protein and carbohydrate fermentation with modifications in the quality of the feces and formation of volatile fecal substances, or inhibition of the local IgA.

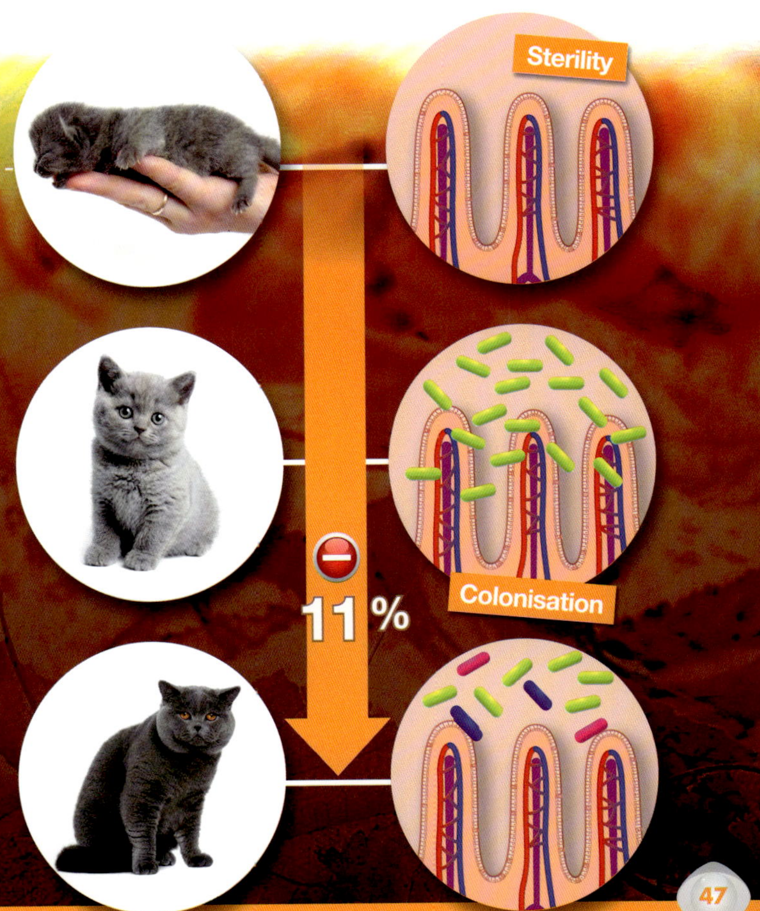

Other systemic

1 Difficulties regulating blood glucose

Older dogs require longer periods of time to regulate their postprandial glycemia. This inability to use carbohydrates makes them prone to moderate diabetes.

It has been observed that a glucose intolerance occurs with age derived from a resistance to insulin.

In the myocardium and the skeletal muscle, this effect is associated with certain changes in the insulin signals and due to a lack of a translocation of the glucose transport protein GLUT-4. In addition, the obtention of energy from non-esterified fatty acids (NEFAs) is decreased due to a lesser expression of the mitochondrial uncoupling protein UCP-3.

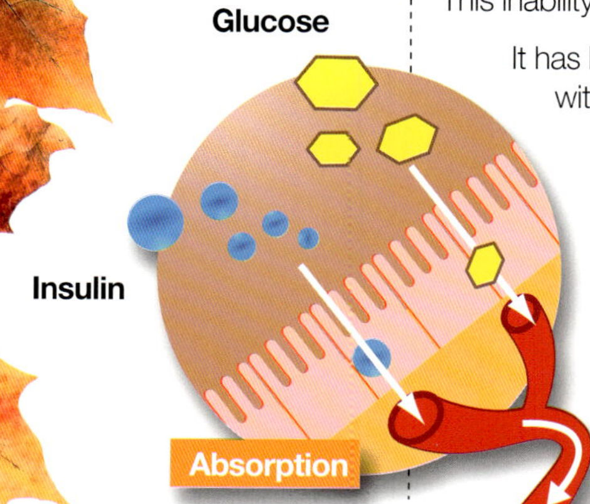

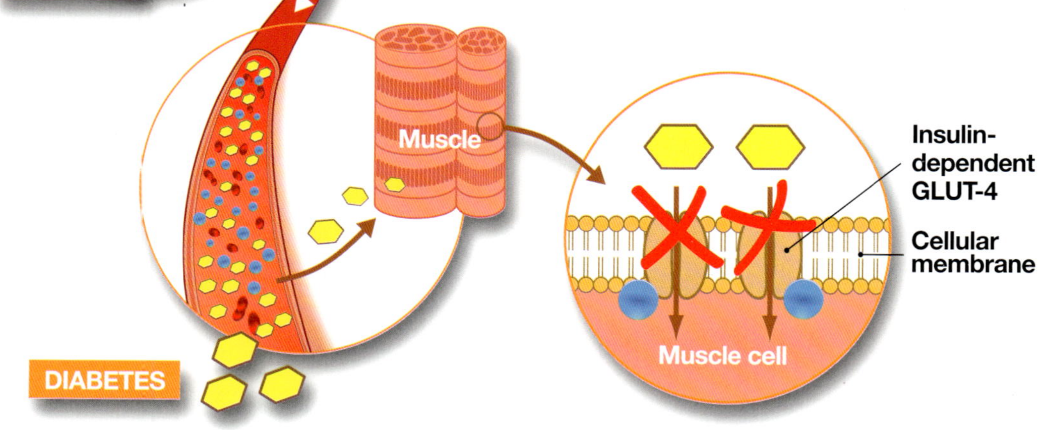

2 Loss of capacity to de-saturate essential fatty acids

The activity of desaturases, especially the Δ-6 desaturase, in the synthesis of eicosapentaenoic acid (EPA) and docosahexaenoic acid (DHA) from α-linolenic acid (ALA), and of arachydonic acid (AA) from linoleic acid (AL), is reduced as a consequence of aging. Therefore, in old dogs, the concentrations of AA and EPA in serum are decreased.

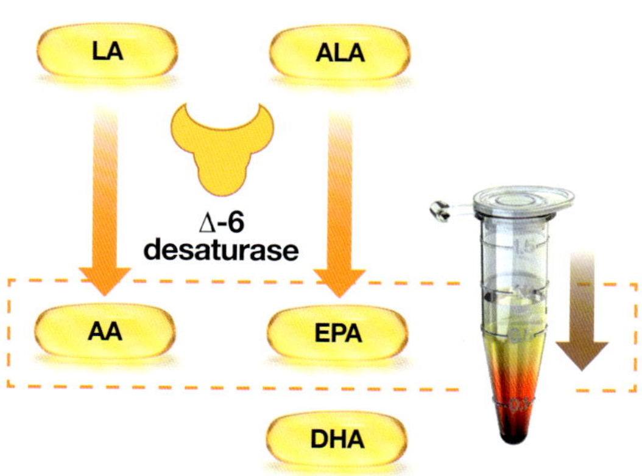

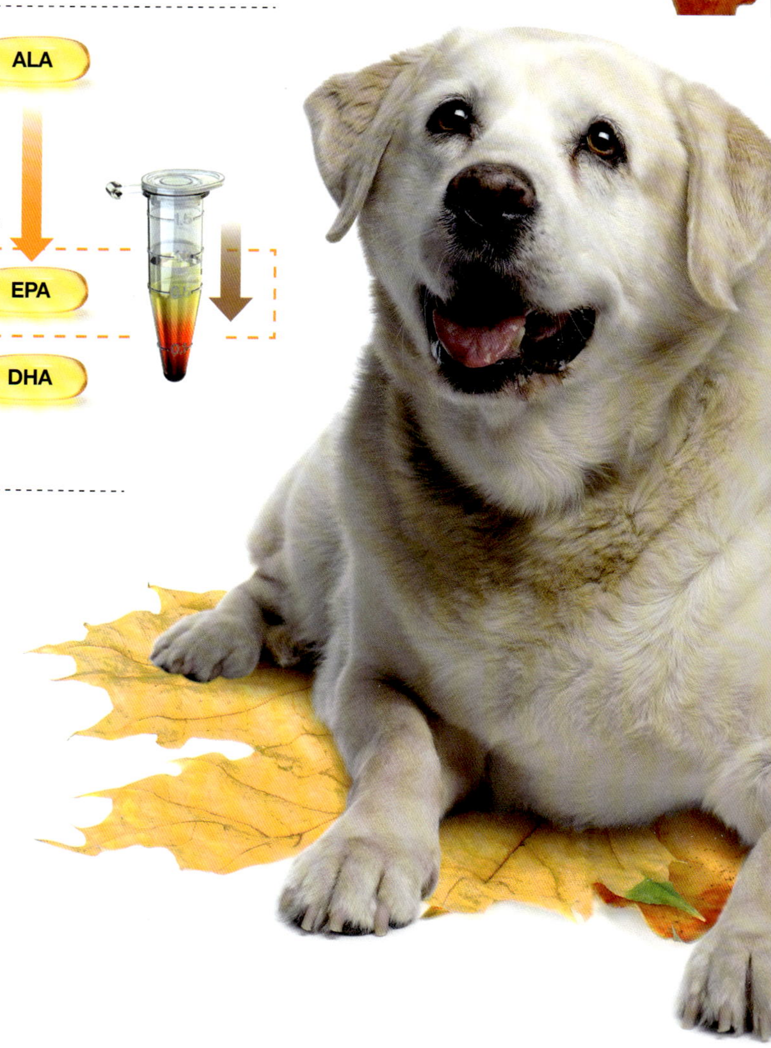

3 Lower response of the immune system

The immune system is also affected by age and sex; especially B and T cells, whose numbers are affected along with their activity (phagocytic, chemotactic and mitogenic) and their lymphoproliferative response. Generally, B cells decrease while T cells, namely CD8 cells, increase.

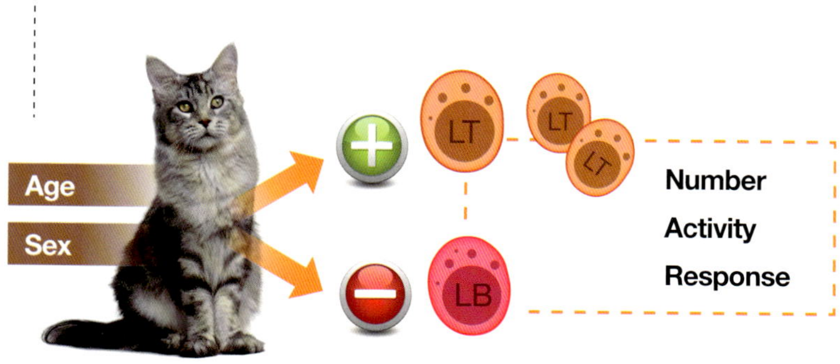

changes of aging

4 Slower basal metabolism and greater deposit of fat

- As a consequence of the changes that take place in the body composition, it has been demonstrated that the basal metabolism gets slower with age.
- On the other hand, with age, muscle mass, bone tissue, and water are lost, while, fatty tissue is deposited.

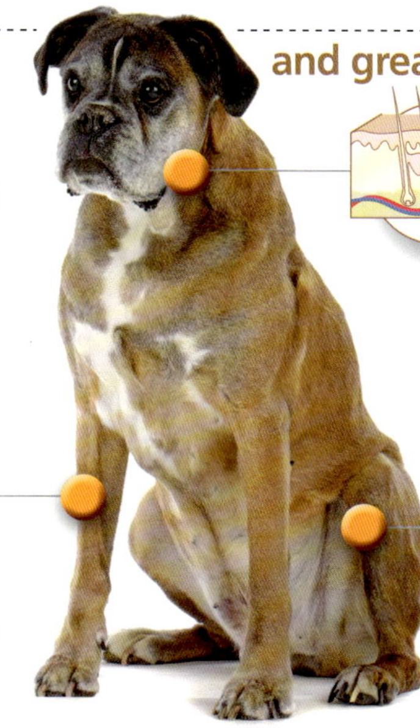

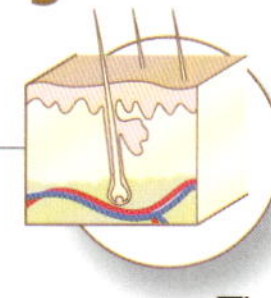

Fur

The fur loses density and color; grey hairs appear due to a lower number of melanocytes and a lack of activity of the tyrosinase (it synthesizes melanin and eumelanin from the amino acids tyrosine and phenylalanine).

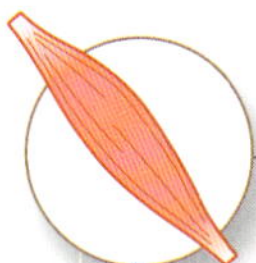

Muscle mass

The decrease in muscle mass could be caused by the loss of motor nerves and lack of activity, leading to the process of cachexia mediated by the ubiquitin-proteasome pathway (system involved in the intracellular protein renewal).

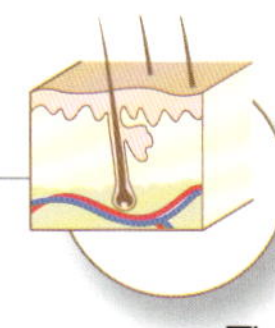

Skin

The skin becomes drier and loses elasticity due to the atrophy of the epidermis and of the follicles.

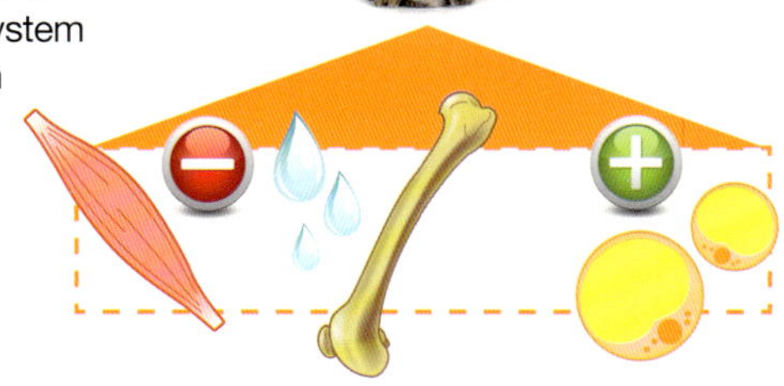

5 Other physiological changes with specific nutritional treatment

Among the most obvious, and those that require the most attention from a nutrition perspective, we find **the loss of the functional capacity of the kidneys and the heart**.

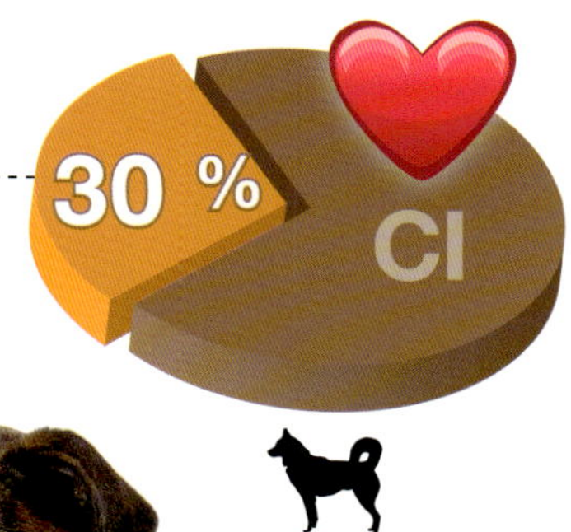

- Chronic kidney disease (CKD) and cardiovascular diseases are within the first three causes of death in senior animals (the other cause is cancer). More than 50 % of dogs and cats that present CKD are older than 10 years of age. Heart failure (HF) affects 30 % of old dogs. The correct management of the patient's feeding slows down the progress of these diseases.

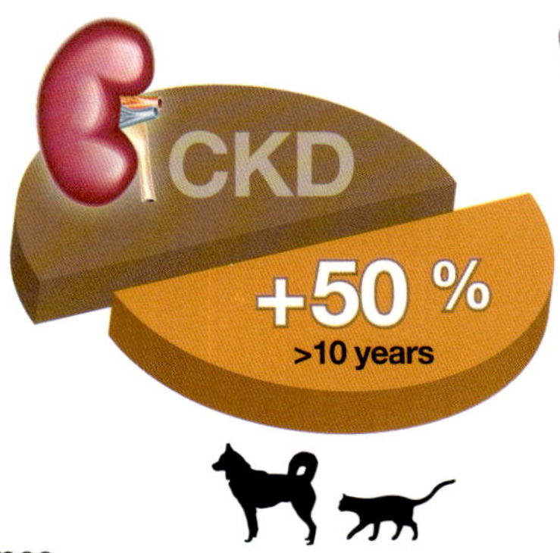

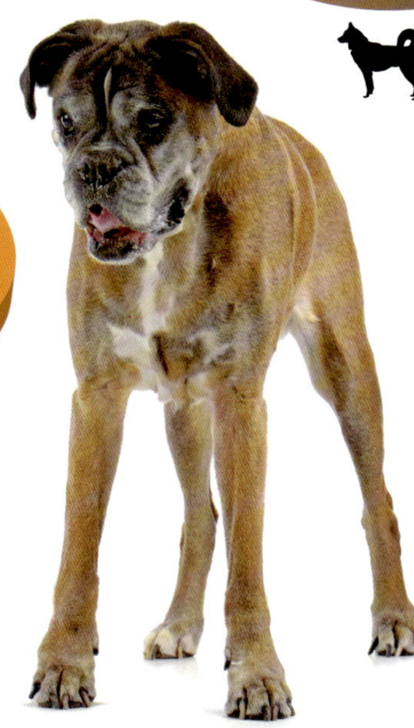

- The loss of elasticity of the joints and the appearance of osteoarthritis and arthritis are common changes associated with aging. Pain and limping will affect an animal's mobility, appetite, and capacity to chew. Certain nutrients are being used (for example, omega-3 fatty acids, antioxidants and chondroprotective agents) to modulate the process.

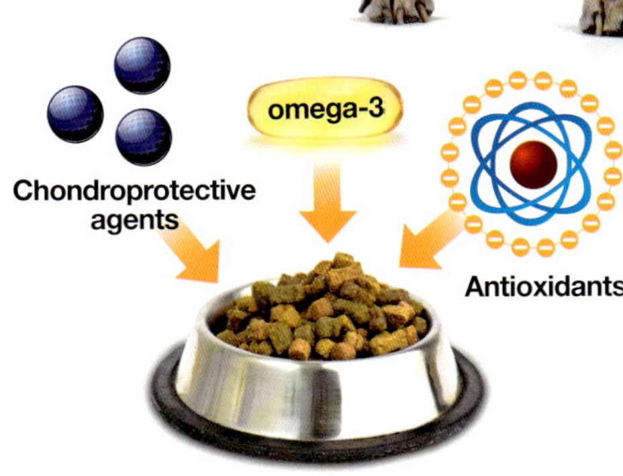

To be taken into account

Although in human medicine osteoporosis is associated with aging, this process is not observed in our pets.

Requirements in

The primary objective of feeding and nutrition in the last stage of life of our pets is to try to prolong their quality of life and life expectancy, delaying the appearance of the symptoms of dysfunction. In this section, we will only discuss the recommendations for healthy dogs and cats of advanced age, that is, that have no pathologies (especially CKD).

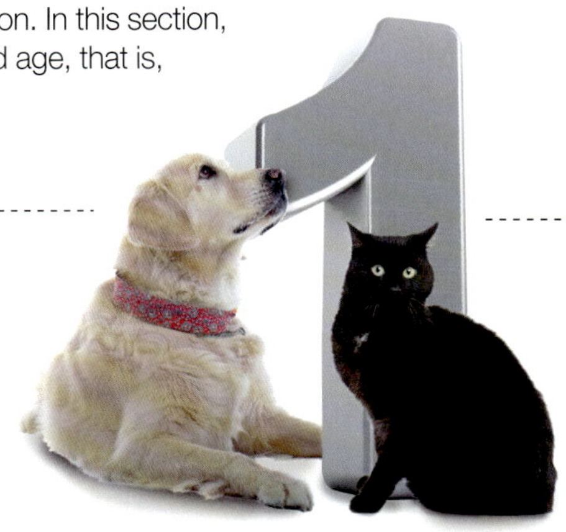

1 Each geriatric patient is unique

The first rule that should always be considered is that each geriatric patient is an individual, due to the great variety of particular situations that appear at these ages. As in other stages of life, it is impossible to generalize: the requirements from the age itself must be considered along with those derived from incipient or concomitant pathologies.

2 The daily energy requirements are lower

In general, in the last third of our pets' lives, and due to the changes that take place in their bodies, including poor functioning of the thyroid gland and less physical activity, the daily energy requirements decrease by between 12 % and 20 % (some authors reference up to 40 %). This effect is somewhat lower in cats, possibly because their physical activity and the changes that take place in their bodies are not as accentuated as those that occur in canines. On average, 15 % is estimated.

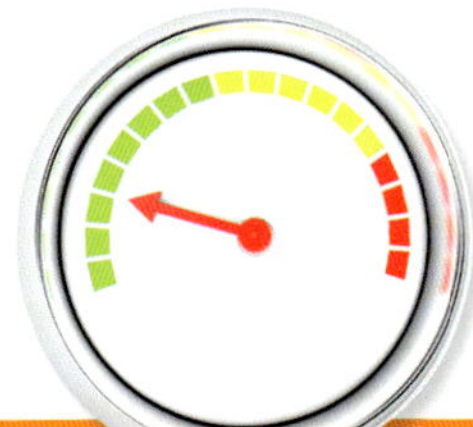

DER = ↓12-20 % (40 %)

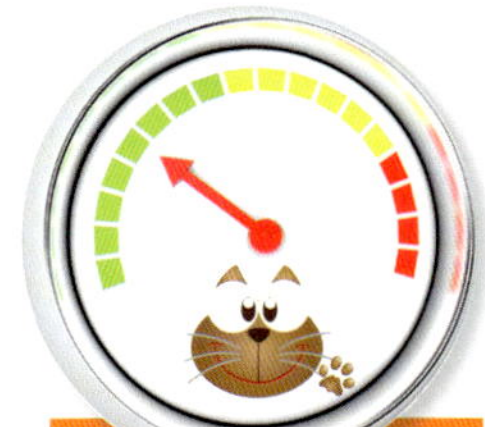

15 %

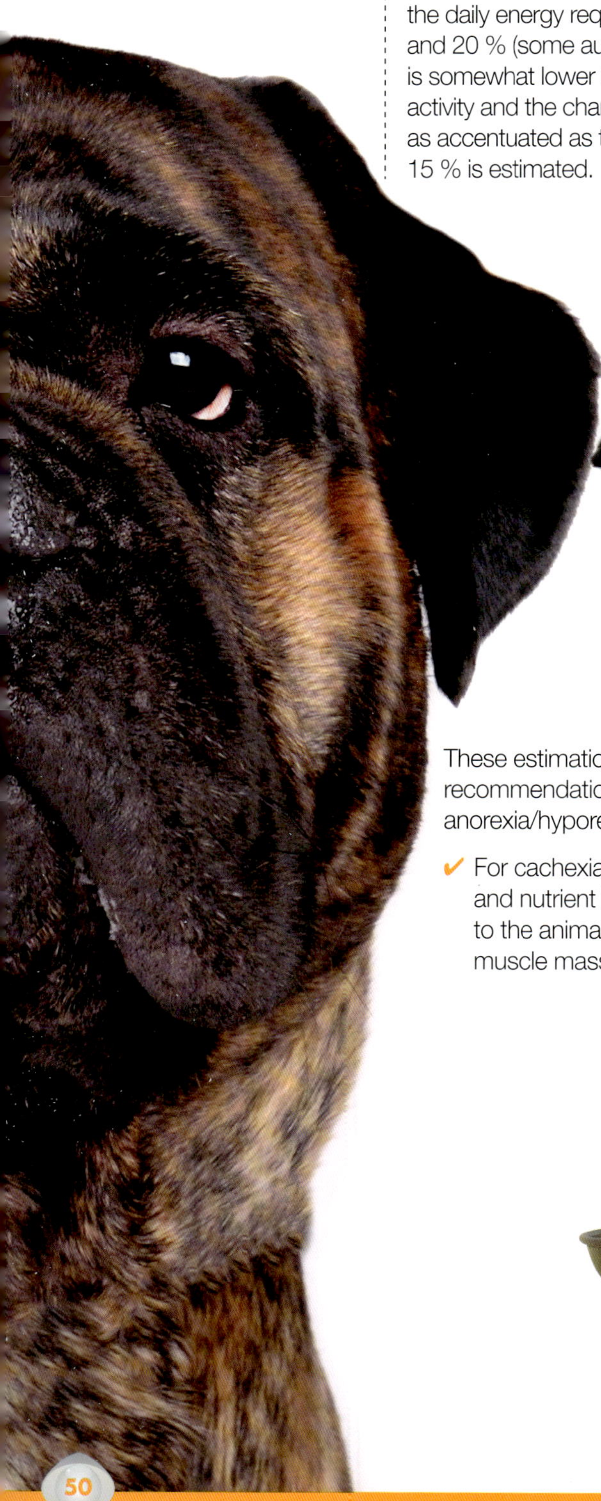

Examples **What are their energy requirements?**

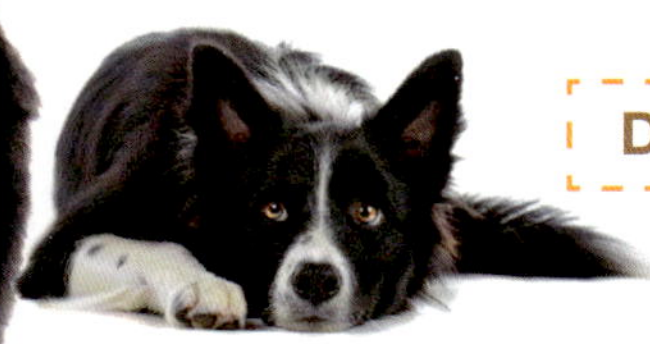

13 years and 12 kg

DER (kcal ME/day) = 85 % × 132 (kcal) × body weight (kg)$^{0.75}$

DER = 112 x 12$^{0.75}$ = 724 kcal ME/day

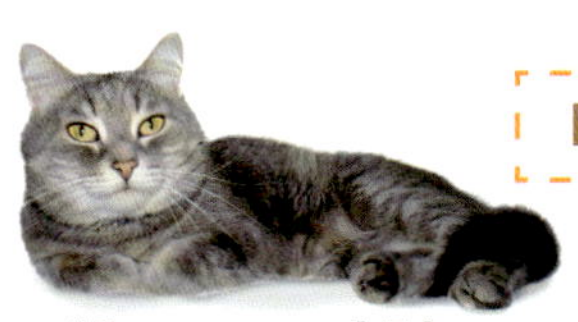

15 years and 5 kg

DER (kcal ME/day) = 85 % × 100 (kcal) × body weight (kg)$^{0.67}$

DER = 85 × 5$^{0.67}$ = 249 kcal ME/day

These estimations are contradictory with the loss of weight and muscle mass in the geriatric phase. Therefore, the energy recommendations will depend on the losses that are produced, differentiating if they are due to a state of cachexia or anorexia/hyporexia.

- ✔ For cachexia, in spite of our efforts to increase the calorie and nutrient intake, it is difficult to achieve improvements to the animal's body condition, especially regarding the muscle mass, although weight can be regained.
- ✔ On the other hand, and given that the fatty tissue continues to deposit itself in the organism, the veterinarian should monitor that food ingestion is correct to prevent the pet from becoming overweight.

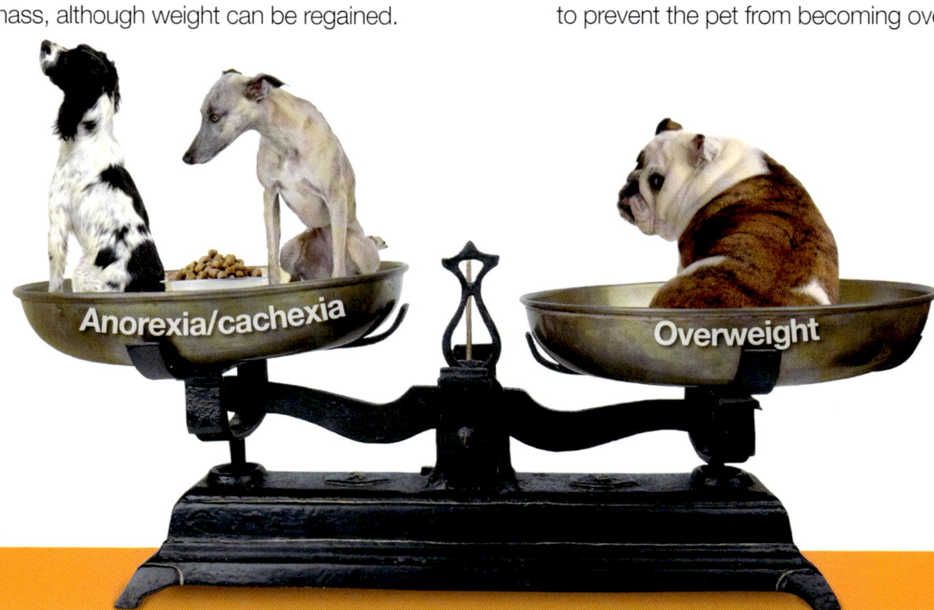

healthy geriatric animals (I)

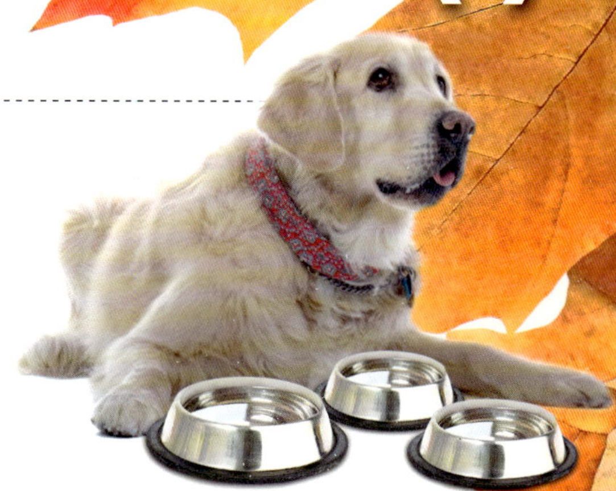

3 Hydric requirements

- According to studies in human medicine, water requirements could be slightly increased as the thirst control and satiety systems are found to be affected by the aging process.
- In controlled environments, the ingestion of liquids is correct, but when these liquids are not available, or due to certain changes in the osmolarity of the liquid (hyperosmolarity), heat or exercise, geriatric patients respond with less thirst and less ingestion of liquids. When faced with this situation, the water requirements and recommendations must be estimated. The best rule to follow is to offer fresh clean water at all times.

4 Be careful with the level of carbohydrates and fiber

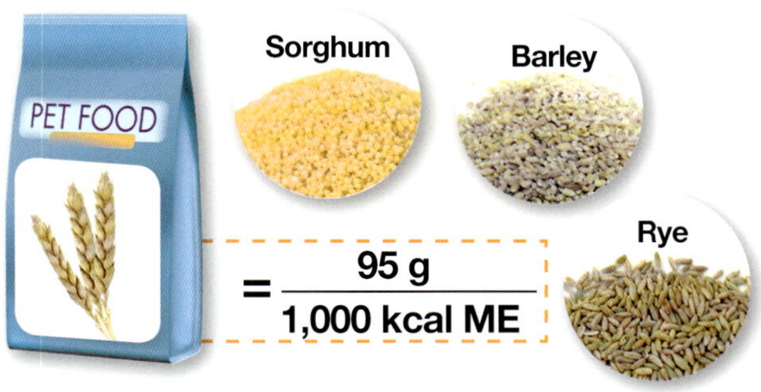

- In old dogs and cats, who may sometimes suffer from senile diabetes, and in the absence of further studies that show the intrinsic mechanisms of this action, using high levels of carbohydrates or ingredients that elevate the glycemic index rapidly is not recommended. Using foods with a moderate amount of starch and rich in fiber is recommended; for example: sorghum, barley and rye.
- There are no specific carbohydrate requirements, but considering their limitations, values close to 95 g/1,000 kcal ME are recommended.
- Regarding fiber and its physiological effects on the digestive process, considering that certain old animals suffer constipation, the type of fiber should be mixed (fermentable and non-fermentable fiber) and the levels incorporated should not be increased. The highest values are reserved for those animals that are less active and overweight.
- At the same time, fiber may help to compensate the changes to the microbiota. Incorporating fiber with prebiotic characteristics determines an increase in the lactobacillus and bifidobacterium populations in the colon and a decrease in the count of fecal clostridium. The following values help to maintain a healthy microbiota.

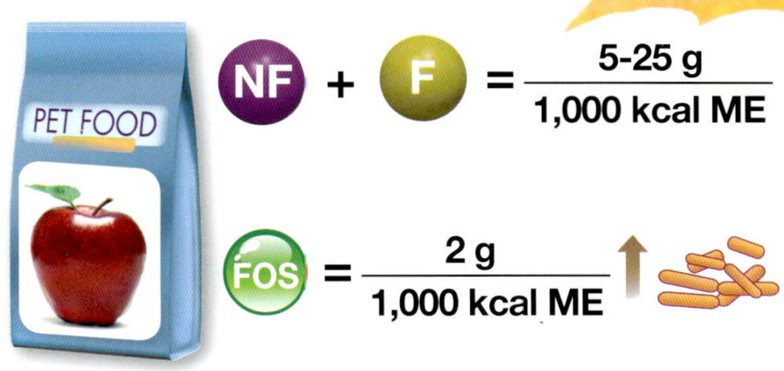

5 More and better quality protein

- Taking into account the changes that take place as a result of aging and the differences in the quality of raw materials, the value shown in (1) is recommended to maintain the nitrogen balance at zero and the immunocompetence in dogs. However, gains in muscle mass are obtained when protein levels are near the value (2). These diets help to:
  - Slow down protein depletion.
  - Collaborate in the response to stress.
  - Re-establish the immune system to values comparable to those found in young animals.
- For cats, it seems that the use of 75 to 110 g of protein/1,000 kcal ME could be sufficient. In both species, it is preferable that the protein be of high quality, with a digestibility greater than 80 %.
- Foods for patients with renal disease and those that include minimal levels of protein or protein of poor quality, are not adequate to feed our healthy geriatric patients.

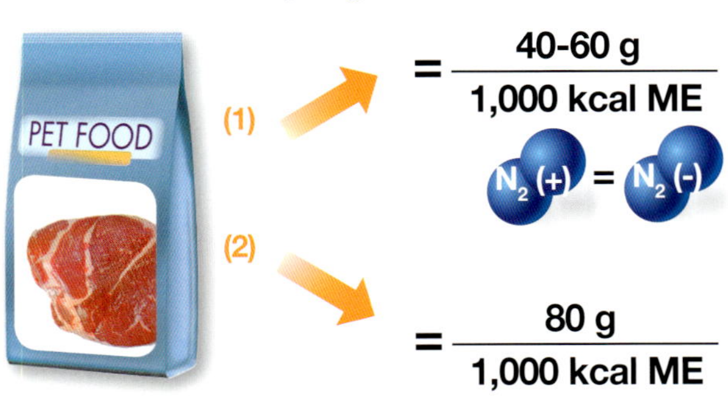

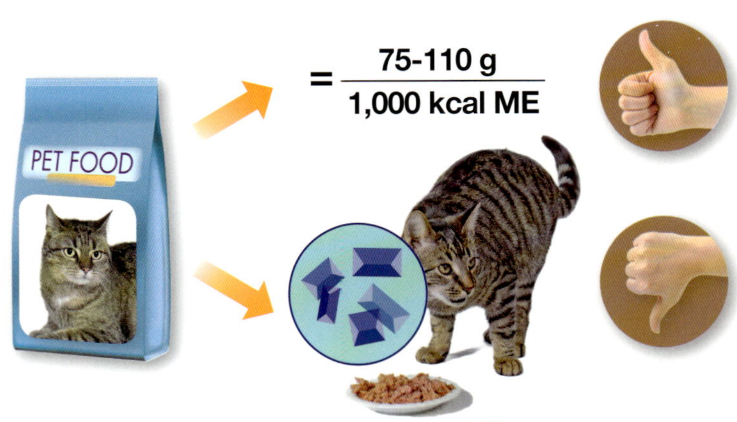

To be taken into account

There is no evidence that supports the idea that reducing the levels of protein ingested delays or avoids CKD in a healthy animal (its effect is only positive when CKD is diagnosed). Therefore, reducing the ingestion of protein or its recommendations is not necessary just because they are old.

Requirements in

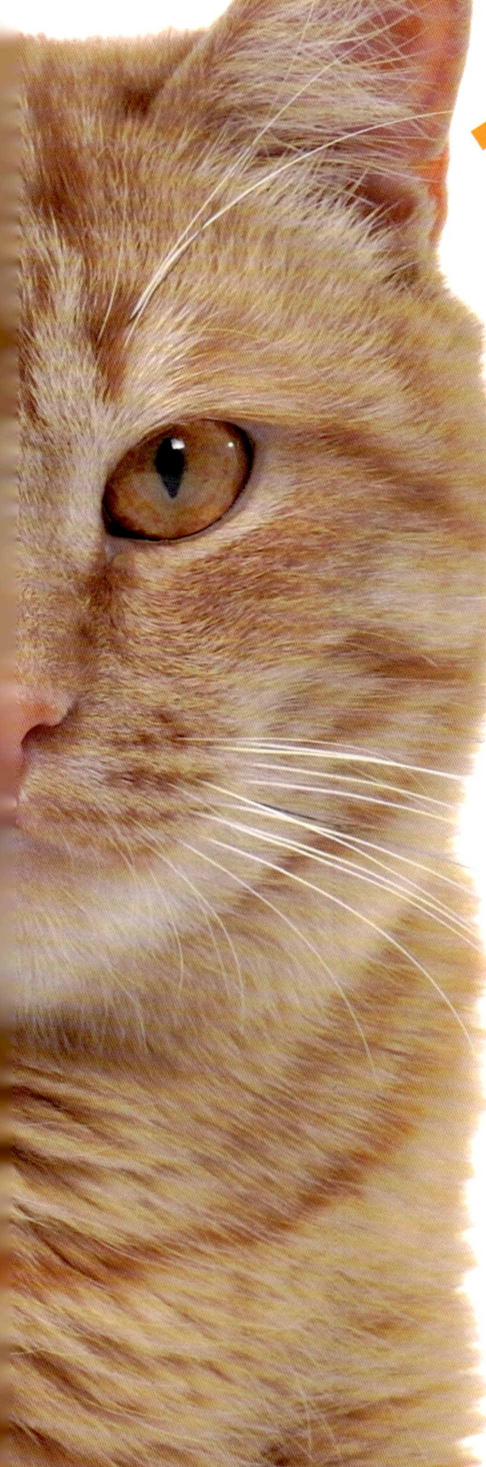

1 Lipid requirements

Energy and palatability

The fat requirements will depend on the patient's body condition. Lipids provide high energetic density and palatability to food rations so that we can improve the consumption and the general condition of our elderly animals, by increasing the concentration of fats in the food rations.

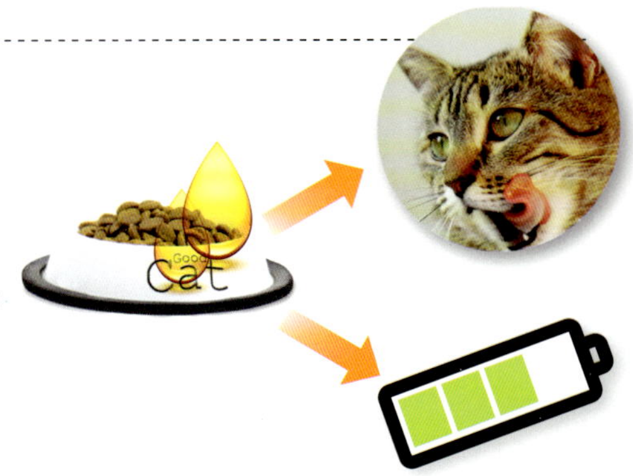

Essential fatty acids

In addition, fats provide EFAs that, as we have already seen, have a limited synthesis in older dogs.

In cats, their requirements do not vary with age

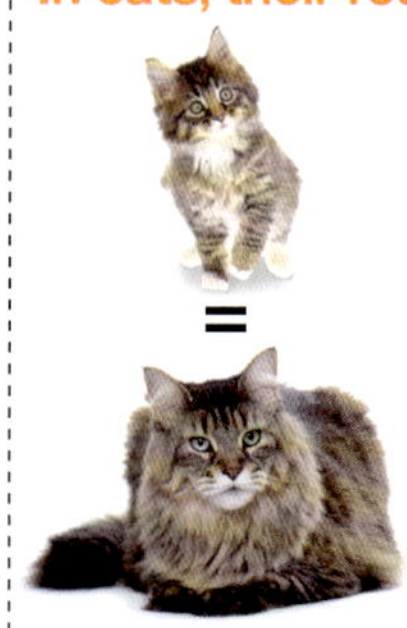

The fat requirements in cats do not change over time with the aging process in spite of the fact that their digestibility is affected.

This fact allows us to increase the levels of this nutrient in the pet's food to compensate for the loss of body fat.

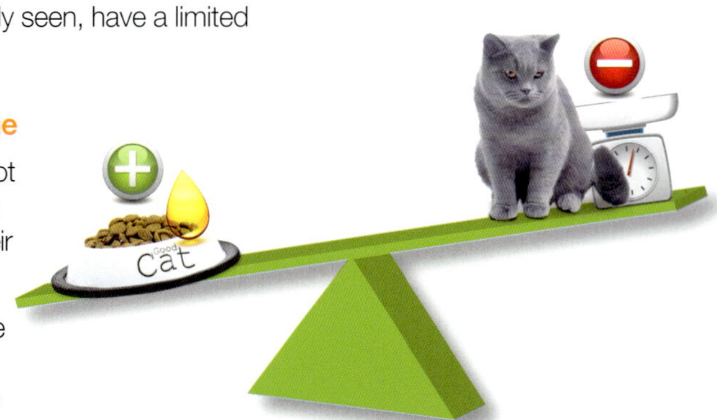

Benefits for skin and fur

Maintaining the recommendations of 25 to 38 g of fat (up to 65 g in cats)/1,000 kcal ME in older, non-obese animals provided benefits on the quality of the animals' skin and fur, body condition and improves ingestion.

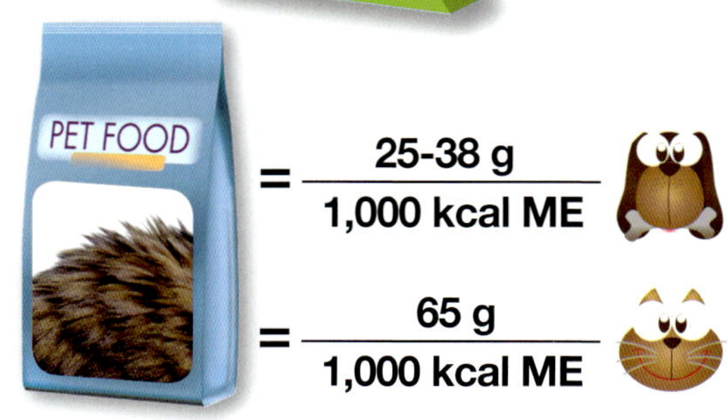

The fat profile is important

It has been documented that an increase in the proportion of saturated fatty acids (>60 %) reduces olfaction. At these levels, the permeability of the membranes is altered, which in turn affects the activity of the sodium-potassium pump in the synapses. A proportion of 25:75 of saturated:unsaturated fatty acids is recommended.

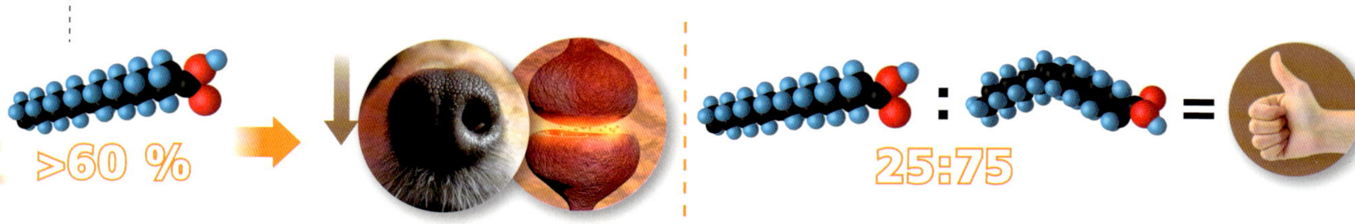

3 Practical management of feeding

- ✔ As a result of the reduction of the senses and the changes in the metabolism, foods for senior dogs and cats should have a high energy content (>4 Mcal/kg DM), and they should be highly palatable and digestible.
- ✔ The texture of the food will depend on the pet's oral health. Softer kibbles or wet food are preferable. When faced with the possibility of an animal developing senile diabetes, semi-wet foods are not recommended given that they use simple carbohydrate humidifying agents.

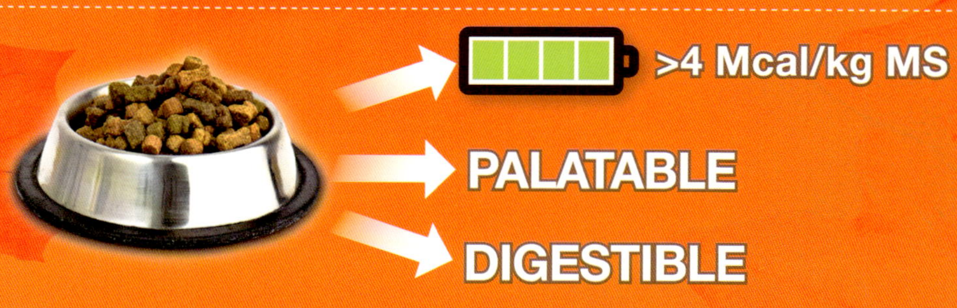

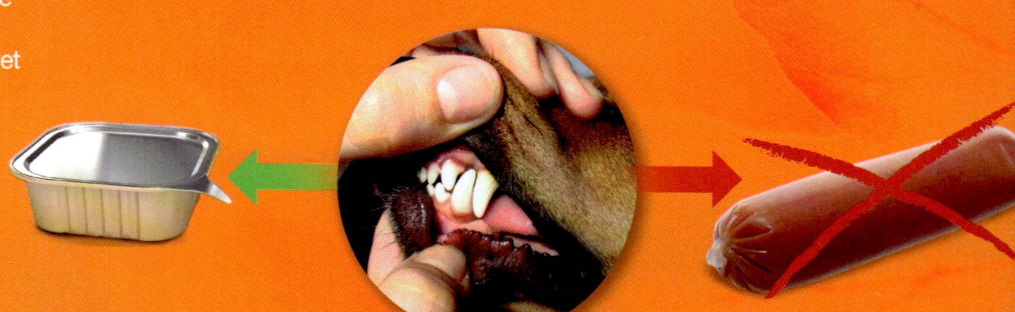

healthy geriatric animals (II)

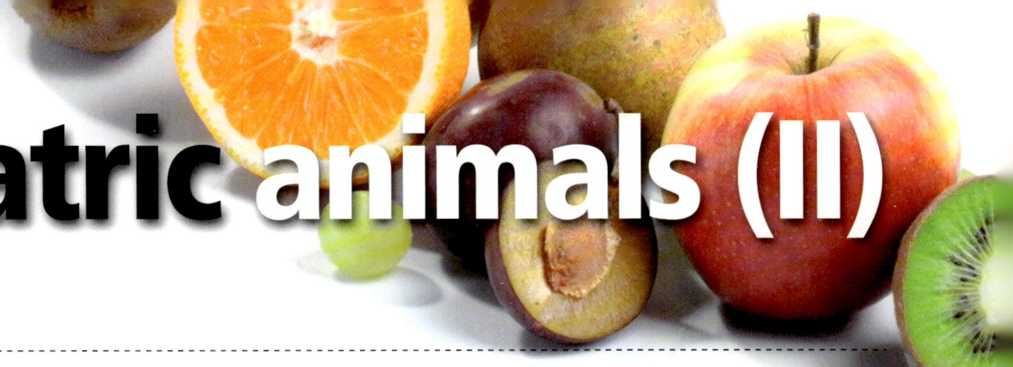

2 Vitamin and mineral requirements

Antioxidants against free radicals

In this stage of life, the vitamin and mineral requirements are not affected in healthy patients. It may be interesting to pay attention to the nutrients with antioxidant activity to compensate for the cellular damage that takes place due to the increase in free radicals from oxidative stress.

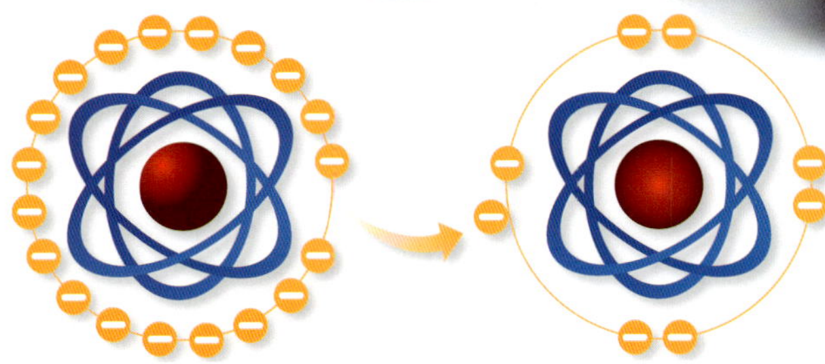

Calcium for correct bone mineralization

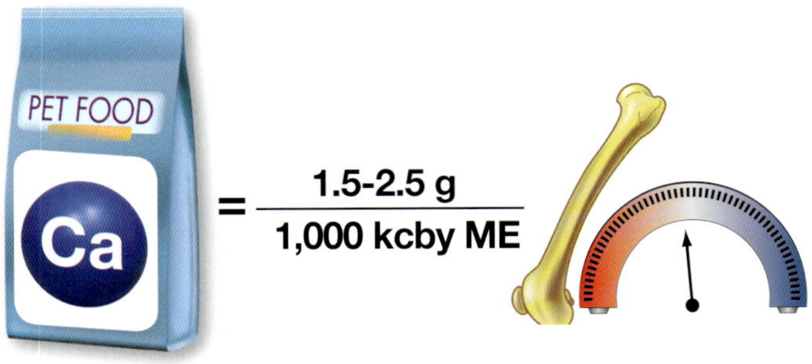

DEB ➔ pH = 6.4-6.6

Slight bone loss occurs in cats and is possibly associated with the decrease in lean mass. There is also secondary bone loss to compensate for metabolic acidosis, with a decrease in the urinary pH, and therefore a predisposition to urolithiasis from calcium oxalate. To avoid these situations and maintain correct bone mineralization, levels of calcium around 1.5-2.5 g/1,000 kcal ME are recommended along with a modification of the DEB (dietary electrolyte balance) that will ensure a pH close to 6.4-6.6.

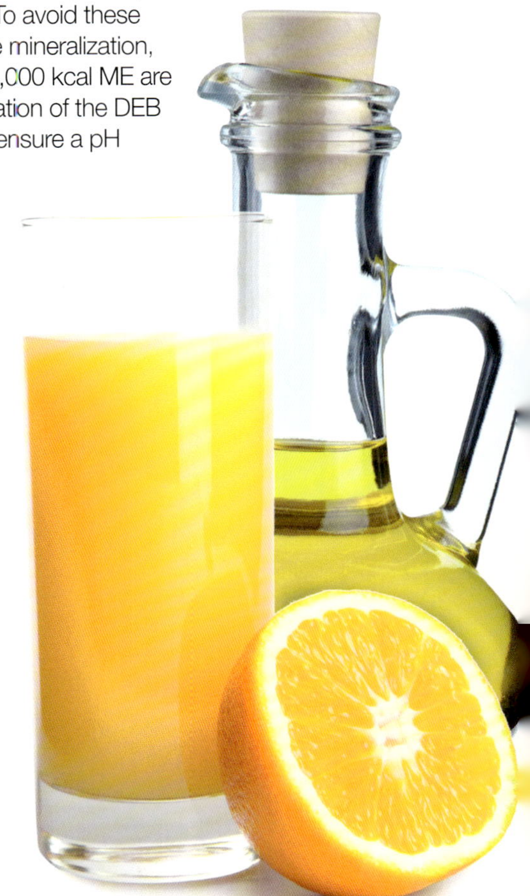

Potassium as a stimulant in feline ingestion?

It has been suggested that increasing the potassium recommendations can stimulate ingestion in older cats (hypokalemia causes nervous system signs and lethargy), but there is no scientific evidence that supports this fact in healthy animals. In commercial foods for senior cats, we can find that potassium may be increased by up to 15 %.

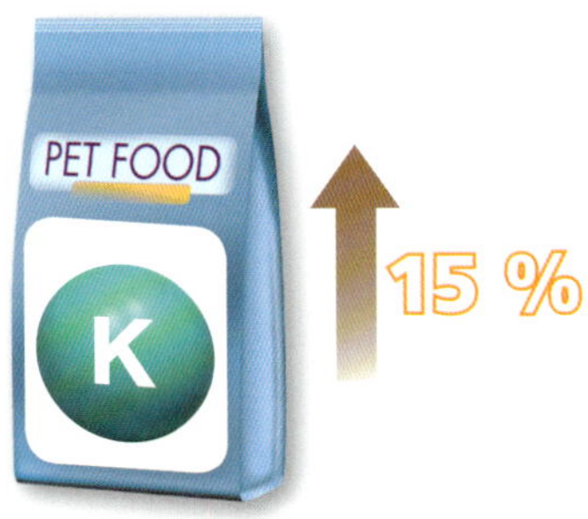

Vitamin A, iodine, or zinc to improve the sense of smell

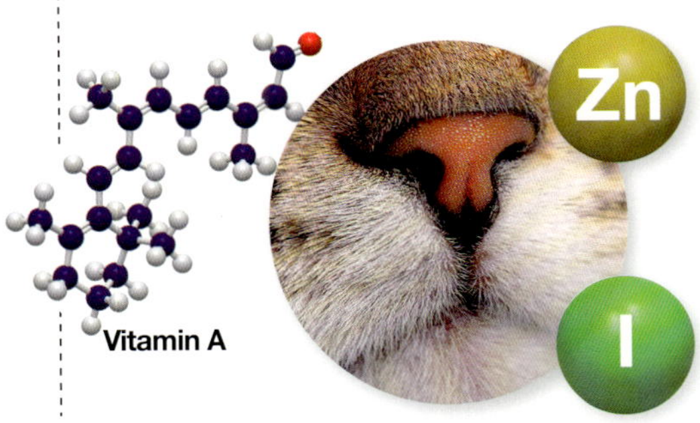

It has been described in human medicine that deficiencies in vitamin A, iodine, and zinc cause a loss of the sense of smell. One of the effects of aging, as we have previously explained, is the loss of the sense of smell. There is no previous research that demonstrates this in pets, but incorporating any of these nutrients may serve to help in the cephalic phase of the digestive process.

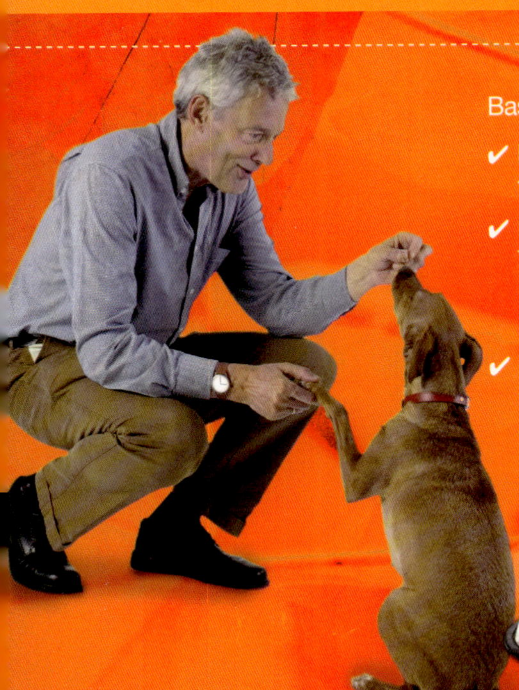

Based on the changes that take place in advanced age pets, attention should be paid to the following points:

- ✔ **Maintain adequate oral health.** Check that the teeth and gums are healthy.
- ✔ **Manage the pet's appetite appropriately.** Try to ensure that the pet ingests their daily ration even if different methods must be implemented to increase ingestion.
- ✔ **Break the total food ration into two or three meals per day.** Large volumes of food are not needed.
- ✔ **Minimize any stressful situations.** For hospitalized animals, we can try to make their hospital environment as similar as possible to their home environment; with care by the most highly trained staff (very friendly and caring with the animals), we can even take them from the cages to other rooms to see if they will eat better there or have the owners come (if possible) during meal times.
- ✔ **Decide at which age** it is recommended that these type of foods be administered.

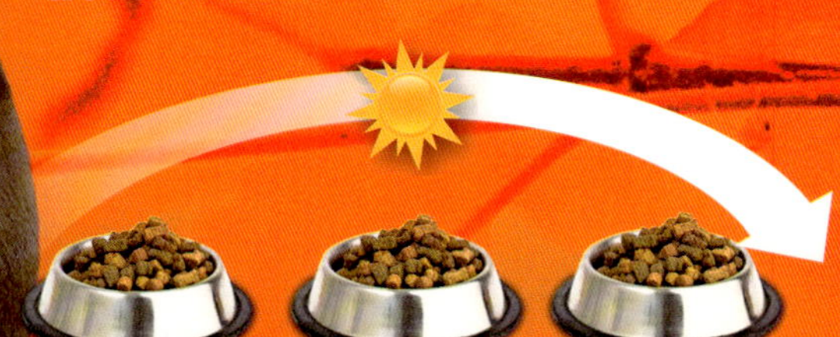

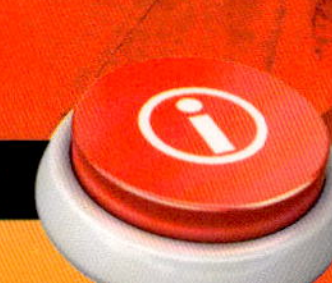

To be taken into account

We must remember that the fat requirements in cats are always higher than those for dogs as a result of their metabolism as strict carnivores.

Cognitive

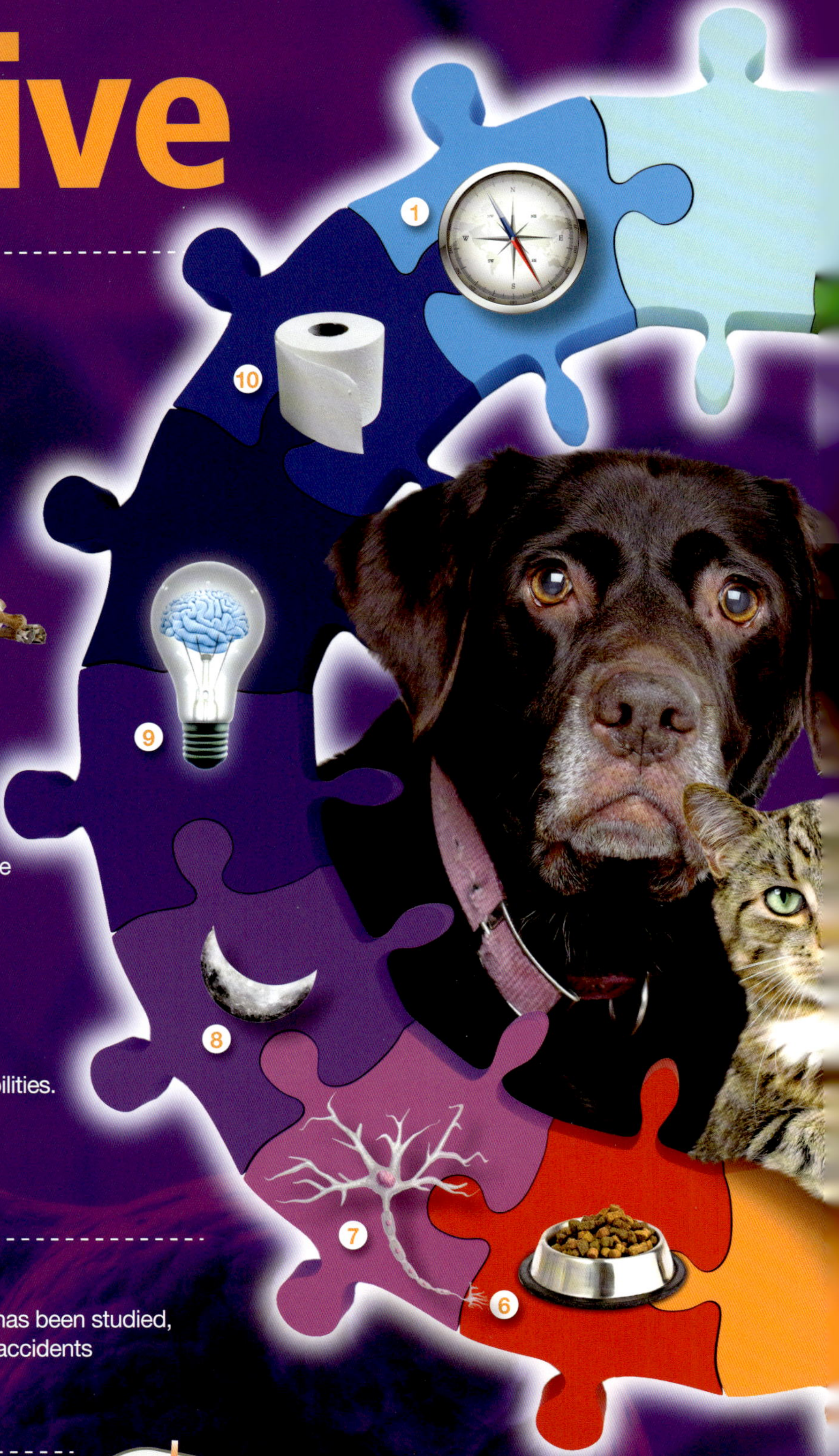

1 Clinical signs of CDS

The cognitive dysfunction syndrome (CDS) is a term used to refer to the behavioral changes of senior pets described by their owners. It affects **one in three animals** aged more than 11–12 years.

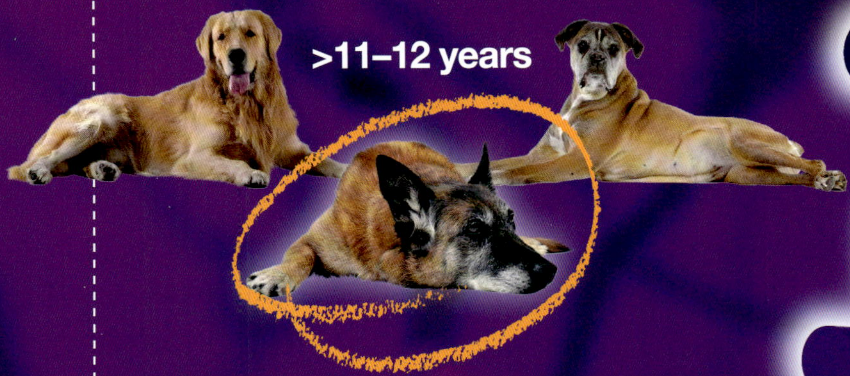

The diagnosis is based exclusively on the signs described by the owner once other medical causes have been ruled out.

1. Confusion and disorientation.
2. Altered relationships.
3. Modified activity patterns.
4. Irritability.
5. Anxiety.
6. Modified appetite.
7. Lack of response to stimuli.
8. Nocturnal activity.
9. Memory loss and loss of learning abilities.
10. Defecating/urinating inside the house.

2 Aging as a risk factor

Aging is currently the only risk factor associated with CDS that has been studied, although the contribution of traumatic injuries or microvascular accidents at a central level has not been ruled out.

3 Gross and microscopic signs

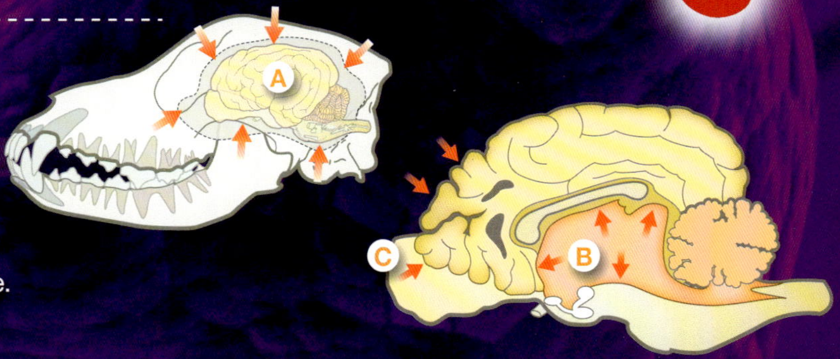

Gross signs

- A. Loss of brain volume.
- B. Enlargement of the ventricles and perivascular space.
- C. Lesions with atrophy of the brain cortex.

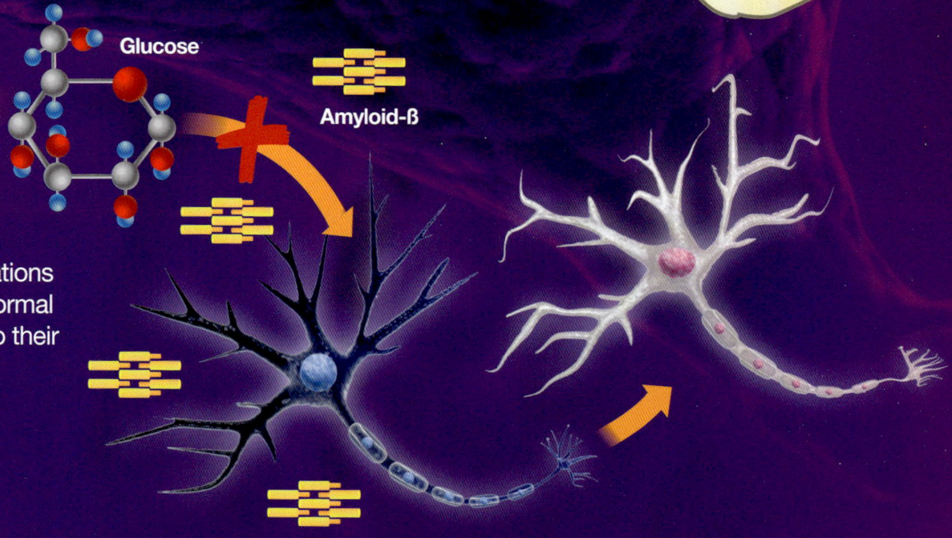

Histologic signs

Accumulation of amyloid-ß on the brain's vascular wall (similar to what occurs in Alzheimer's disease). Amyloid-ß deposits in different regions of the cortex cause modifications in the blood-brain barrier, interfering with the normal transport of nutrients to neurons, which leads to their degeneration: glucose metabolism in the brain is reduced.

dysfunction syndrome

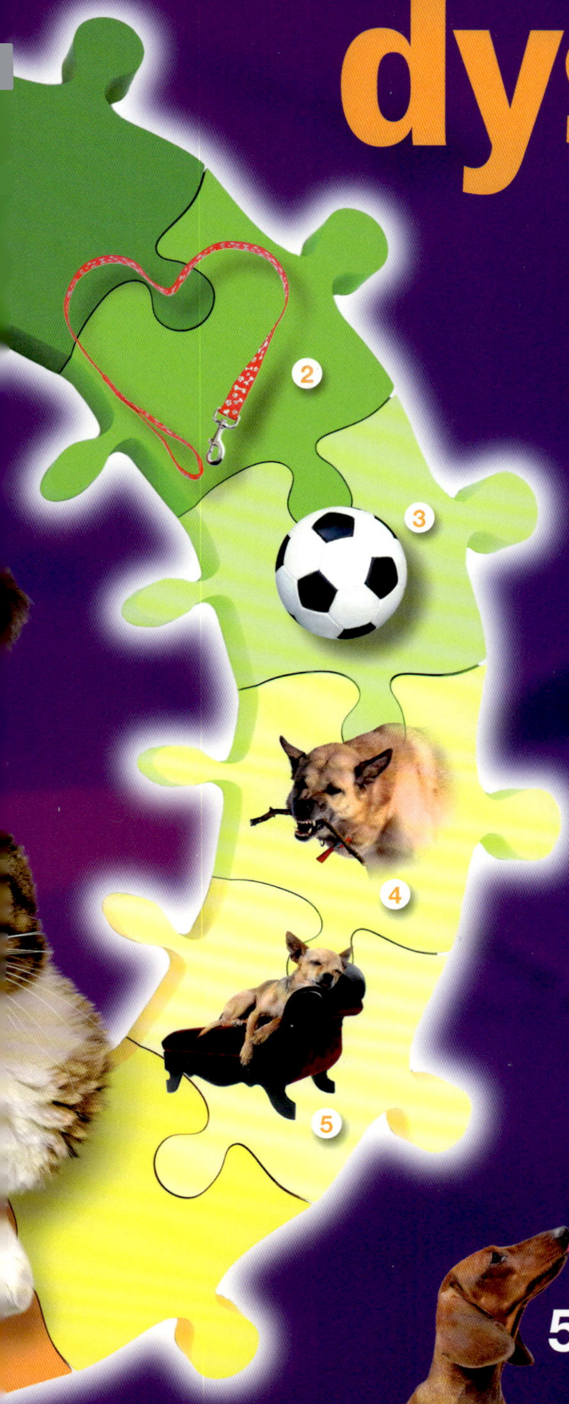

4 Oxidative damage

- ✔ Aging causes the deterioration of the mechanisms responsible for the production, control and detoxification of the by-products of aerobic metabolism, named reactive oxygen species (ROS).
- ✔ The main by-product is superoxide anion (O_2^-), which is controlled by superoxide-dismutase.
- ✔ ROS cause oxidative damage to proteins, lipids and nucleotides, which, at central level, produces lesions and death of the neurons.

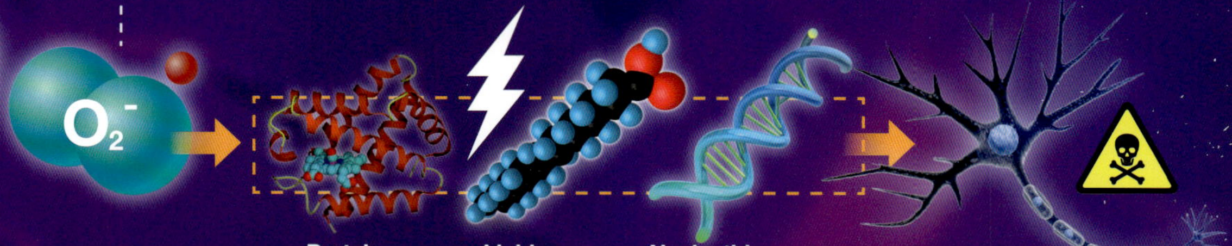

5 Fighting ROS through diet

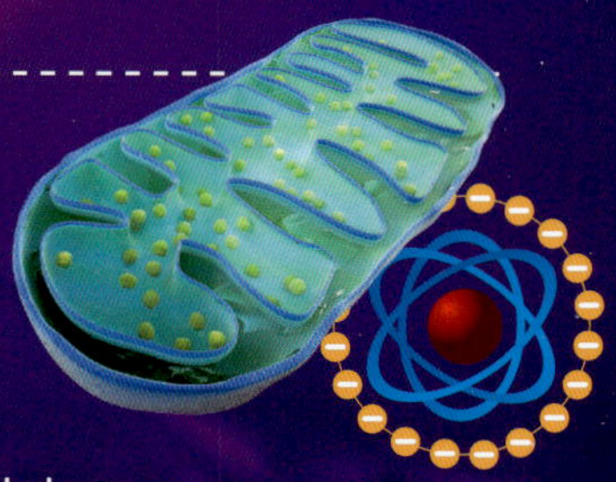

Dietary management of CDS involves the use of antioxidants and mitochondrial cofactors, which will increase the function of aged mitochondriae. The objective is to reduce the production or increase the capacity to eliminate ROS in order to delay the progression of age-related pathological changes.

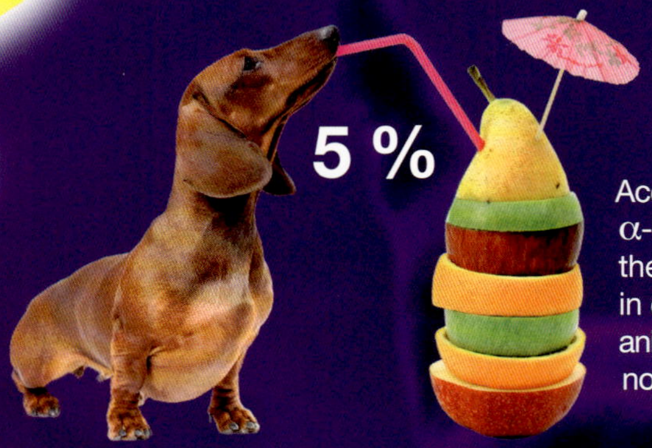

According to a study, vitamin E, vitamin C, selenium, α-lipoic acid, L-carnitine and fruit/vegetables (for 1 % in dry matter, they provide 5 % of bioflavonoids) in diets for dogs with CDS, in combination with stimulation programs, improved these animals' behavior and prevented histopathological changes but did not reverse the effects of the disease.

6 Lesion distribution depends on the age

It is worth highlighting that lesions appear in different areas at different ages. In Beagle dogs (medium-size breed), alterations can already be seen in the prefrontal cortex at 8–9 years old, while amyloid-ß starts depositing in the parietal and entorhinal regions when animals are more than10 years old. This will condition the appropriate time to start dietary modifications if we want to prevent this disease.

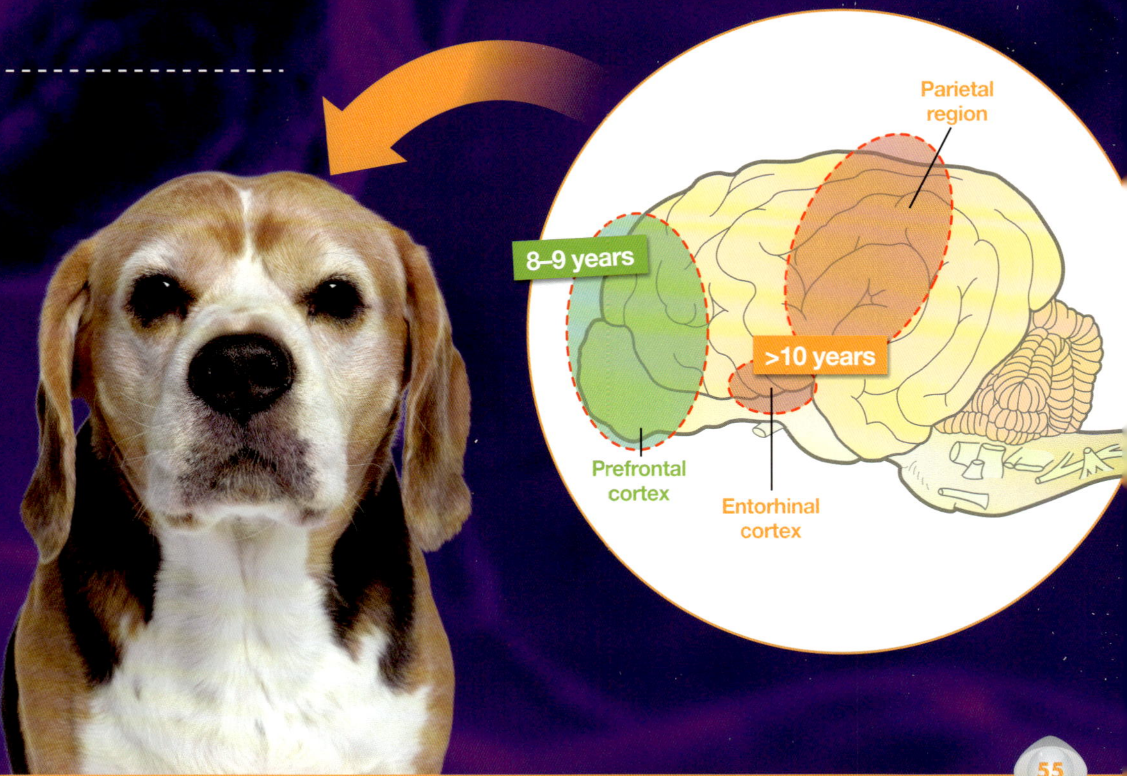

Nutrients

Antioxidants: Vitamins C and E

Vitamin C (ascorbic acid)

Vitamin C, or ascorbic acid, is not essential in pets given that it is synthesized in the liver from the metabolism of glucose and with the intervention of L-gulono-γ-lactone oxydase, although the capacity of cats and dogs to synthesize this vitamin is only a fourth of that of other mammals.

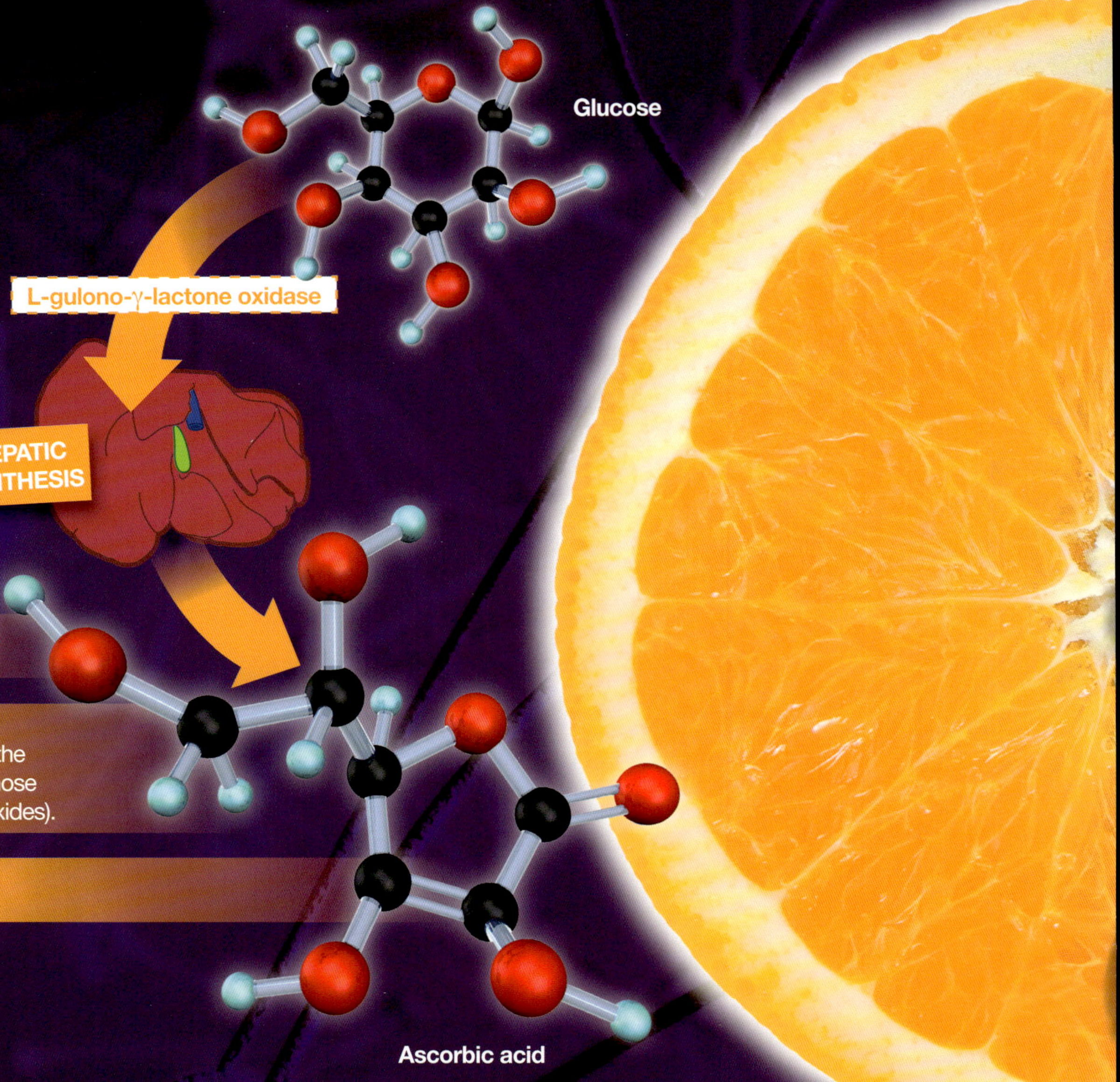

Some of its functions include the following:

- ✔ Regeneration of oxidized vitamin E, glutathione and flavonoids.
- ✔ **Redox factor:** captures the intra- and extracellular ROS, including those from the metabolism of cancer cells, as well as those derived from the N_2 (peroxynitrites, nitroxides).
- ✔ Maintains transition metals in their reduced form.

The ingestion of high levels acts like a pro-oxidant, which facilitates the oxidation of the membrane lipids. In this case, the ingestion of vitamin E should be increased.

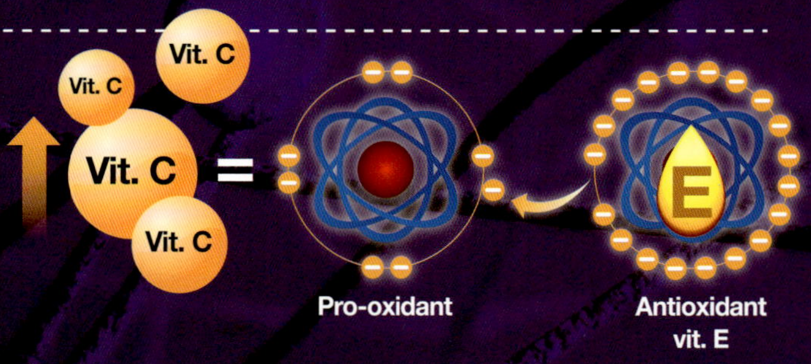

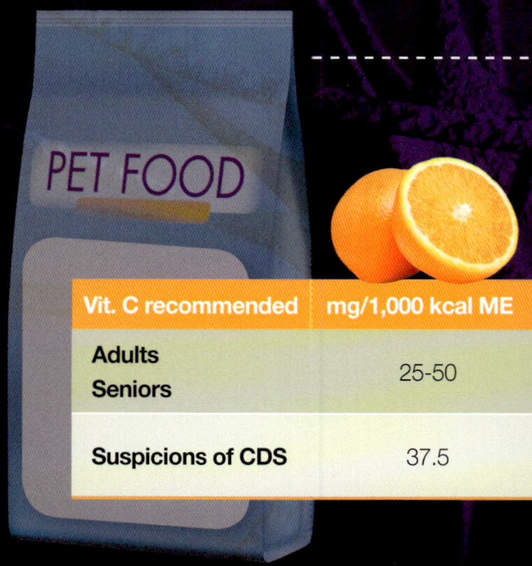

Vit. C recommended	mg/1,000 kcal ME
Adults Seniors	25-50
Suspicions of CDS	37.5

Due to its effect on the urinary pH, this should be evaluated in senior cats when the recommended levels of vitamin C are surpassed.

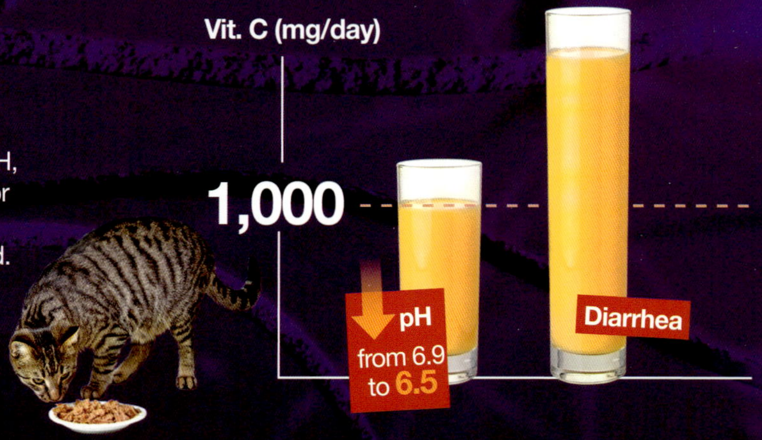

to fight CDS (I)

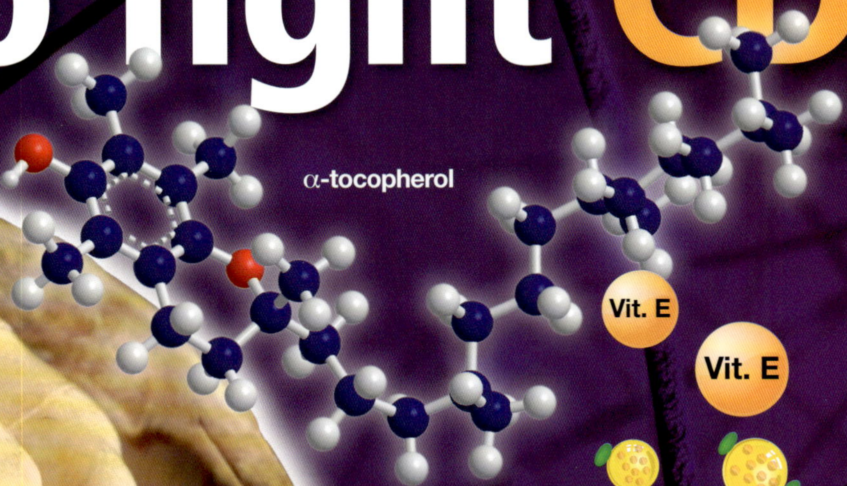

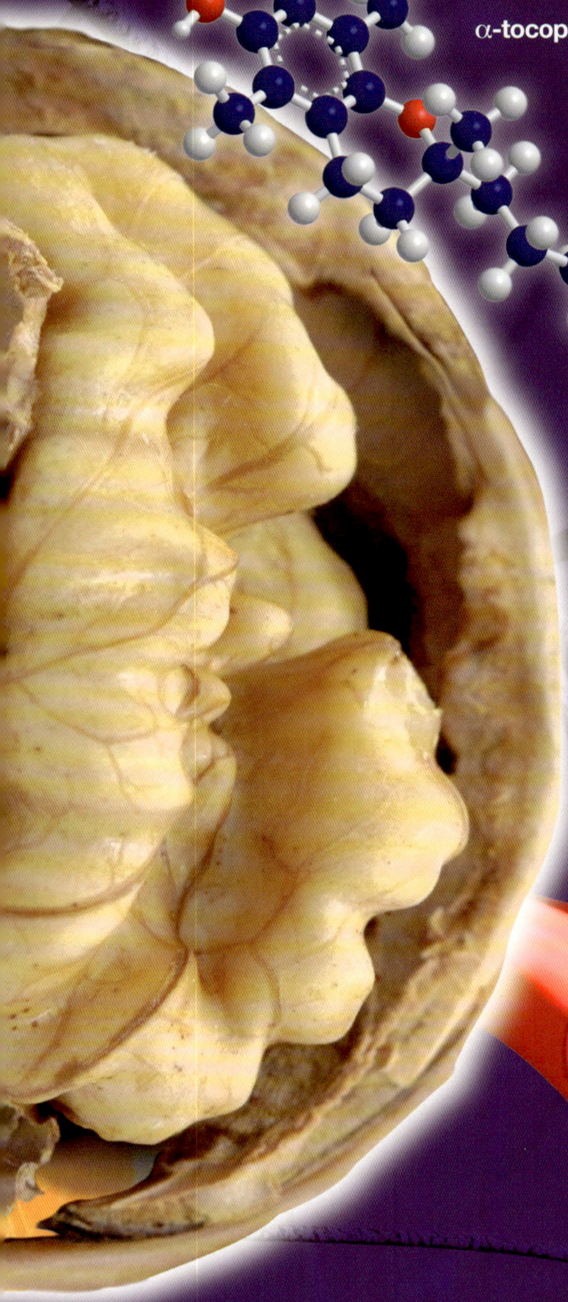

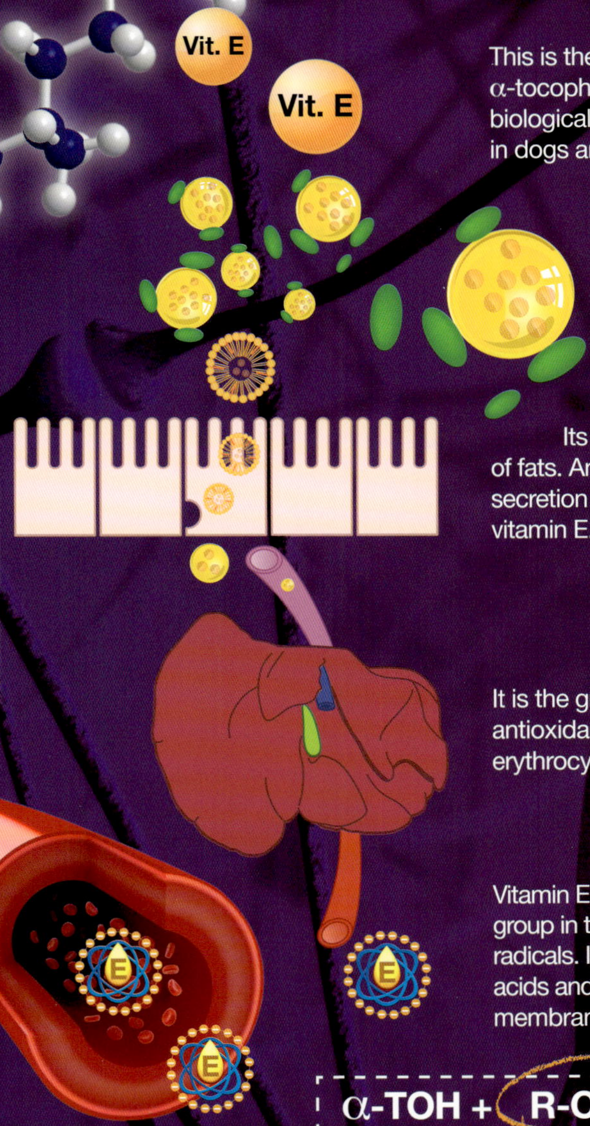

Vitamin E

This is the generic name for tocols and tocotrienols. α-tocopherol is the isomere with the greatest biological activity, although it has not been tested in dogs and cats.

Its absorption and metabolism is linked to that of fats. Any factor that affects pancreatic or biliary secretion will alter the efficiency of the intestinal use of vitamin E.

It is the greatest fat-soluble antioxidant present in plasma, erythrocytes and tissues.

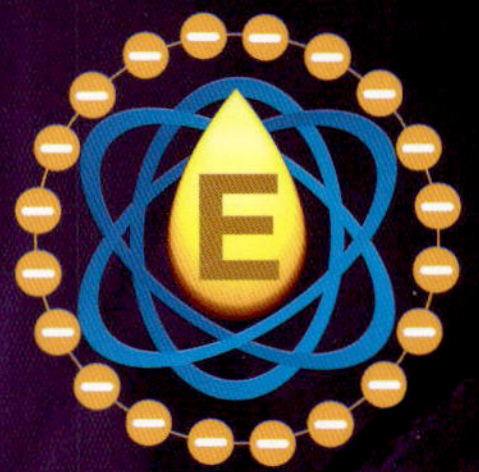

Vitamin E acts as a donator of hydrogen from the 6-OH group in the presence of free radicals, especially peroxide radicals. It prevents oxidative damage to the nucleic acids and to the poly-unsaturated FAs of the lipoprotein membranes.

$$\alpha\text{-TOH} + \text{R-COO}^- \rightarrow \alpha\text{-TO}^- + \text{R-COOH}$$

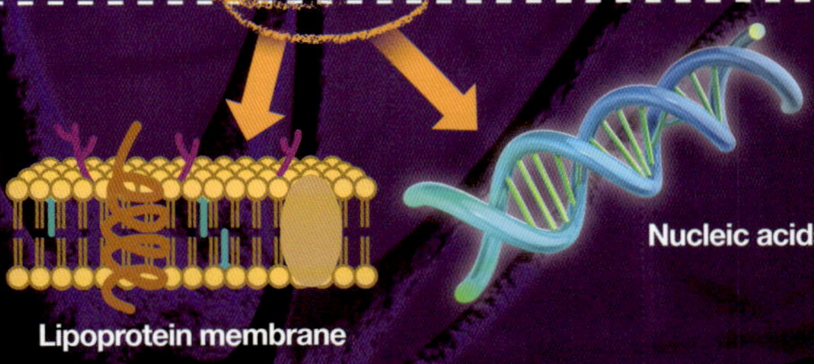

It has low toxicity, but high levels interfere in the metabolism of vitamins D and K. Its safe upper limit is between 13-20 times higher than its recommendations.

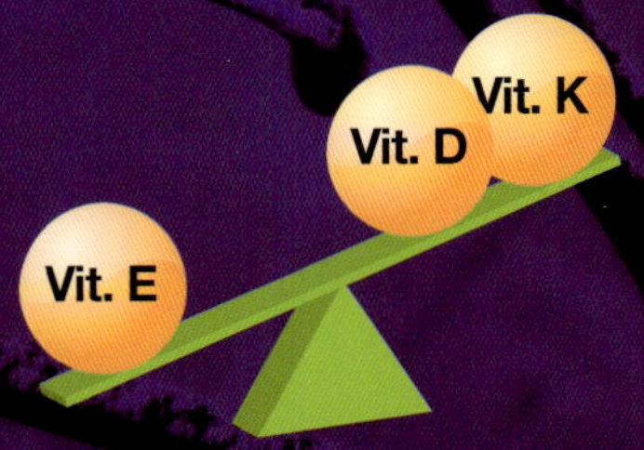

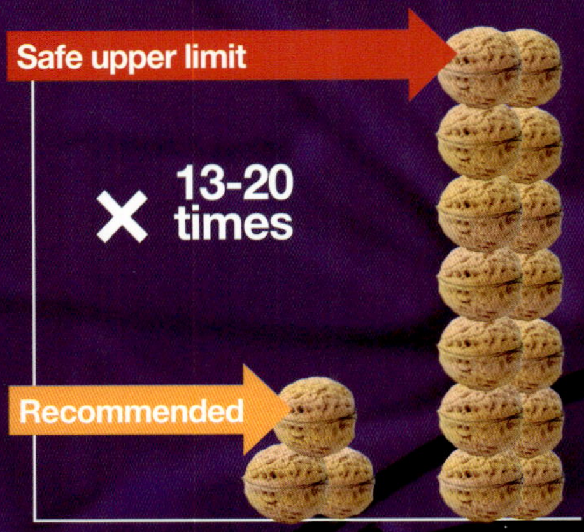

Vit. E recommended	mg/1,000 kcal ME
Adults Seniors	120-125
Suspicions of CDS	120-125 × 2
Benefits to the immune system	140; 500

In general, the levels of inclusion surpass the recommendations by more than 10 times, possibly due to the differences in the biological potency of the different isomeres and due to the losses associated with manufacturing.

Its use should always be in association with other antioxidant substances, such as vitamin C, given that on certain occasions it temporarily turns into radical α-tocopherol, with pro-oxidant activity.

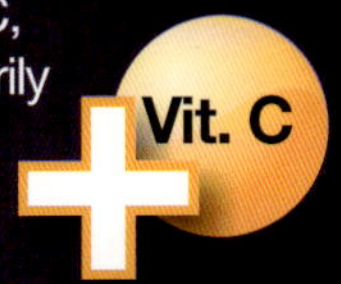

Nutrients to

Other antioxidants

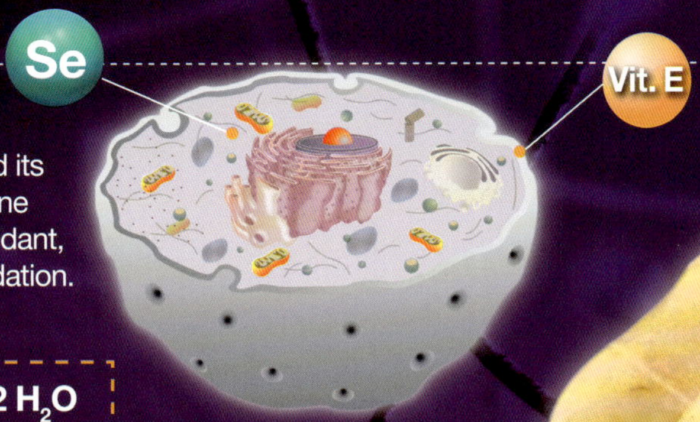

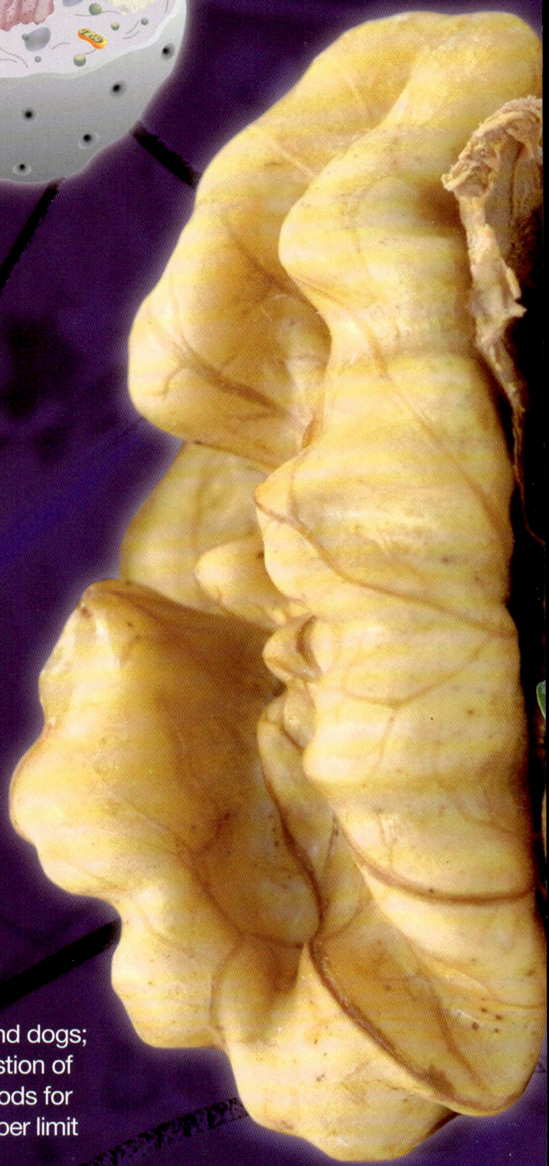

1 Selenium

This micromineral forms part of the **glutathione-peroxidase** and its deiodinase and reductase isoforms. Unlike vitamin E (a membrane antioxidant), this enzyme is a powerful intracytoplasmatic antioxidant, representing the second line of defense when faced with peroxidation. The reaction would be as follows:

2 glutathione + H_2O_2 → glutathione sulfide + 2 H_2O

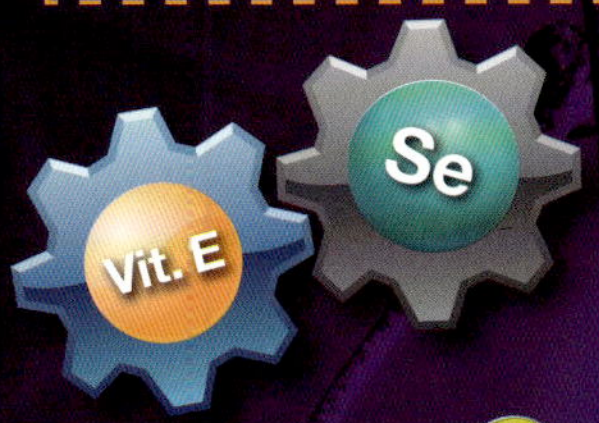

This enzyme and vitamin E work synergically to reduce the effects of oxidative reactions.

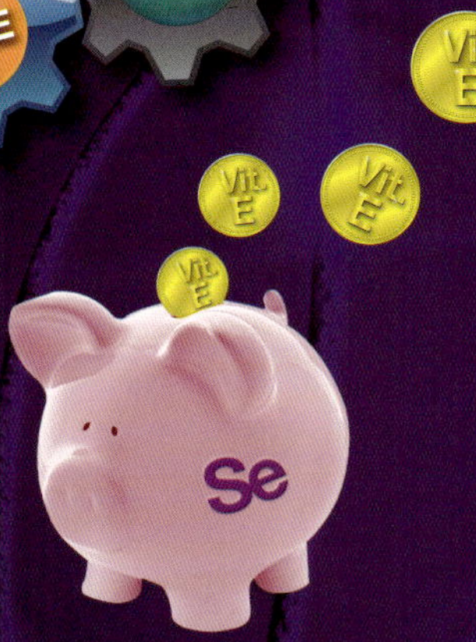

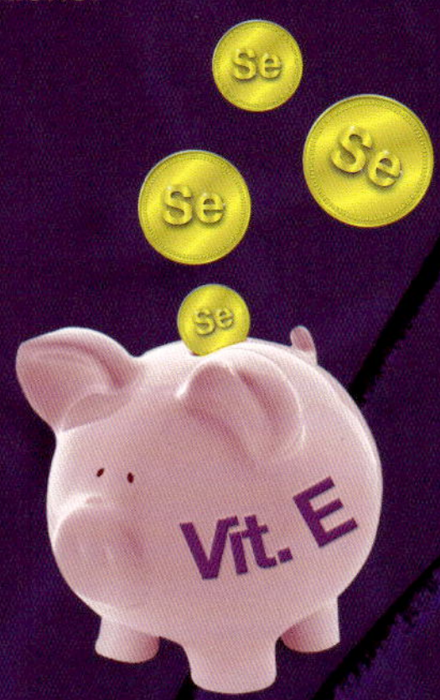

Selenium is a vitamin E saver for various reasons:

- ✔ It maintains the integrity of the pancreas, which is needed to digest fats.
- ✔ It reduces the vitamin E requirements via glutathione-peroxidase.
- ✔ It retains vitamin E in plasma.

Vitamin E itself reduces the selenium requirements in two ways:

- ✔ It maintains and avoids losses.
- ✔ It prevents the destruction of the membrane lipids (and the formation of ROS), therefore decreasing the requirements of the selenium-dependent enzyme.

There is no available data regarding the recommendations for this mineral in adult cats and dogs; it is considered that the recommendations for puppies and kittens ensure adequate ingestion of selenium. The recommendations for treating CDS are the same as the dose present in foods for healthy adult and senior animals (see table). Although it does not exist as such, the safe upper limit is established at 0.5 mg/1,000 kcal ME.

It seems that cats are more tolerant than dogs and other species to this micromineral; its concentration in plasma is 40-60 % higher. The nature of this effect is unknown.

Tolerance and concentration in plasma

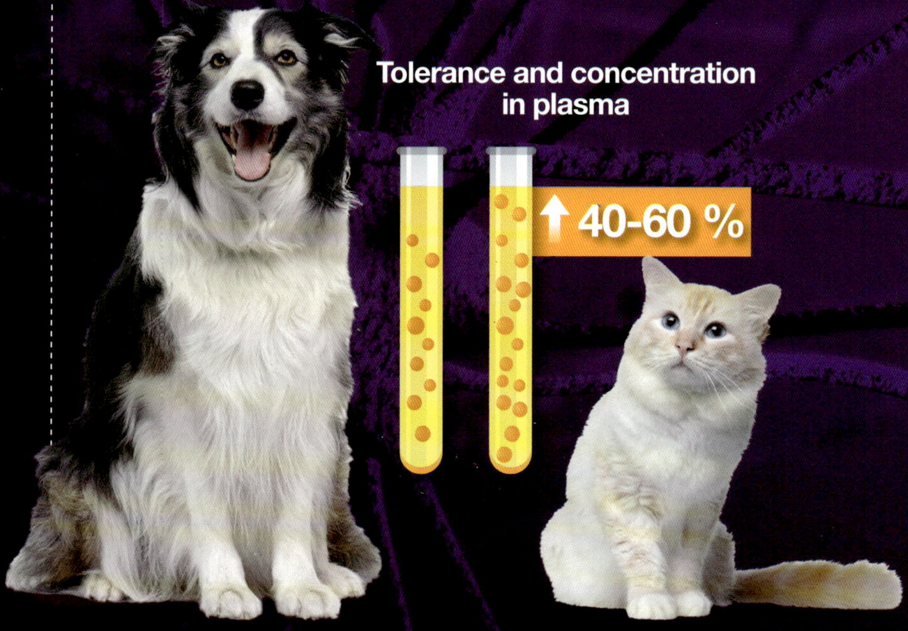

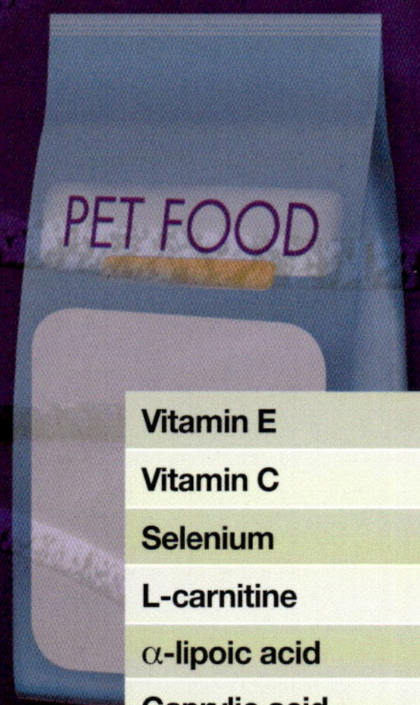

	CDS treatment Nutrient/1,000 kcal ME
Vitamin E	200-250 mg
Vitamin C	37.5 mg
Selenium	0.125-0.325 mg
L-carnitine	62-185 mg
α-lipoic acid	32 mg
Caprylic acid	11.32 mg

fight CDS (II)

Supplements for mitochondrial activity

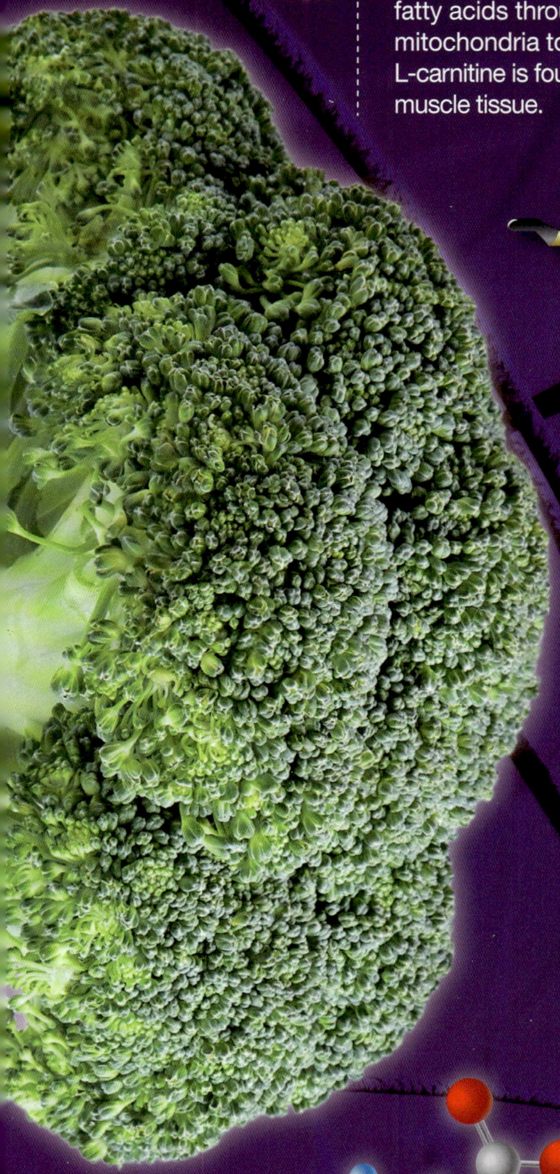

2 L-carnitine

This substance transports long-chain fatty acids through the membrane of the mitochondria to be oxidized. Most of the L-carnitine is found in the skeletal and heart muscle tissue.

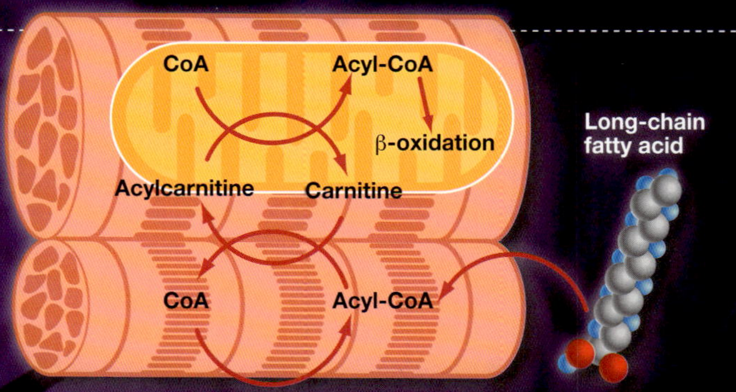

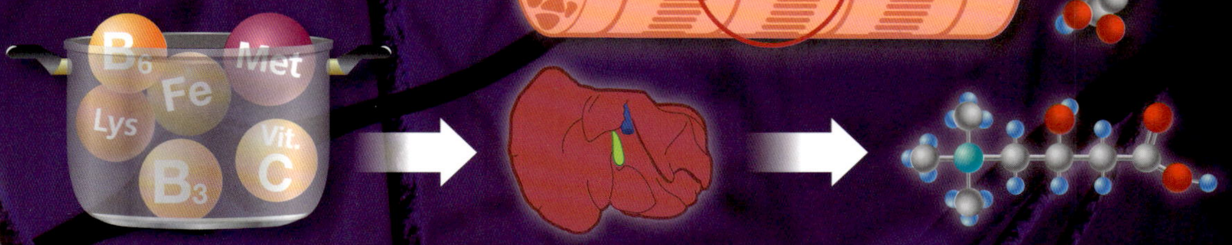

Its synthesis is endogenous in the liver, using the following as substrates: lysine, methionine, ascorbic acid, iron, vitamin B_6 and niacin. The supplements of this nutrient attempt to reduce ROS by increasing mitochondrial function efficiency. No specific dose for use has been described.

3 Medium-chain triglycerides and α-lipoic acid (AAL)

α-lipoic acid is derived from caprylic acid (octanoic acid).
Its antioxidant effects are not clear.
There are two theories:

- ✔ They are due to its reduced intracellular form (dihydrolipoic acid), which eliminates ROS.
- ✔ They modify the genetic signals that allow for an improvement of the antioxidant state of the cell.

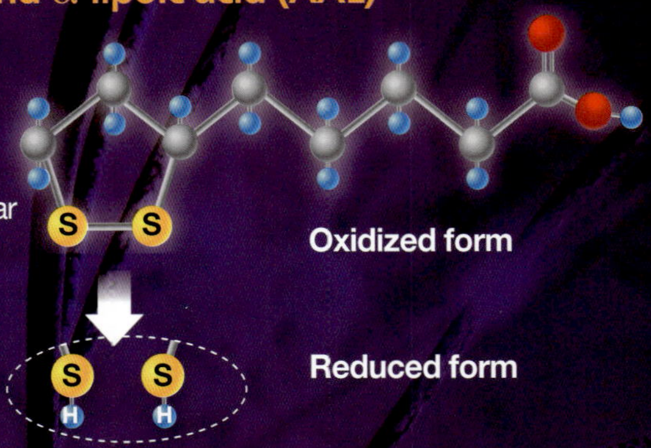

Also, incorporating medium-chain FAs such as caprylic acid (11.32 mg/1,000 Kcal ME) in food rations for sick dogs represented benefits in the different evaluation tests. This FA is converted into ketones (β-hydroxybutyrate) in the liver, and these are the alternative substrate to glucose for the astrocytes. The habitual substrate for neurons is glucose, but with age, the capacity to metabolize it and obtain ATP is reduced.This explains the relationship between CDS and metabolic alterations.

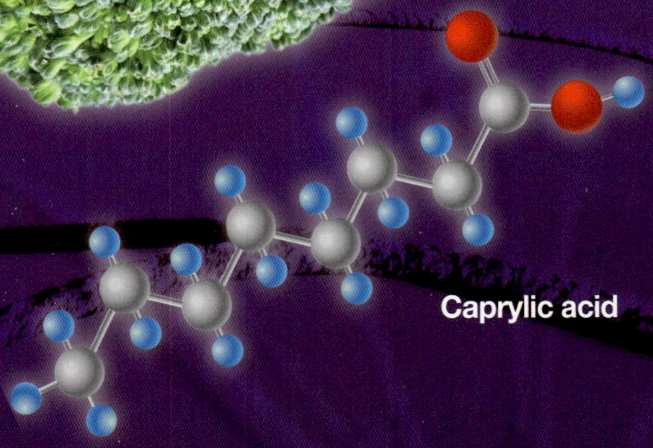

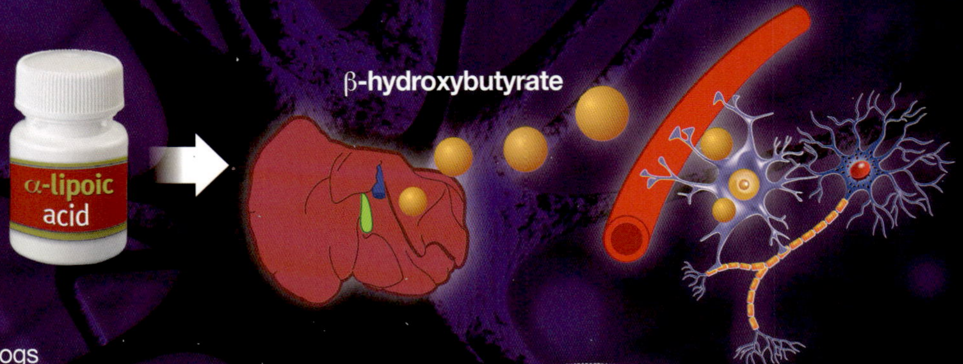

Be careful with α-lipoic acid in cats

- ✔ It cannot be used at the same doses as those used with dogs or other species, such as humans or rats, as it would be toxic for cats.
- ✔ The maximum tolerable dose is 13 mg/kg of body weight (almost 10 times less than in dogs). At a dose of 30 mg/kg, non-specific semi-acute hepatitis can already be observed. The hepatic changes are evident due to an elevation of blood urea nitrogen (BUN) and a decrease in the ratio between branched and aromatic amino acids. It is not entirely clear if the cause of the toxicity is due to the accumulation of α-lipoic acid favored by the entero-hepatic circulation or due to a defect in the enzymes responsible for detoxification.

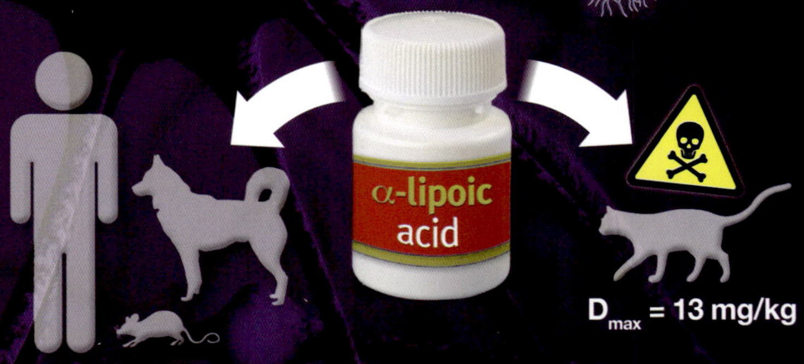

Sporting dogs

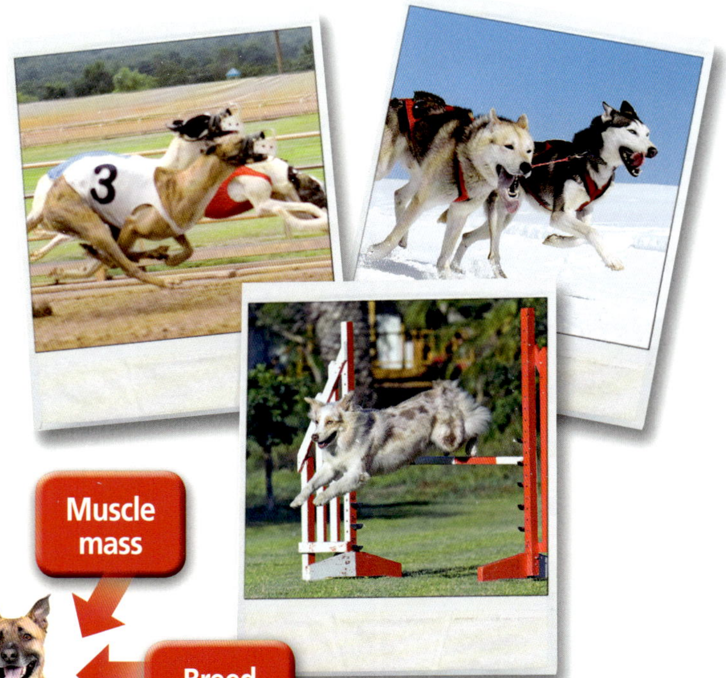

1 Athletic breeds

Dogs can perform different tasks

Their training, exercise, and feeding will depend on the activity that they carry out.

Sporting competitions are popular right now

Sporting competitions with dogs have become popular over the last few years. This species represents one of the largest exceptions among mammals due to their extensive variability regarding their weight and body condition, as well as their athletic capacity.

Variables that affect their nutritional requirements

We can find different types of foods for dogs on the market depending on their age and body weight. However, there are other variables that can affect their nutritional requirements. The body mass index, muscle mass, body composition, resting metabolism and breed of the dog are all factors that modify their requirements.

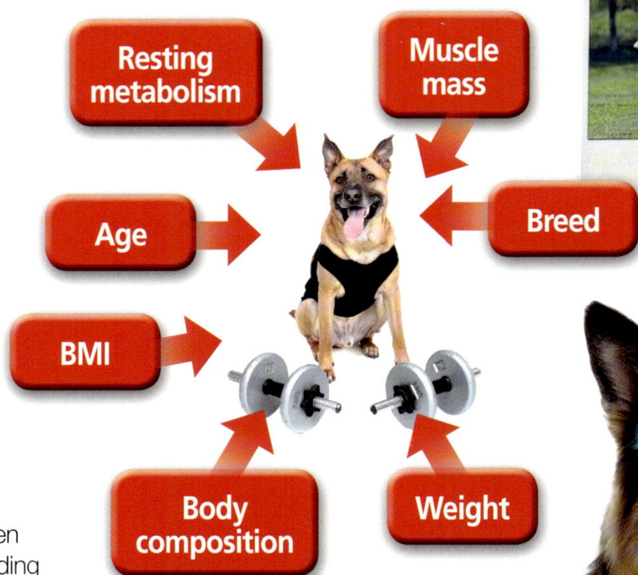

The genetics of breeds

Currently, dog breeds (more than 400 have been described) have already been classified in at least four groups, according to their genetic proximity. They are as follows:

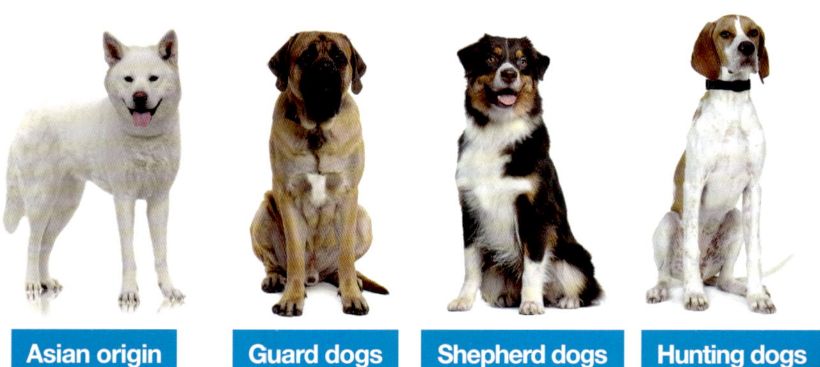

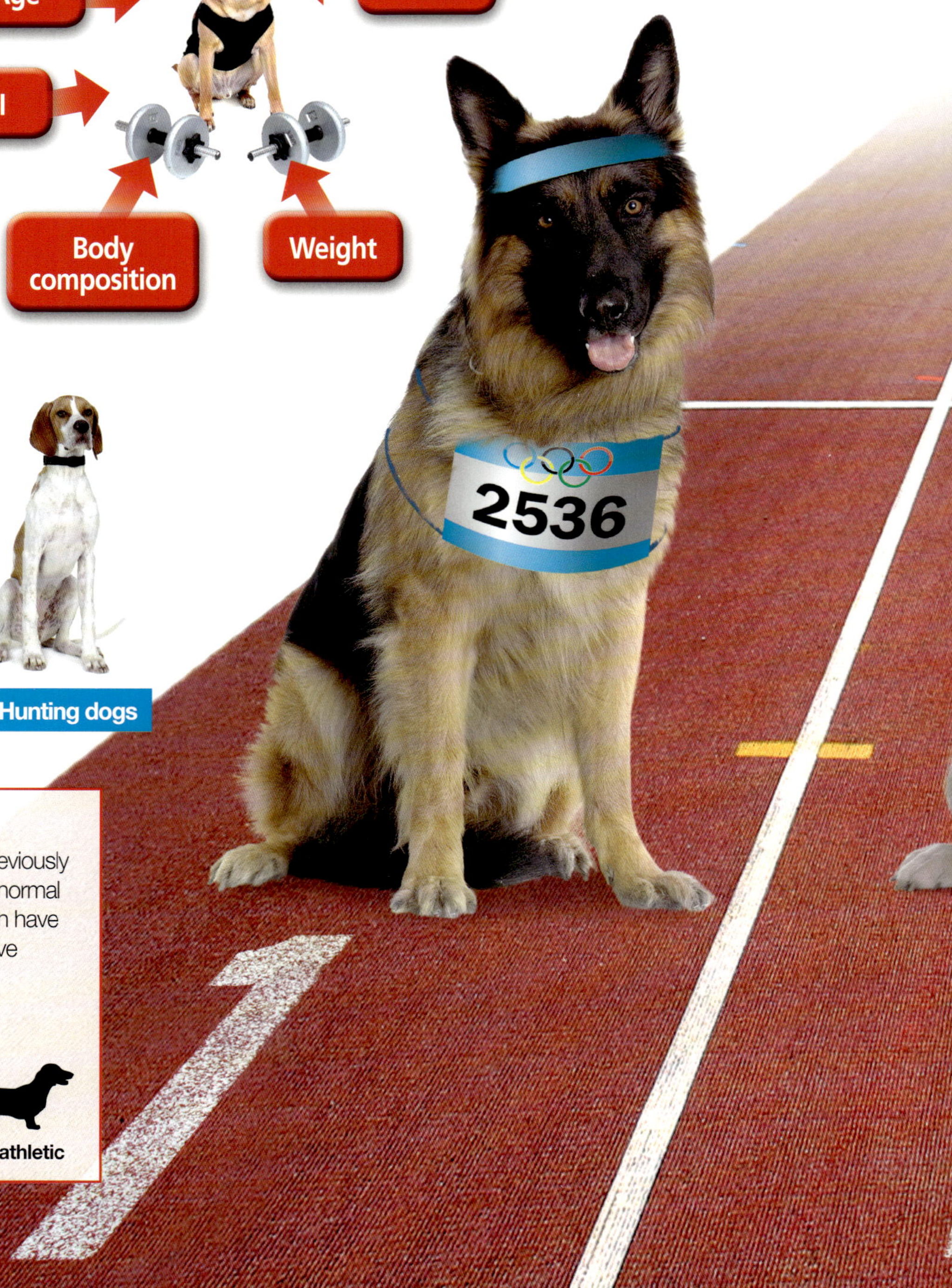

Division between athletic dogs and normal dogs

From a feeding perspective, and taking into account all of the previously mentioned factors, we can subdivide dogs into two categories: normal and athletic. The breeds included within the athletic conformation have a higher resting basal metabolism rate (RBMR) and therefore have greater energy requirements.

It has been estimated that the RBMR is 57 % greater compared to breeds with non-athletic conformation.

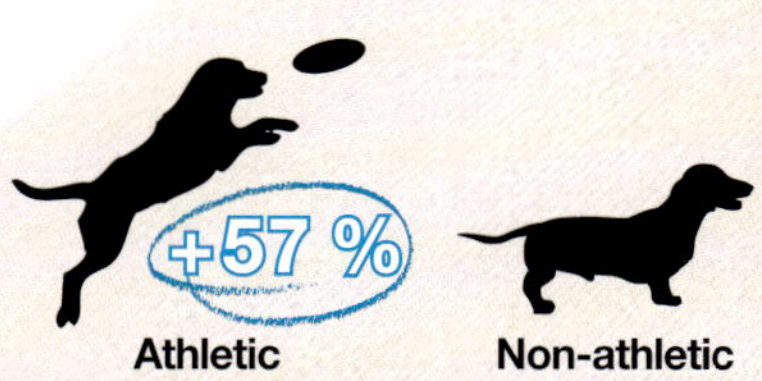

2 Morphology of athletic breeds

Some authors have attempted to morphologically define athletic dogs from a series of characteristics:

Body mass index (BMI) **BMI <90 kg/m²**

✓ $BMI = Ideal\ BW\ (kg)/WH(m)^2$

Thorax:abdominal circumference ratio **TC:AC>1.5**

High body surface area (BSA) per kilogram of body weight ratio.

✓ $BSA = 10.1 \times [BW\ (kg)^{0.67}/100]$

The lighter the animal, the greater the BSA:kg ratio.

Adipose:muscle tissue ratio **Fat:muscle <1**

Percentage of fatty tissue in the organism **<10 %**

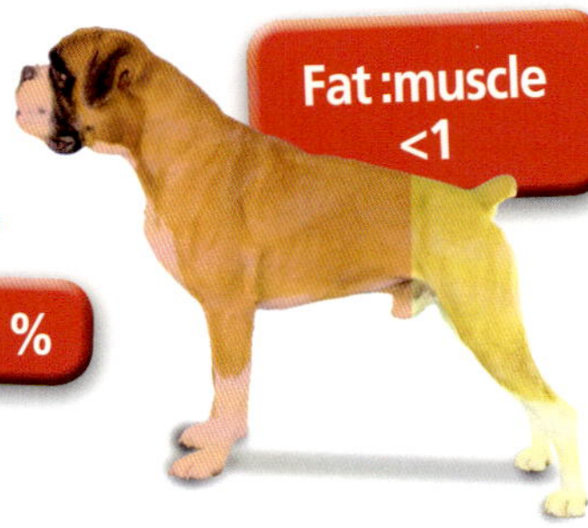

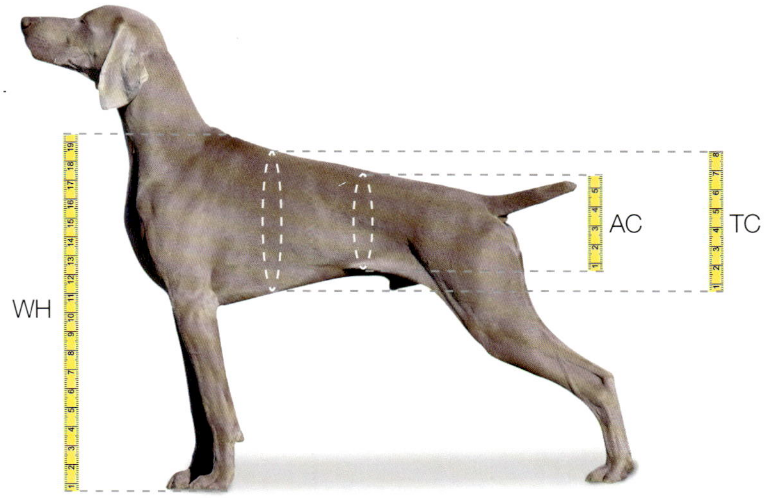

BW: body weight (kg).

WH: withers height (m).

TC: thorax circumference at the level of the ribs 9-11 (cm).

AC: abdominal circumference at the level of the lumbar vertebra 5-6 (cm).

Certain breeds classified as athletic would be, for example, the following: Yorkshire Terrier, Springer Spaniel, Fox and Airedale Terrier, Pointer, German Short Hair, English Setter, Greyhound, Husky, German Shepherd, and Bobtail. However, the following are not considered as athletic: French Bulldog, Beagle, Rottweiler, Labrador, and Golden Retriever.

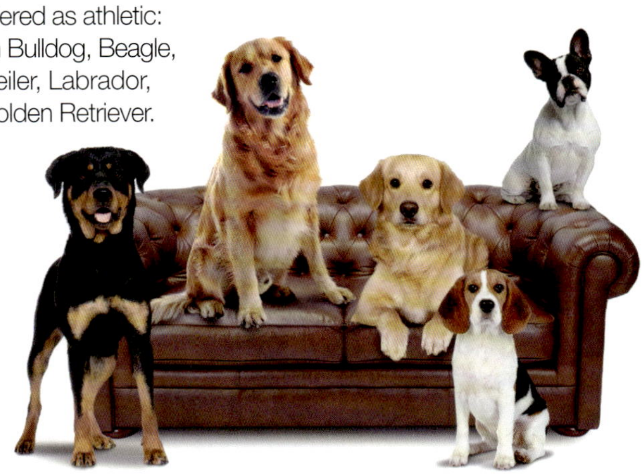

Non-athletic breeds

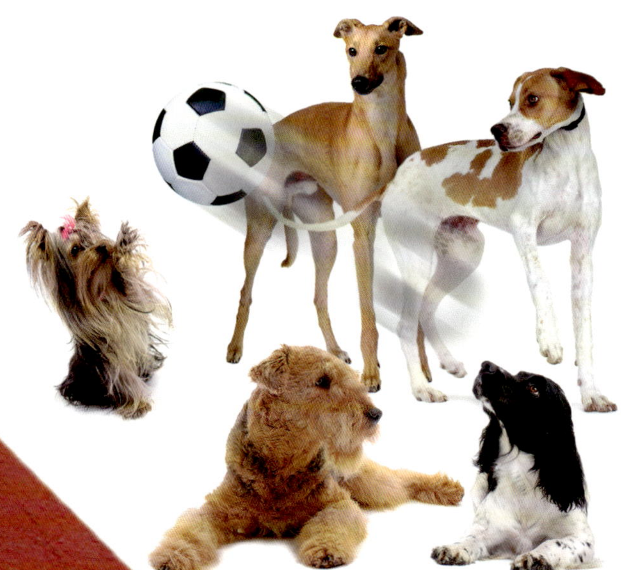

Athletic breeds

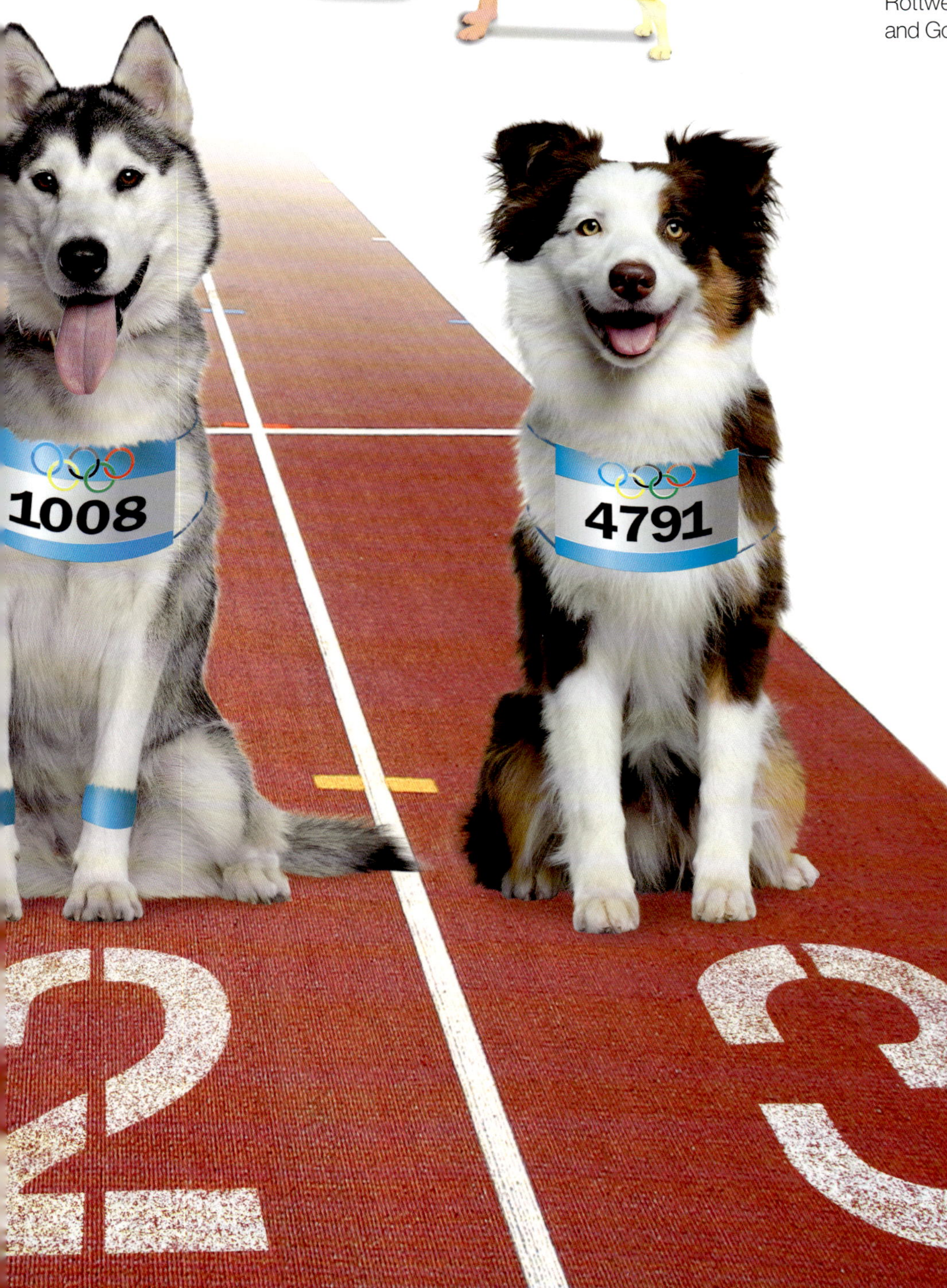

Effects of
on digestion and

Changes in the digestive physiology

When dogs exert themselves physically 20 % less than their maximum capacity, a series of changes take place in the digestive physiology that are not observed at maximum capacities. The mechanisms are not well understood.

Exertion ≈ 80 % of the maximum capacity

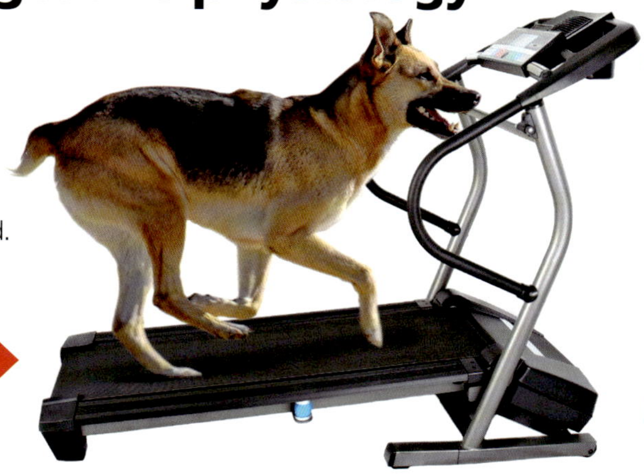

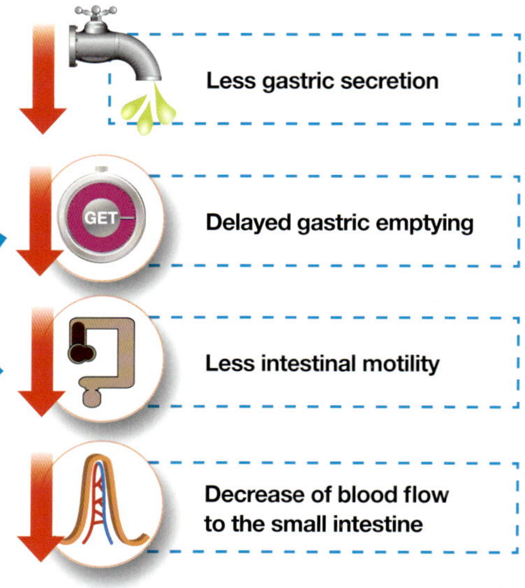

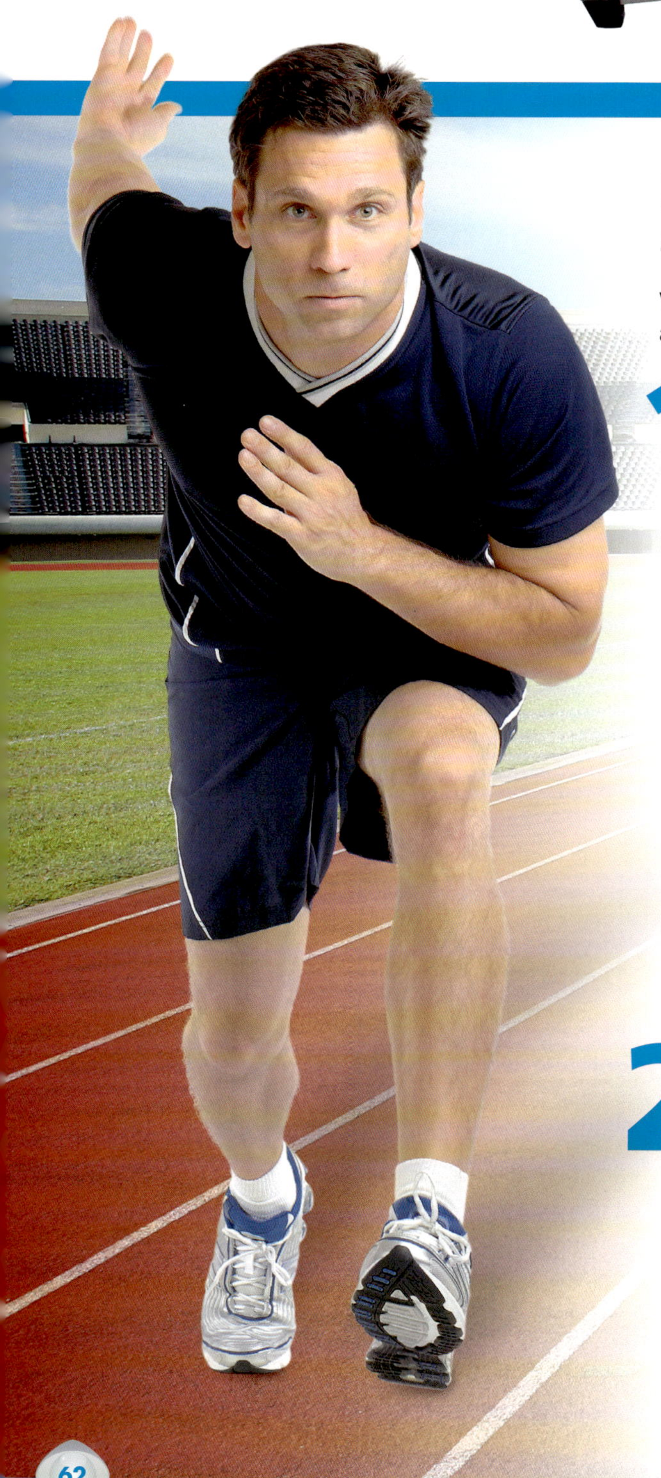

Differences between human and canine athletes

We cannot extrapolate the results from human athletes to our dogs as the efficiency of the use of nutrients is different in each species.

1 They obtain energy from body fat

- During exercise, the obtention of energy to maintain activity is done using body fat.
- In these dogs, an increase in the lipoprotein-lipase of the muscle tissue and an increase of triglycerides in plasma have been observed. This makes us think, and it has thus been demonstrated, that in the resistance training tests, the free fatty acids (FFAs) from the food rations are the primary source of energy for the muscle (they provide between 70-90 % of the energy): the concentration of FFAs in plasma increases, a greater assimilation of the chylomicrons and a lesser reuptake and synthesis of triglycerides (TGs) take place.
- This fact is confirmed by an increase of the plasmatic glycerol, a decrease in the FFA:glycerol ratio in plasma and by the reduction in the use of glycogen.

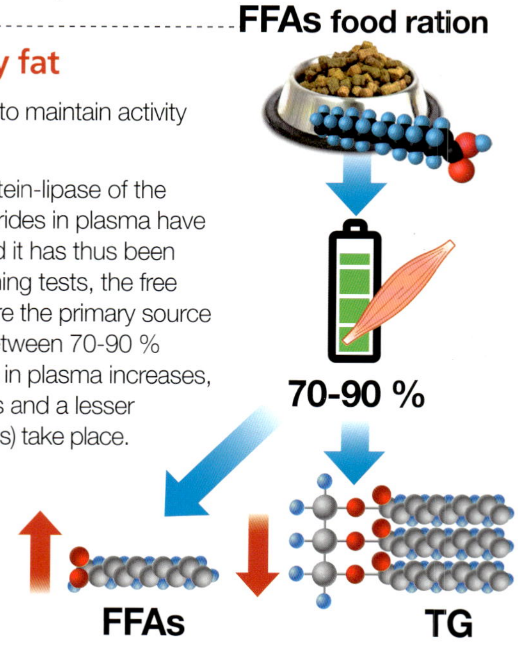

2 Benefits of high quality proteins

The administration of high quality protein immediately after intense exercise provides benefits. The synthesis of protein lost during physical exertion is twice as fast and protein catabolism is reduced by half. In this case, it is not very clear when is the best moment to carry out replacement.

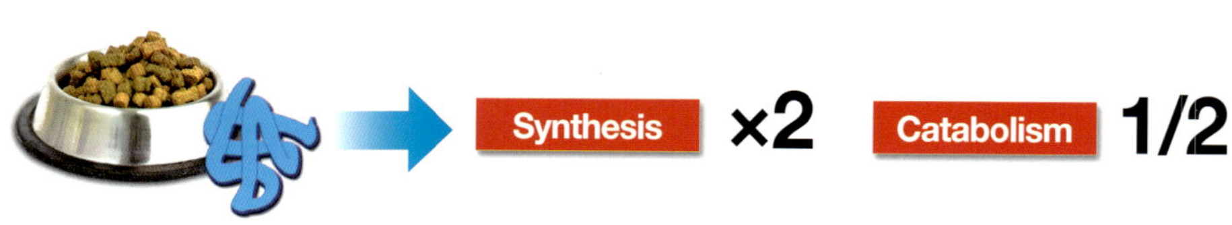

exercise
the metabolism

Cease in the myoelectric activity

- ✔ The mechanism responsible for the digestive changes seems to be a cease in the myoelectric activity that controls peristaltic waves.
- ✔ It has been seen that the digestive resting time is related to the composition of the food ration and not to its energy concentration. The myoelectric activity is abolished for a longer time with fats > sugars > dairy proteins.
- ✔ For this reason, and depending on the volume of the food ration, it is recommended that 8-16 hours pass after ingesting a food ration rich in fat before exercising.

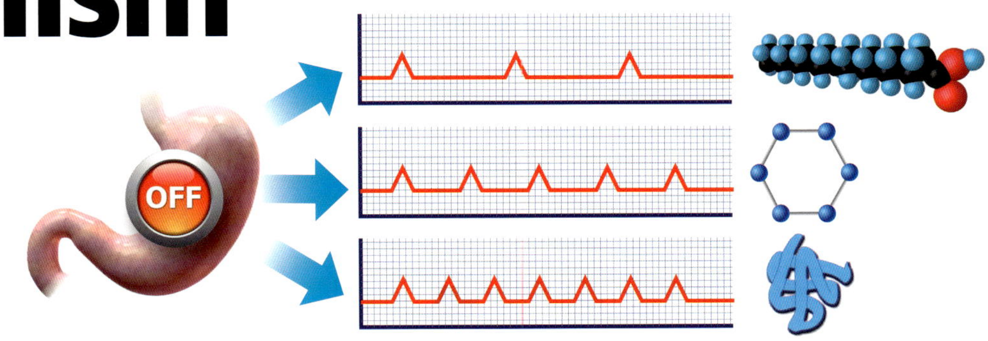

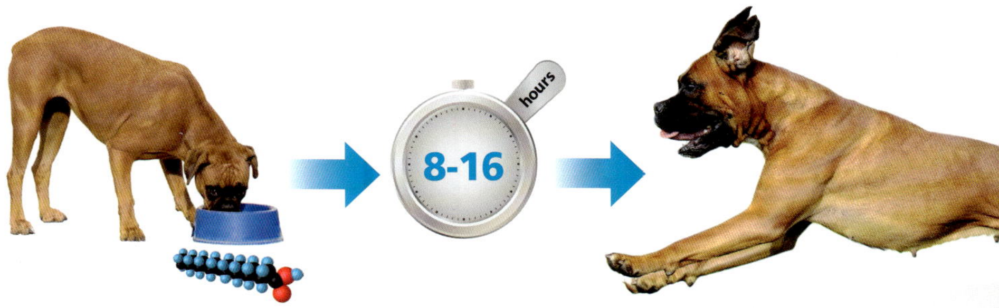

Be careful with digestibility and minerals

- ✔ The changes that take place in the composition and the amount of food offered to working dogs can lead to episodes of diarrhea. The primary cause is using food rations that are hard to digest, given that the digestibility of the dry material and of the principal nutrients is not affected by exercise. Likewise, some mineral-rich solutions produce the same effect.

3 Benefits of carbohydrates

- ✔ Administrating glucose immediately after intense work enables the recovery of glycemia and the levels of muscular glycogen to values similar to those before exertion. Between 30 and 120 minutes after finishing the exercise, this recovery is maximum. After 120 minutes, the repletion of glycogen decreases to half. Glucose in the portal circulation sends a signal that stimulates the synthesis of hepatic glycogen but inhibits muscular synthesis.

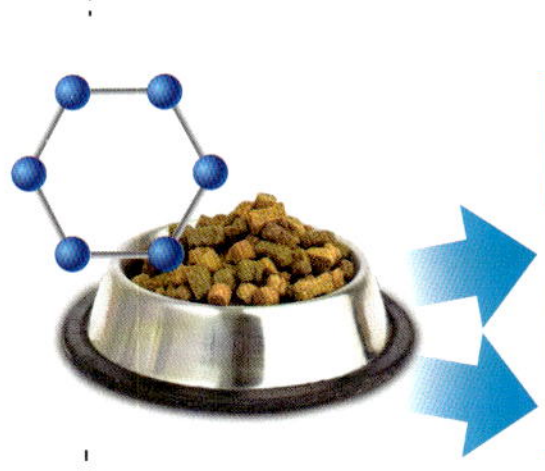

	Recovery of glycemia and glycogen levels
30-120 minutes	✔
>120 minutes	✘

- ✔ It seems that the intestinal absorption of glucose in this immediate period of time is faster and has no inhibitory effect, allowing for a greater synthesis of muscular glycogen (up to three times greater). However, in dogs that are not in ideal physical shape, their metabolism is primarily anaerobic, and thus it is important to provide them with glucose before, during and after exercise.

4 They do not present hypoglycemia after exercising

The occurrence of post-exercise ketosis and hypoglycemia is not common in dogs. They are capable of performing resistance training tests after having been in fasting conditions for five days, without receiving any water while running (although their resistance is increased by more than 70 % when we provide them with water during exercise), and show normal glycemia levels at the end of the test.

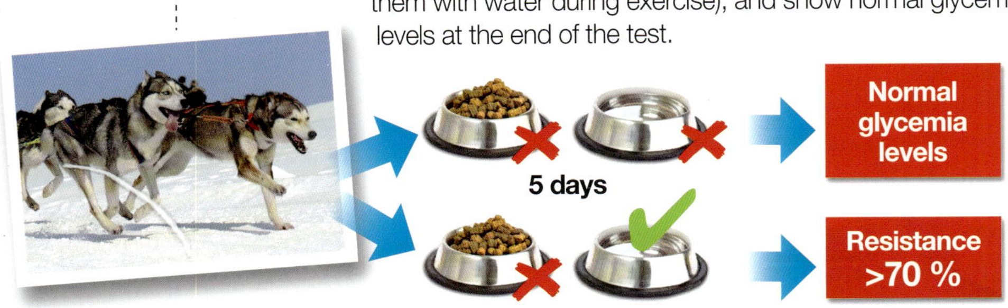

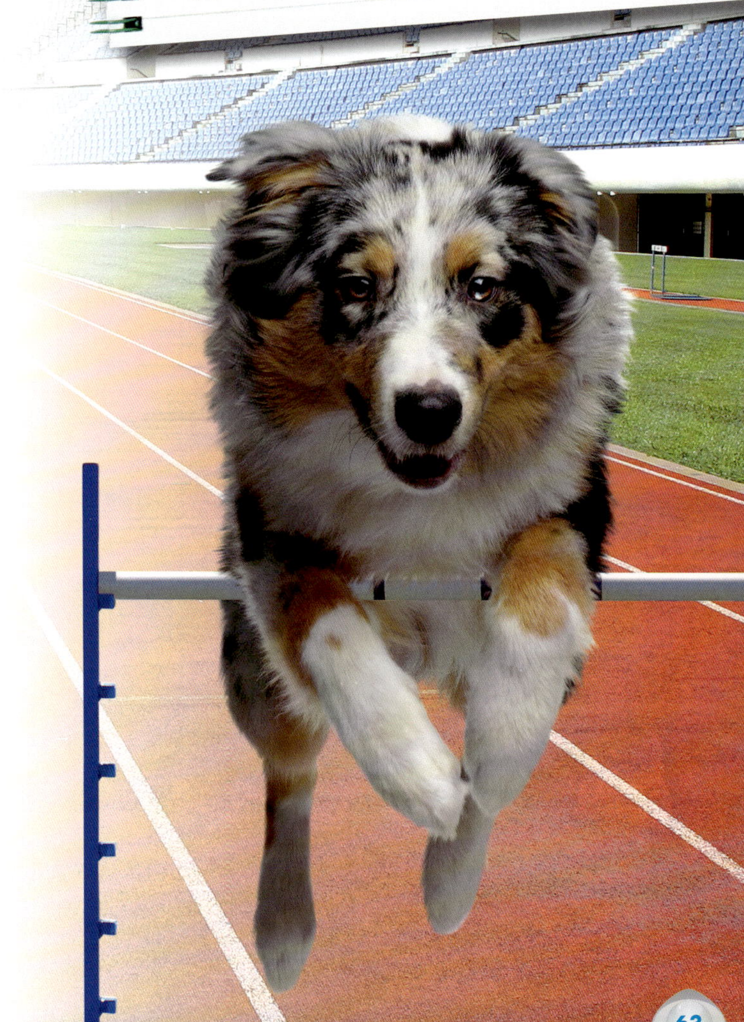

Changes associated

Different studies have highlighted the changes that take place as a result of exercise, although genetics also plays a very important role. The following should be mentioned:

1 The musculoskeletal system

✔ **Muscle hypertrophy**

This is the most perceivable change. The musculature of the forelegs, diaphragm and tongue increases up to 600 %. Their metabolism increases up to 20 times.

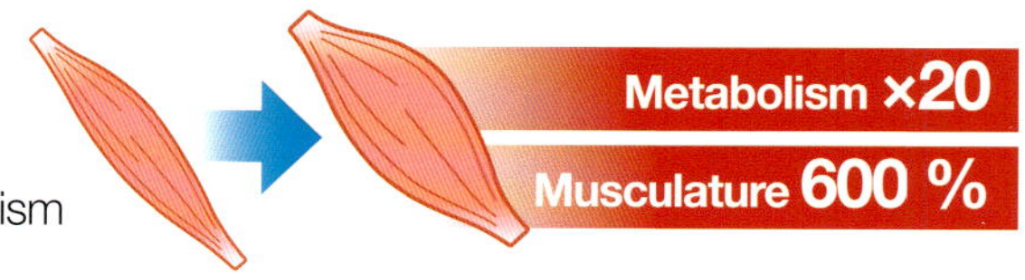

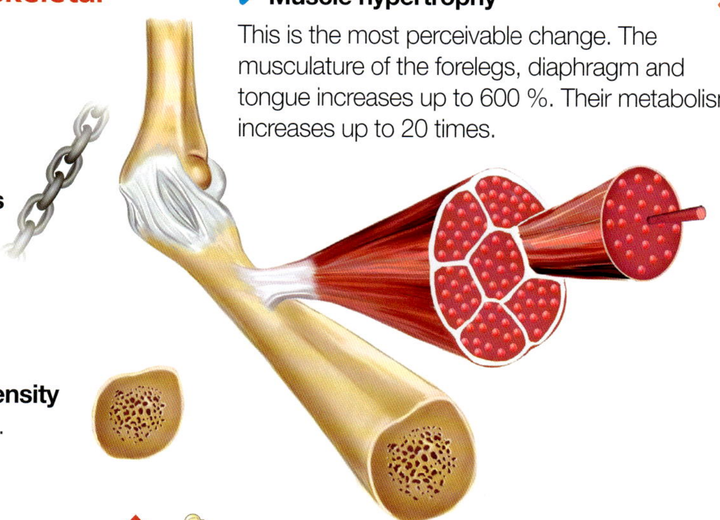

✔ The **collateral knee ligaments** become more resistant.

✔ **Better efficiency in the use of energy by the muscle**; the volume and the number of mitochondria increases.

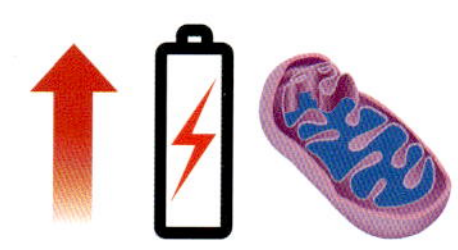

✔ **Lower bone density** of the flat bones.

✔ Increase in **growth of the long bones**. They also have a greater relative weight (10 %).

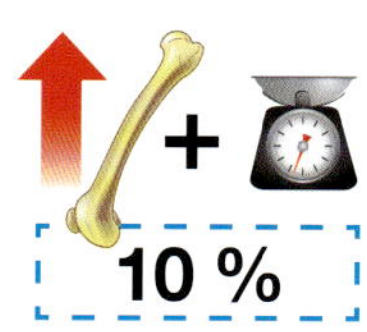

✔ **The bone metabolism is increased**; the levels of plasma alkaline phosphatase (ALP) are double. The plasma calcium is also increased.

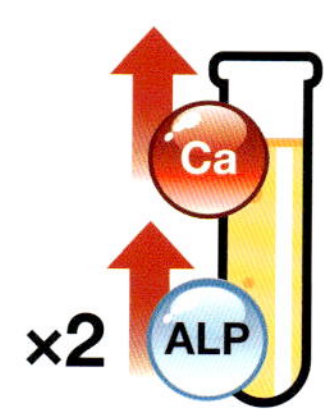

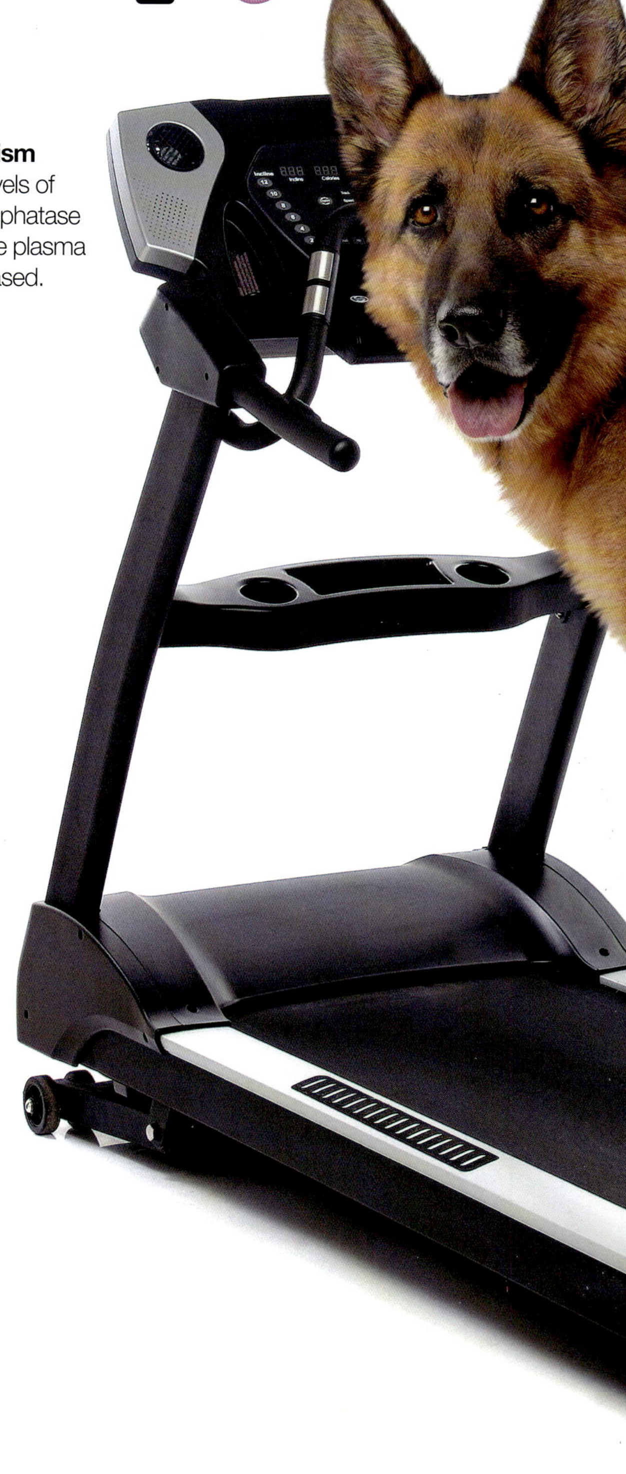

Types of muscle fibers

There are two types of muscle fibers, depending on their contractile properties: type I and type II. The predominance of one type or another depends on the genetics and exercise makes modifications possible. The different populations of type II make dogs tireless runners. The exercise that most of them perform is a mixture of both, but there is a slight predominance of type I fibers compared to the others.
The table summarizes their properties:

Parameter	Type of muscle fiber	
	Type I	Type II
ATPase activity	No	II-A, II-Dog and II-C
Type of response	Slow	Fast
Metabolism (place)	Aerobic (mitochondria)	Anaerobic (cytoplasm)
Primary substrate	Fats, carbohydrates and amino acids	Glycogen/ glucose
Size of the fiber	Short	Long
Type of exercise and breed example	Resistance	Intense and brief

with training

2 Energy required for muscle contraction

- The energy for muscle contraction comes from adenosine triphosphate (ATP) and is proportional to the level of performance. There is a direct relationship between the level of performance by the dog (km/h), which varies between breeds, and the energy requirements (kcal/h).

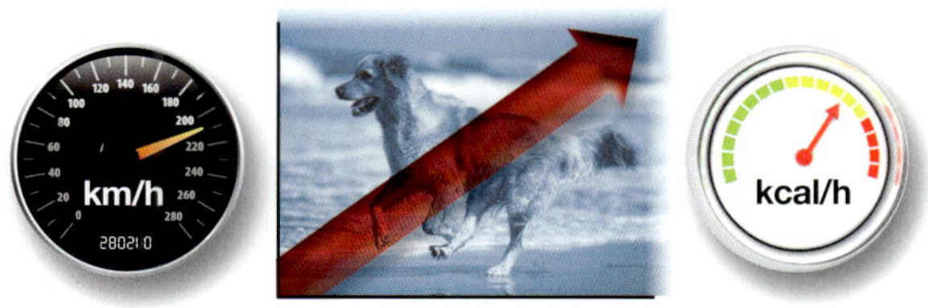

- To evaluate the energy required during exercise, the oxygen consumed has been used. According to this relation, we can classify the intensity of the exercise in three categories (see table).
- The consumption of O_2 is maximum when reaching 80 % of the maximum velocity. Greater exertion, with the highest velocities (100 %), is absolutely dependent on the anaerobic metabolism.

Parameter	Intensity of the exercise		
	Low	Medium	High
O_2 consumption (% of maximum)	<30 %	30-50 %	>70 %
Velocity (% of the maximum)	25 %	40 %	>50 %
Metabolism	Aerobic	Aerobic	Anaerobic
Substrate	Fatty acids	FAs and glycogen	Glycogen
Concentration of lactate in blood	Low	Low	High

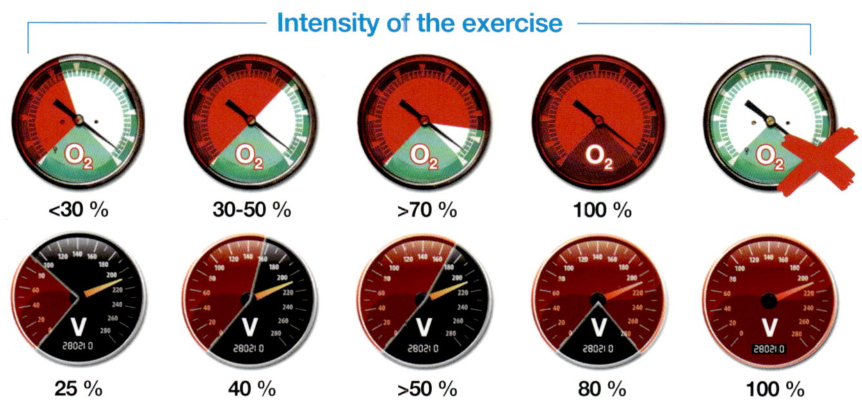

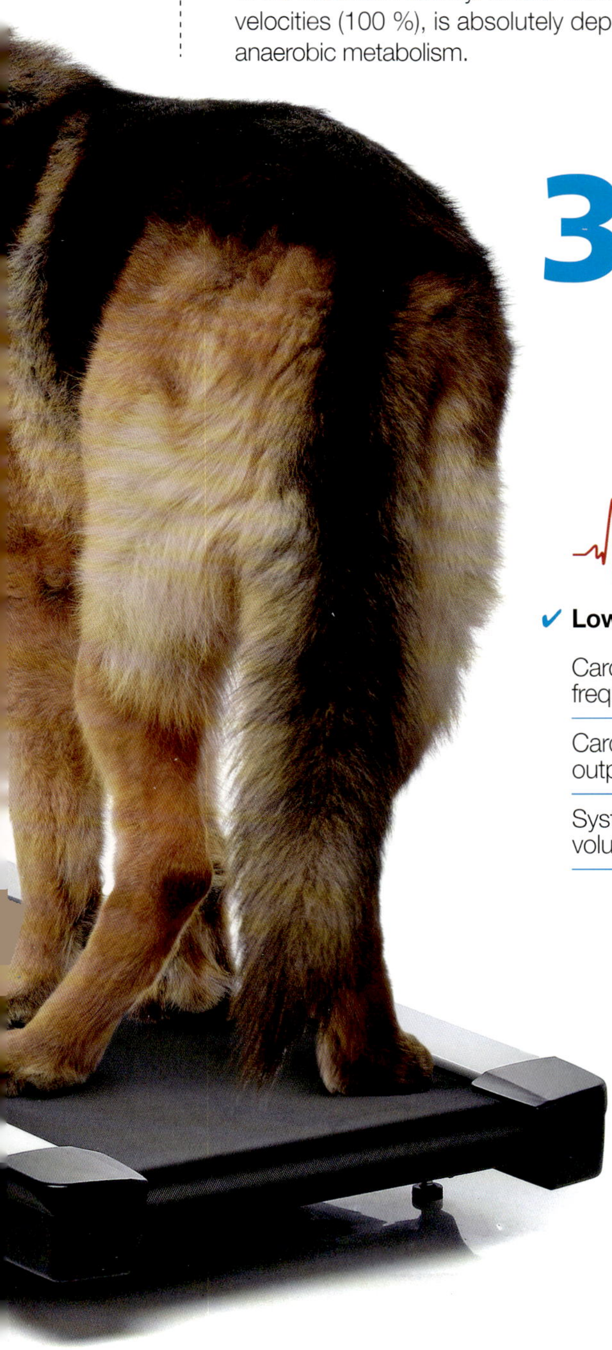

3 The heart and circulatory system

- **Increase in the respiratory function (frequency and volume)**. This way, the use of O_2 is increased and the heat and CO_2 generated are eliminated.

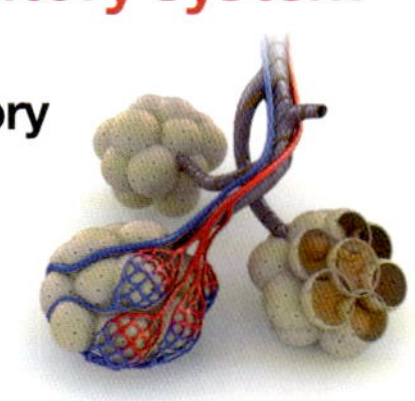

- The **relative size of the heart** is greater; it increases up to **24 %**.

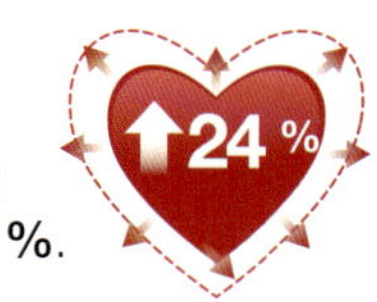

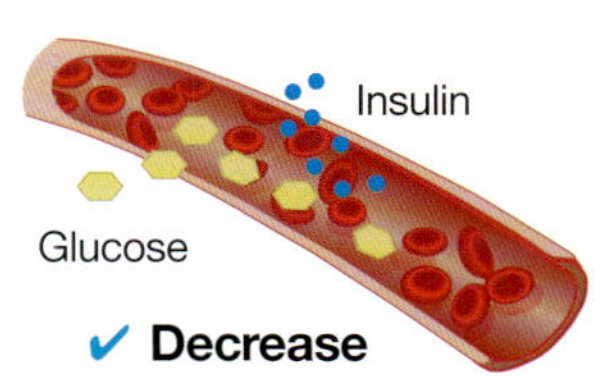

- **Decrease in the levels of glucose and insulin** in blood.

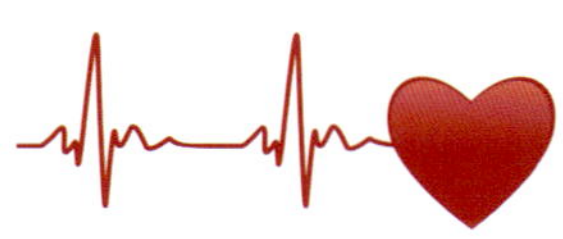

- **Lower cardiac exertion**

Cardiac frequency	↓ 12 %
Cardiac output	↑ 27 %
Systolic volume	↑ 14 %

- Increase of **hematocrit**, in more than **25 %**, due to the contractions of the spleen and the decrease of the plasma volume.

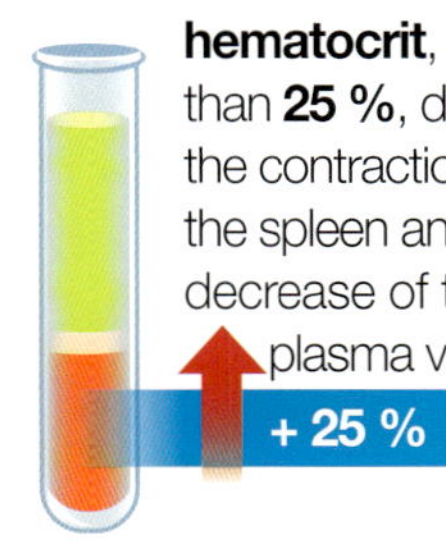

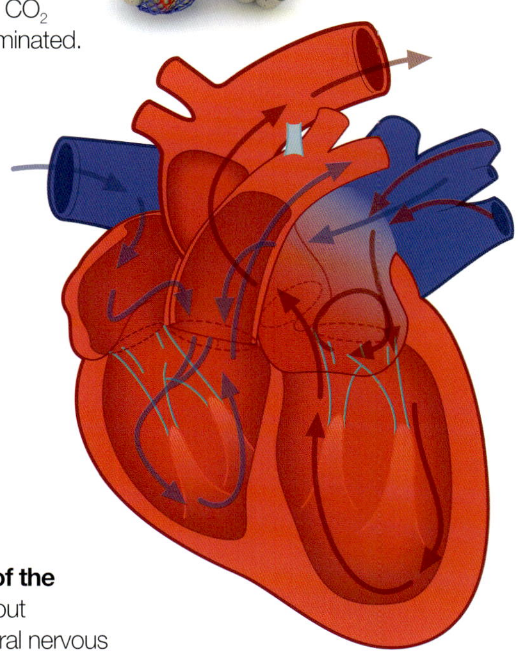

- **Redistribution of the blood flow** without affecting the central nervous system. Those muscles and organs that are not necessary for exercise receive less blood.

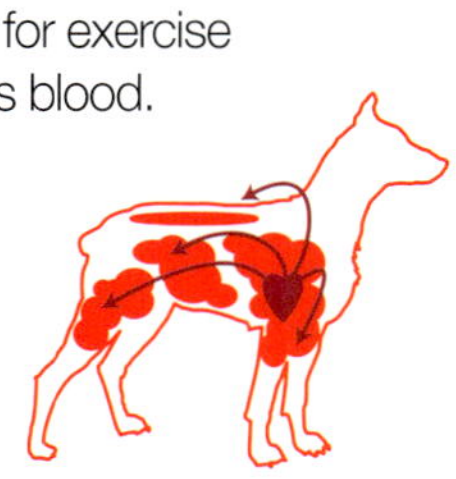

- **Decrease of the plasma volume** by:
  1. Hydrostatic effect.
  2. Osmotic efect.

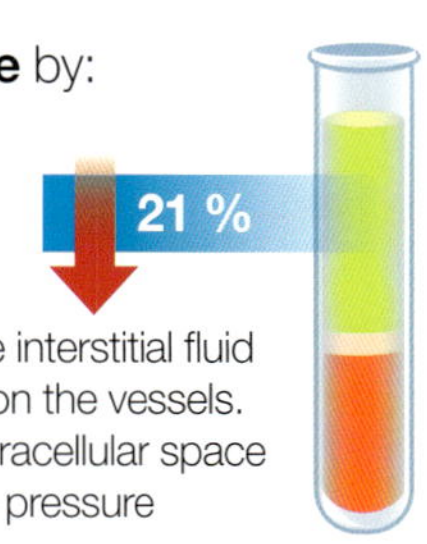

1. Passage of the ntravascular fluid to the interstitial fluid due to the muscular pressure exerted on the vessels.
2. Passage of the nterstitial fluid to the intracellular space compensating the intracellular osmotic pressure increased by the muscular activity.

Obtaining ATP

1 The muscle has few ATP reserves

The concentrations of ATP in the muscle are low and not sufficient to cover the needs of the cells during prolonged periods of physical exertion. Therefore, obtaining energy in the form of ATP comes from the following:

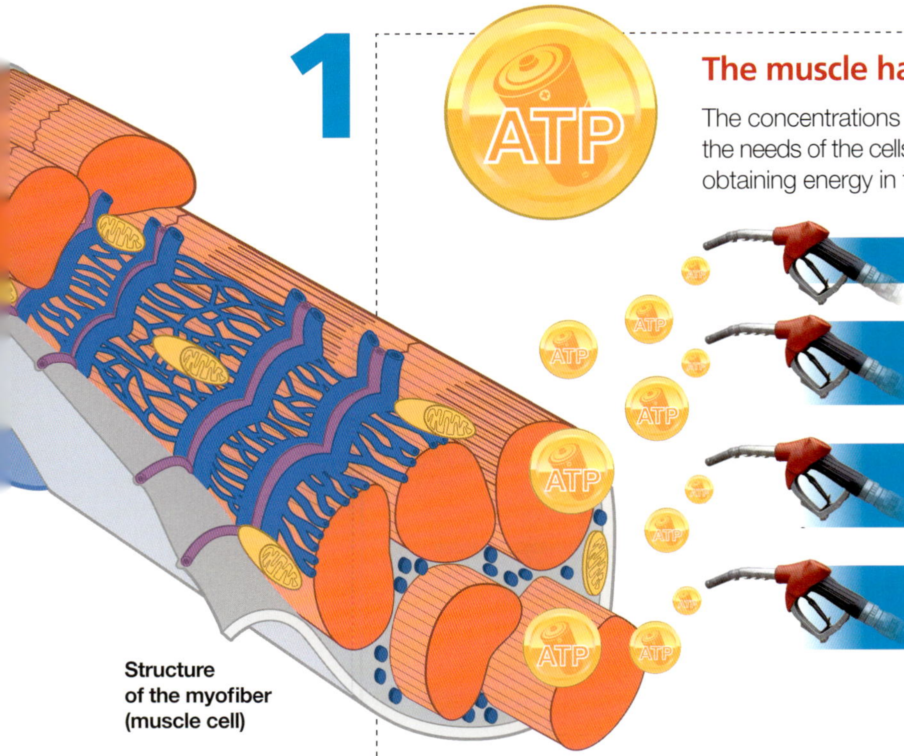

Structure of the myofiber (muscle cell)

- **Anaerobic metabolism** (glycolysis)
- **Aerobic metabolism** (tricarboxylic acid or Krebs cycle)
- **Endogenous substrates** (phosphocreatine or creatine phosphate and glycogen)
- **Exogenous substrates** (hepatic glycogen, adipose tissue and structural proteins)

The proportion of glycogen in the organism is 10 times less than that of fatty tissue (up to 20 % of the body weight).

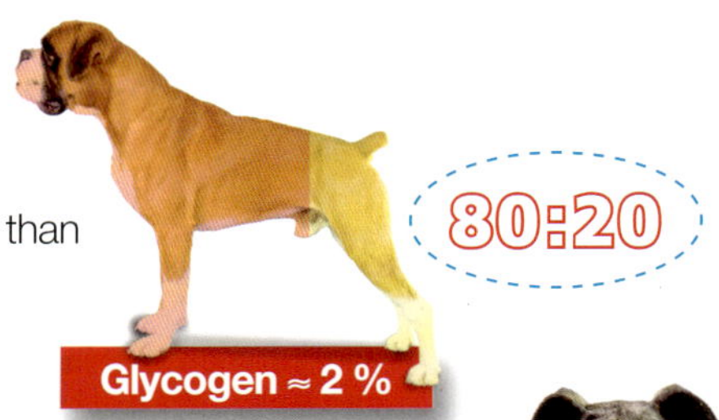

2 Obtaining ATP by anaerobiosis

Creatine phosphate (CP) and glycogen are used anaerobically for the rapid obtention of ATP (μmole ATP/g muscle/minute). Their use for physical exertion varies from seconds (CP) to times under 10 minutes (glycogen). However, its efficiency (mole ATP/mole substrate) is very low: lower than 3. This is the choice route for Greyhounds, sporting dogs that carry out intense and brief physical exertion (minutes).

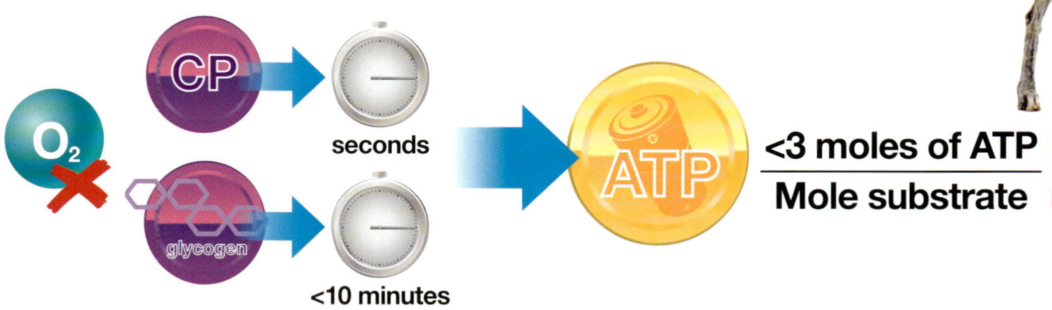

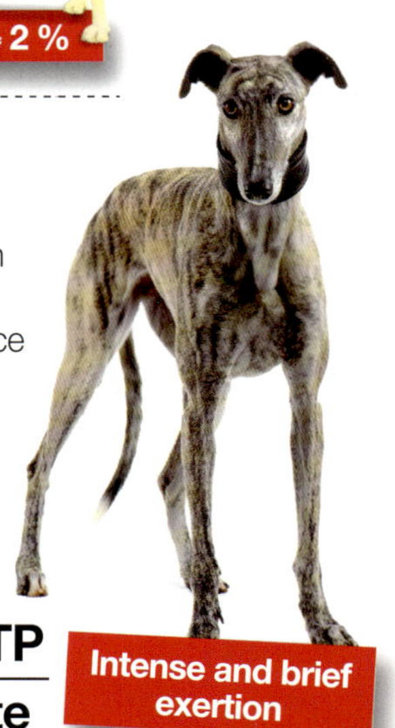

3 Obtaining ATP by aerobiosis

Obtaining ATP by aerobiosis is slower but more efficient: it varies between 18-400 moles, depending on the substrate. If we classify the substrates by their performance (from lesser to greater), the order is:

Lactate > proteins > glucose > glycogen > fatty acids > triglycerides

This route allows dogs to perform more prolonged exertion over time depending on the substrate.

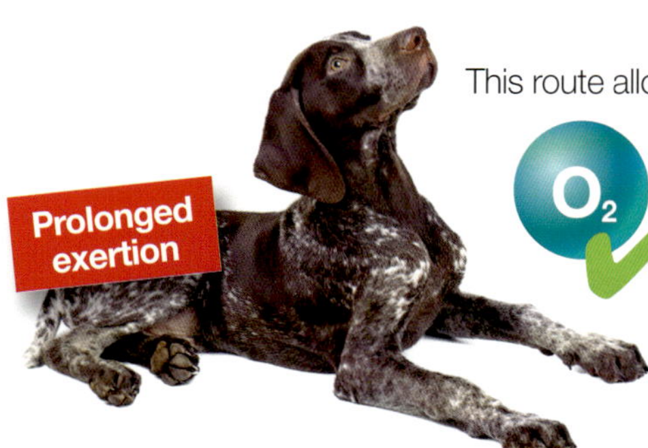

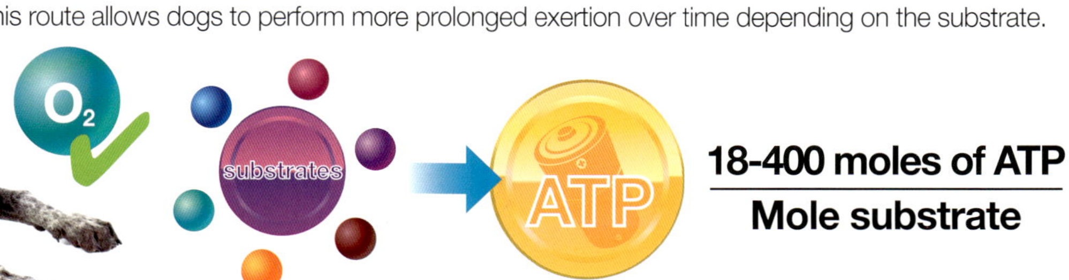

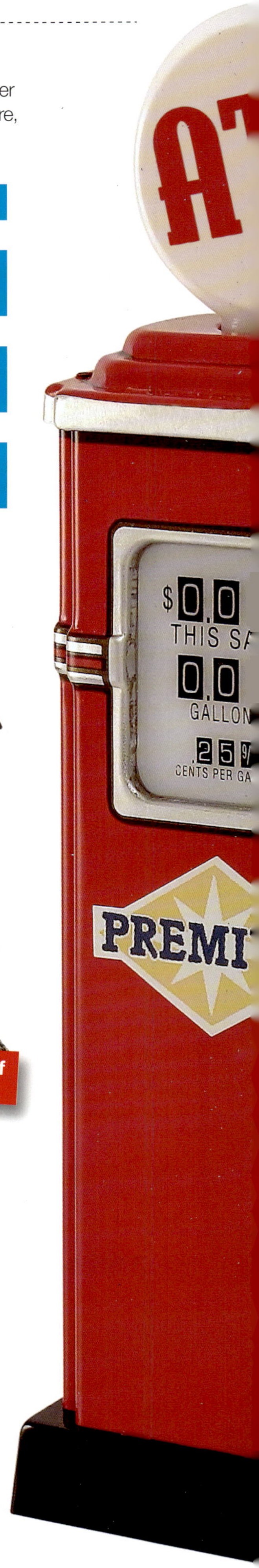

for exercise

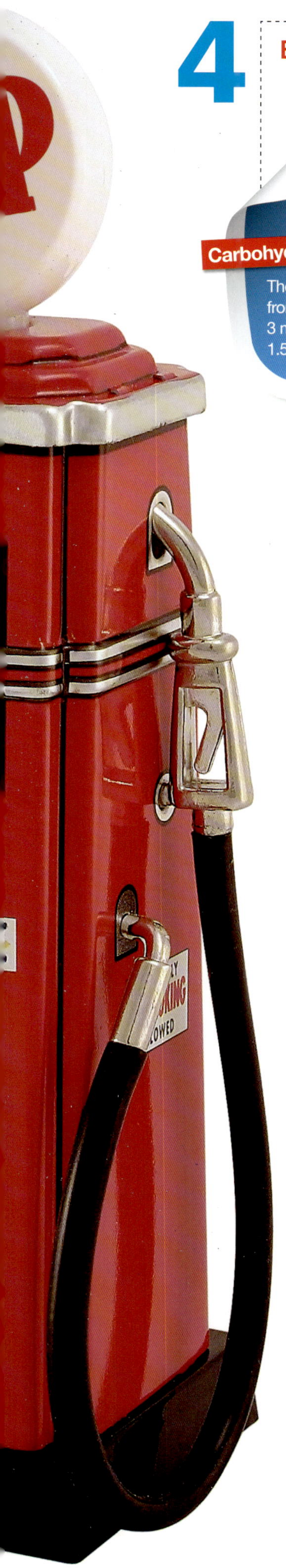

4 Energy from carbohydrates, fats and proteins

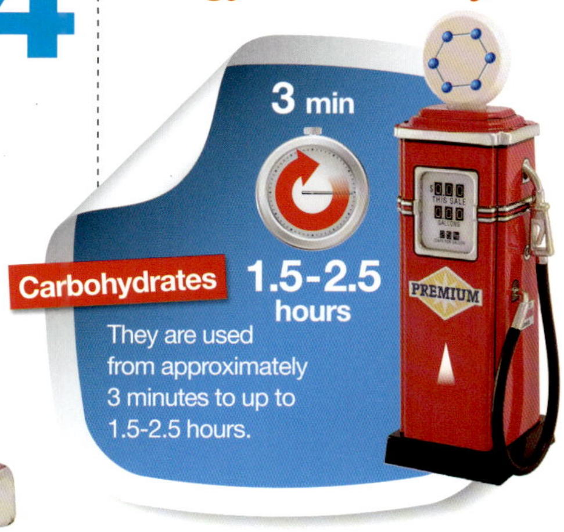
3 min
Carbohydrates
1.5-2.5 hours
They are used from approximately 3 minutes to up to 1.5-2.5 hours.
PREMIUM

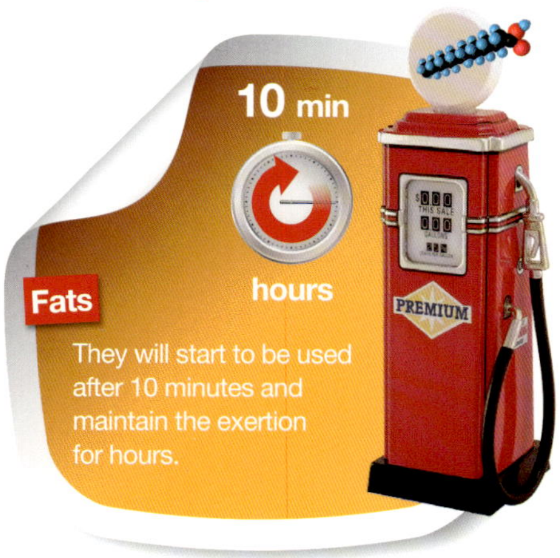
10 min
Fats
hours
They will start to be used after 10 minutes and maintain the exertion for hours.
PREMIUM

As the duration of the exercise increases, the participation of fats as a source of energy also increases. It is the choice route for hunting dogs and sled dogs where the intensity varies from moderate to intense and is maintained over time (hours).

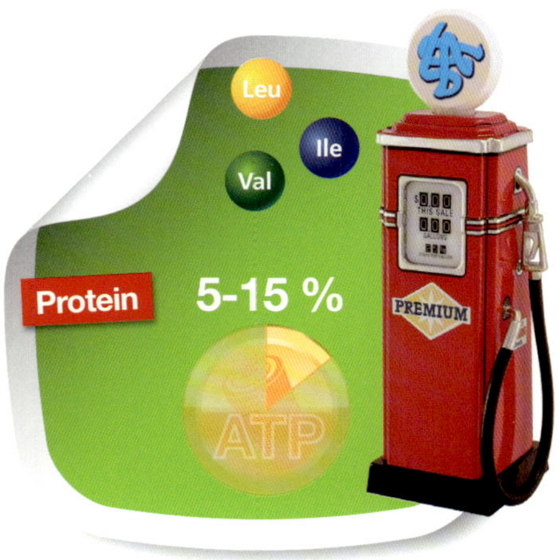

Oxidation of the proteins, from the metabolism of the branched amino acids leukin, isoleukin and valine, contributes with 5-15 % of the energy required during the physical exertion.

5 Changes associated with training and exercise

Lower lactic acid concentrations. The elevated levels of lactate (>4 mmol/l) limit the duration of the exercise. In Greyhounds, their values after exercise can reach levels 8-15 times greater.

Increased creatine kinase concentrations in serum. Its level varies with the type of exertion, and is greater in animals that perform shorter and more intense sprints or races (Greyhounds).

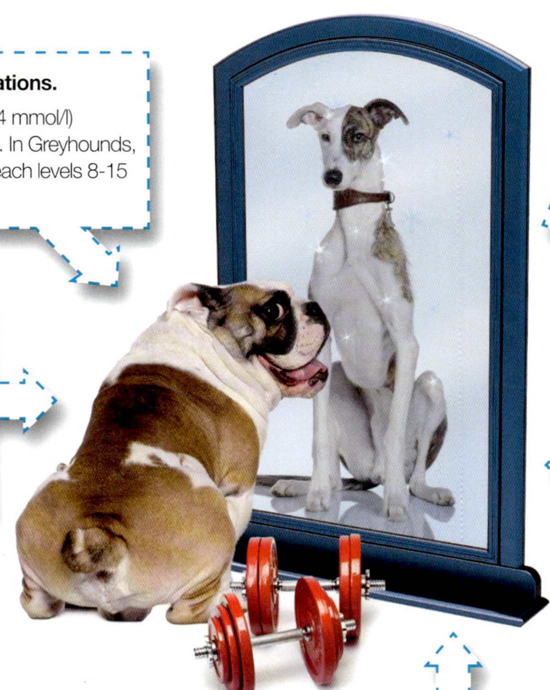

Less proteolysis of the skeletal musculature, as greater control of the ubiquitin-proteasome pathway is produced.

Increase of gluconeogenesis. The synthesis of glucose from glycerol (lipolysis) and from glutamine increases 9- and 4-fold during exercise, respectively.

Increase in the concentrations of muscular glycogen during the 3 first weeks of training until reaching maximum values.

Physiological adaptation to exertion

Training, therefore, allows for better physiological adaptation to maintain the exertion. The perfect understanding of these physiological changes allows us to be one step ahead of them and establish sporting and nutritional strategies that will optimize performance. Generally, we rarely have dogs that train daily; most are occasional athletes (for example, hunting, agility, dog frisbee, freestyle...). Training means exercising over a long period of time.

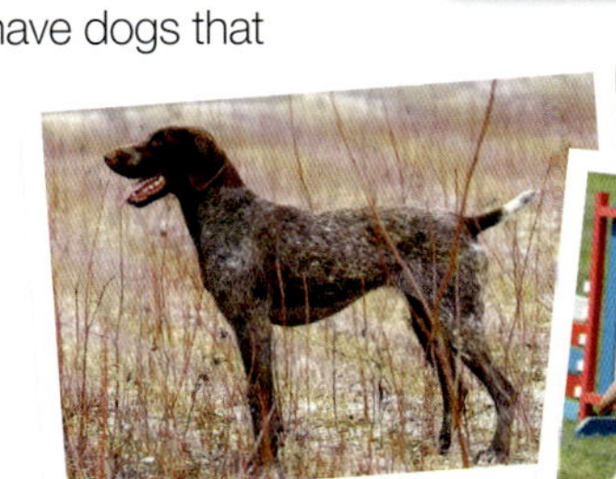

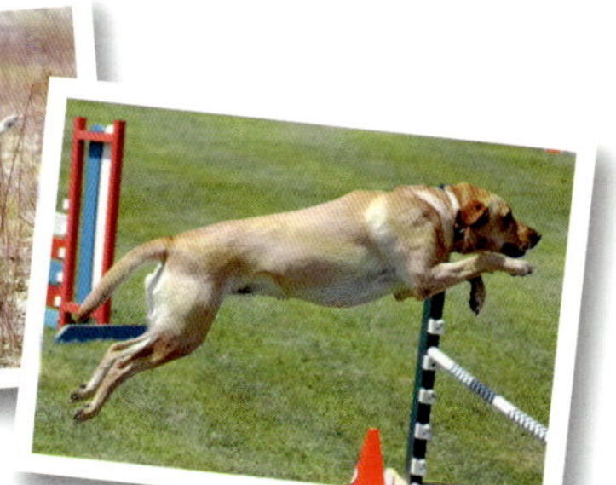

How much energy

1

Specially designed diets

Food rations for sporting dogs are designed for a specific job. The indiscriminate use of this type of food ration outside of their initial purpose leads to the excessive ingestion of potentially toxic substances.

In a practical sense, we can see that not all nutrients should be increased in the same manner as energy; with certain microminerals, their safe upper limit should be reduced up to eight times to avoid toxicity problems.

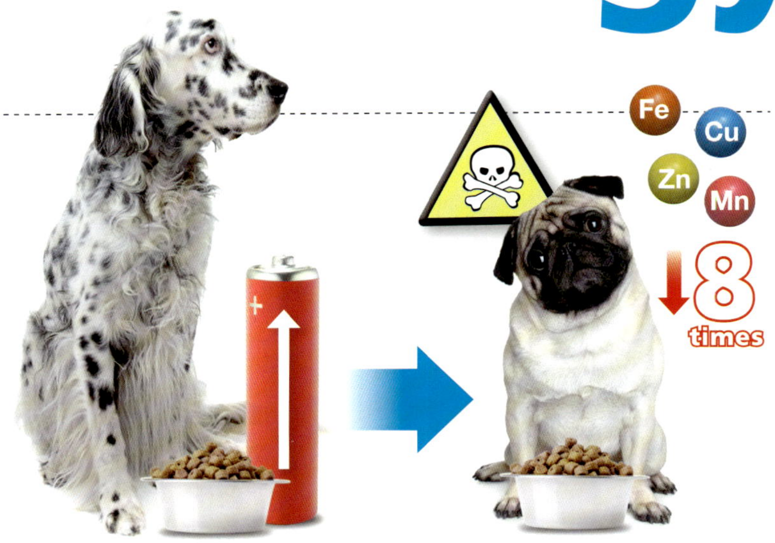

3

Calculations and examples

The following equation allows us to estimate the energy needed for a running dog (ER: energy requirements):

$$ER_{running}\ (\text{kcal ME/day}) = 1.77 \times \text{distance (km)} \times \text{BW (kg)}^{-0.4} + 1.25 \times \text{BW (kg)}^{-0.25}$$

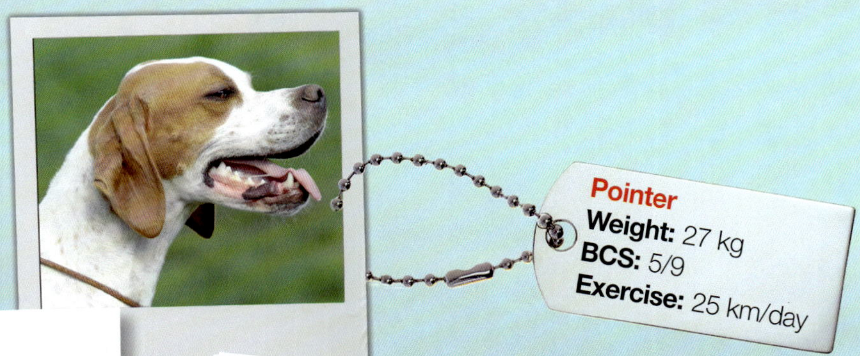

Example

What are this animal's energy requirements for the exercise?

$ER_{running} = 1.77 \times 25 \times 27^{-0.4} + 1.25 \times 27^{-0.25}$

$ER_{running} = 334.5$ kcal ME/day

And the daily requirements?

$$DER = ER_{running} + MER$$

$MER = 132\ (\text{kcal/kg/day}) \times 27\ (\text{kg})^{0.75}$

$MER = 1{,}563.5$ kcal ME/day

$DER = 334.5 + 1{,}563.5$

$DER = 1{,}898$ kcal ME/day

According to the tables on the following page and following with the previous example:

What are this animal's daily energy requirements?

$MER = 1{,}563.5$ kcal ME/day

$ER_{running} = 21\ \%$ of MER

$ER_{running} = 328.33$ kcal ME/day

$DER = 1{,}563.5 + 328.33$

$DER = 1{,}891.83$ kcal ME/day

Or:

$DER = MER \times 1.21 = 1{,}891.83$ kcal ME/day

As we can see, the differences are insignificant (<1 %) compared to the exact calculations.

The energy requirements of a dog running are only slightly modified compared to the daily requirements for maintenance. The larger the animal, the more reduced the energy requirements as a consequence of a smaller exertion while walking (biomechanical effect).

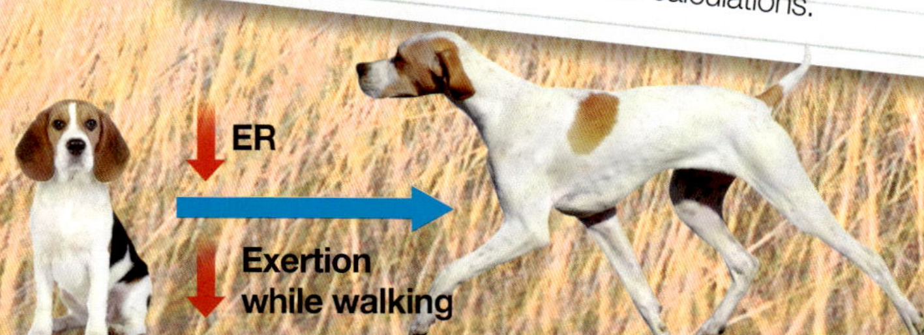

does a dog spend when running?

2 Occasional athletes

The energy requirements for the different exercises are perfectly determined depending on the exertion performed. In this sense, we can classify our dogs as follows:

- ✔ Racing dogs (less than 2-3 minutes).
- ✔ Intermediate resistance.
- ✔ High resistance (more than 2 hours per day).

As we previously mentioned, our pets are generally occasional athletes (once or twice weekly) and by seasons (certain times of the year).

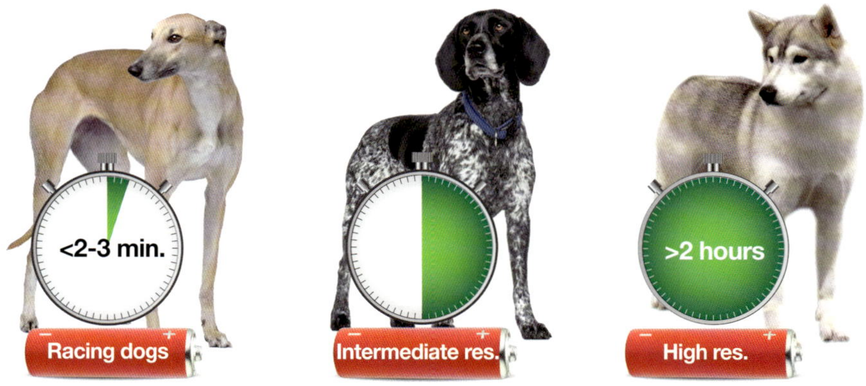

Distance	Increase regarding MER
<10 km	<12 %
15 km	15 %
30 km	>30 %

For distances lower than 10 km and with a moderate intensity (up to 40 % of the maximum velocity), proportional to the size of the breed, the energy expenditure is less than 12 % of the maintenance requirements. The exception takes place in middle distances; at distances greater than 15 km, the average energy expenditure is 15 %, reaching more than 30 % when the distance covered is 30 km or greater.

Due to the fact that the equation is complex, for our clinical practice, it is easier to increase the daily requirements according to the following table:

	Distance covered (km)								
	<5	10	15	20	25	30	50	100	150
Weight (kg)	kcal ME as % of maintenance								
<10	2-6	12	17	22	29	33	55	109	162
11-20	2-5	10	15	18	23	28	45	89	133
21-30	2-5	9	13	18	21	26	42	83	124
31-40	2-5	9	13	17	20	24	40	79	118
41-50	2-5	9	12	16	20	24	39	76	114
>50	2-5	8.5	12	16	19	23	37	74	111
	As multiples of maintenance (MER)								
× MER	1.05	1.10	1.14	1.18	1.23	1.27	1.44	1.88	2.31

Reality shows us that the values as multiples of the MER are somewhat lower in distances greater than 15-20 km, given that the breeds involved are over 25 kg and have biomechanical advantages when moving. We could therefore apply the following correction to the previous table:

	Distance covered (km)					
	20	25	30	50	100	150
Dogs >25 kg	As multiples of maintenance (MER)					
× MER	1.17	1.21	1.25	1.41	1.80	2.20

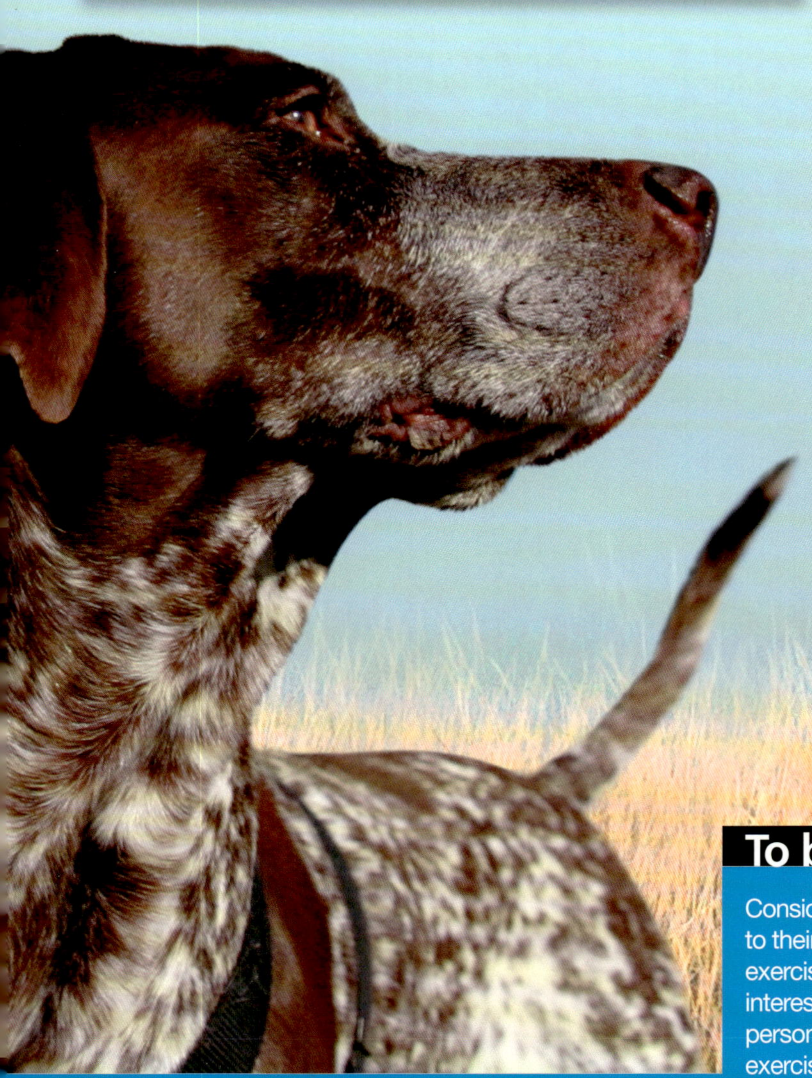

To be taken into account

Considering these results, most of our canine patients will not need any modifications to their food rations for the normal exercise that they perform, nor does this moderate exercise lead to weight loss when the patient is obese. These estimations are only of interest for our non-professional occasional sporting dogs. Elite sporting dogs need personalized treatment. The values will be modified depending on the frequency of exercise.

Factors increasing

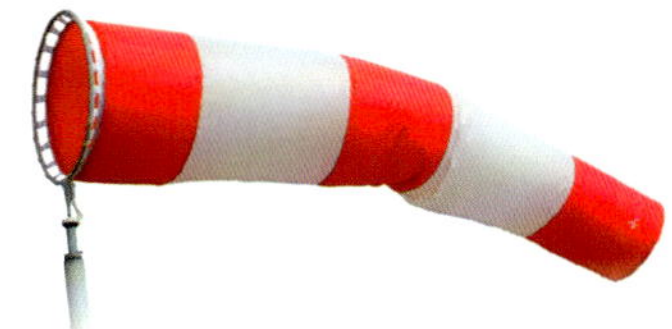

1 Running surface and wind

Other factors that can increase energy needs when running are:

Rough surface

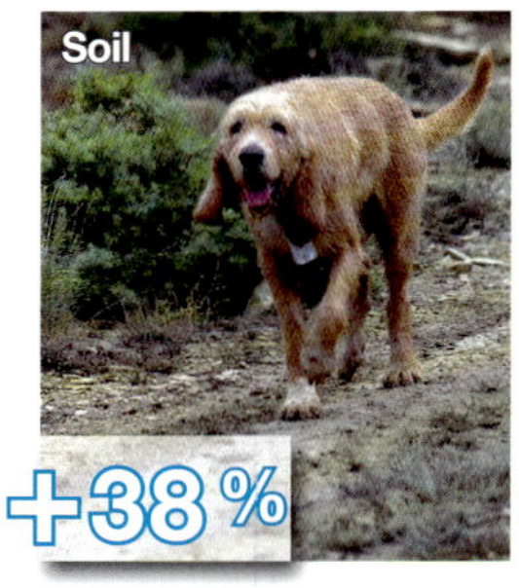
Soil

Wet surface

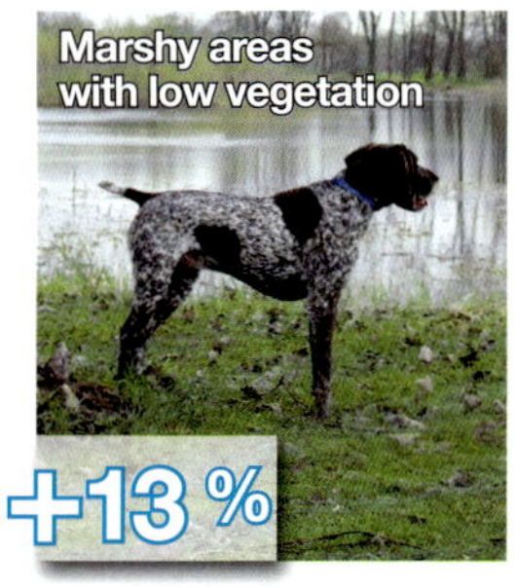
Marshy areas with low vegetation

Snow

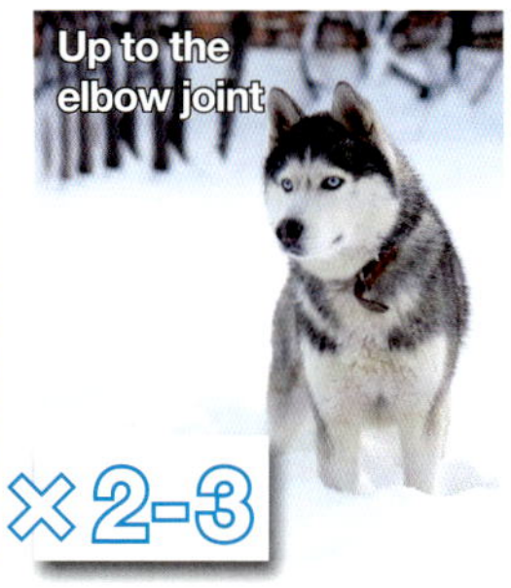
Up to the elbow joint

Snow

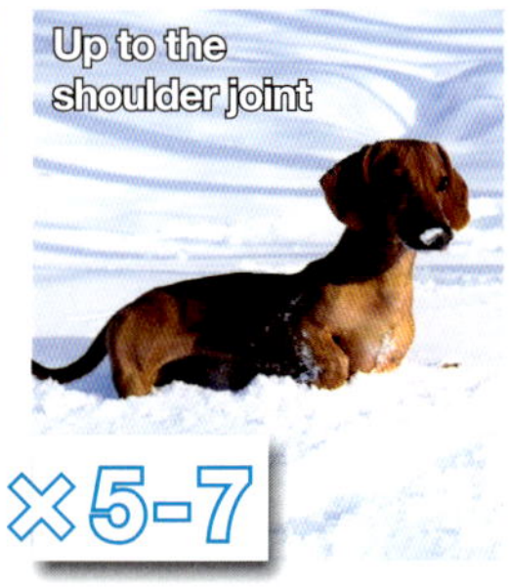
Up to the shoulder joint

DEN = +38 % | +13 % | ×2-3 | ×5-7

With headwind, needs vary according to wind speed:

	Wind speed (km/h)		
	18	36	65
Increase in DER*	+8 %	+15 %	+70 %

* Data obtained in humans. It may be slightly lower in dogs since their resistance is lower as they walk on four legs.

3 Calculations and examples

✔ Reality shows that they can carry weights of more than 30 % their body weight. Prediction equations are:

$$ER_{load\ pulling}\ (kcal\ ME/day) = ER_{race} \times \%\ increase\ in\ weight^*$$

$$^*\ \%\ increase\ in\ weight = \frac{load\ weight}{body\ weight} \times 100$$

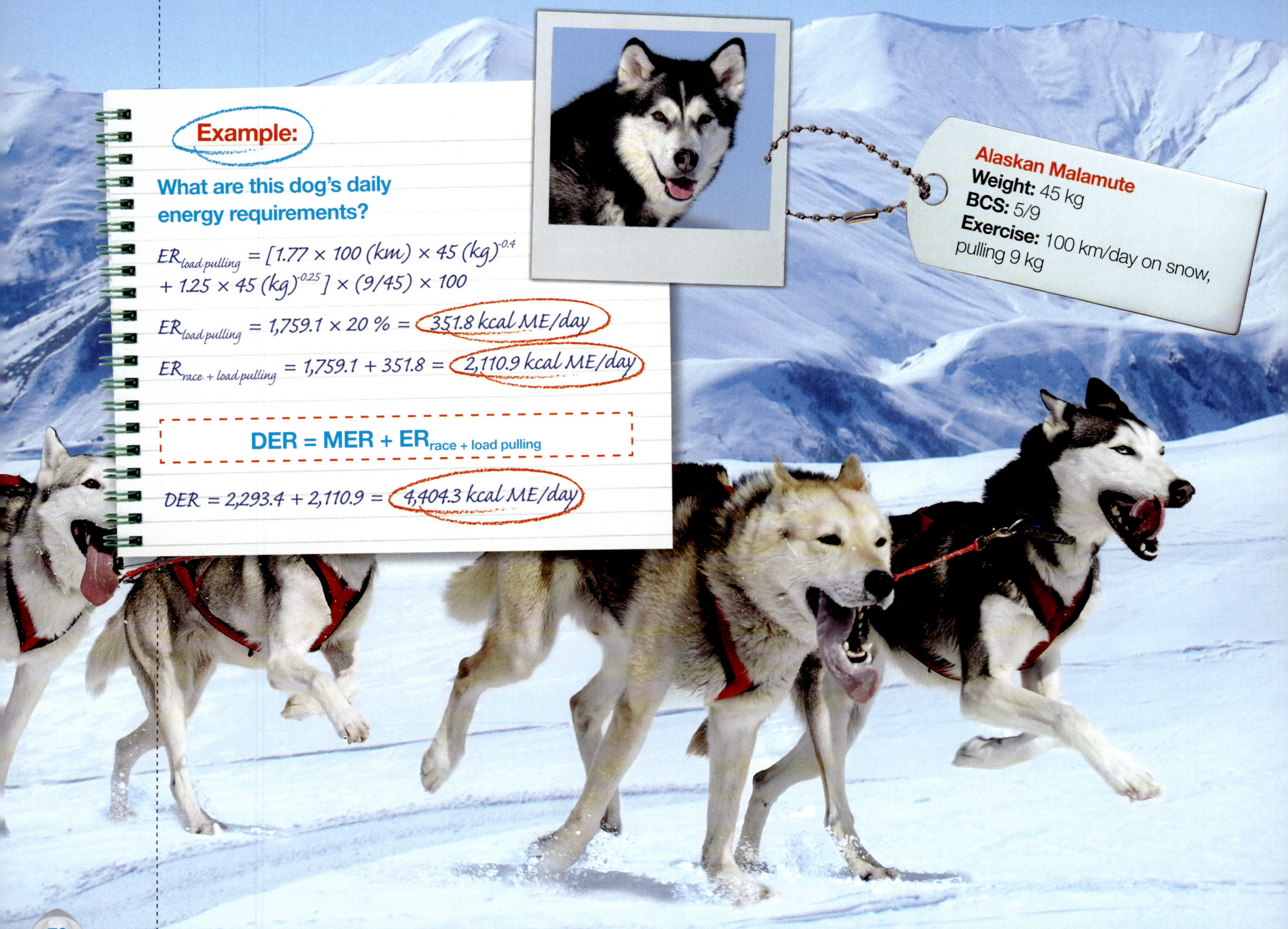

Example:

What are this dog's daily energy requirements?

Alaskan Malamute
Weight: 45 kg
BCS: 5/9
Exercise: 100 km/day on snow, pulling 9 kg

$$ER_{load\ pulling} = [1.77 \times 100\ (km) \times 45\ (kg)^{-0.4} + 1.25 \times 45\ (kg)^{-0.25}] \times (9/45) \times 100$$

$$ER_{load\ pulling} = 1{,}759.1 \times 20\ \% = 351.8\ kcal\ ME/day$$

$$ER_{race\ +\ load\ pulling} = 1{,}759.1 + 351.8 = 2{,}110.9\ kcal\ ME/day$$

$$DER = MER + ER_{race\ +\ load\ pulling}$$

$$DER = 2{,}293.4 + 2{,}110.9 = 4{,}404.3\ kcal\ ME/day$$

ER when running

2 Load pulling

- This same exercise can be modified when dogs carry or pull loads ($ER_{load\ pulling}$).
- O_2 consumption (that is, needs in kcal) changes in proportion to the weight of the load and the percentage of body weight it represents.

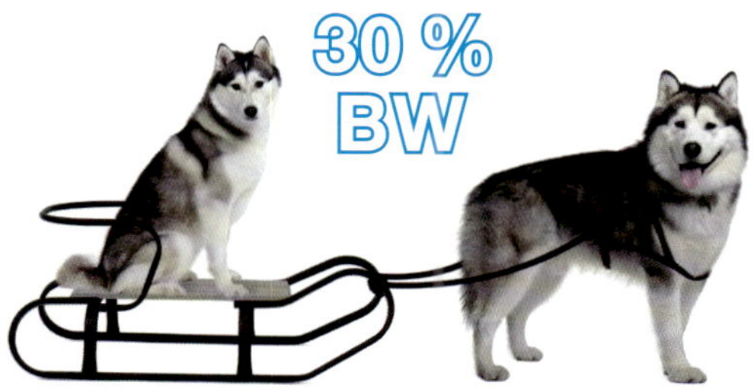

- The maximum weight dogs can carry without any consequences on their biomechanics is 30 % of their body weight. Based on the similarity between pulling a load on a smooth surface and carrying the same weight, this value also seems applicable.

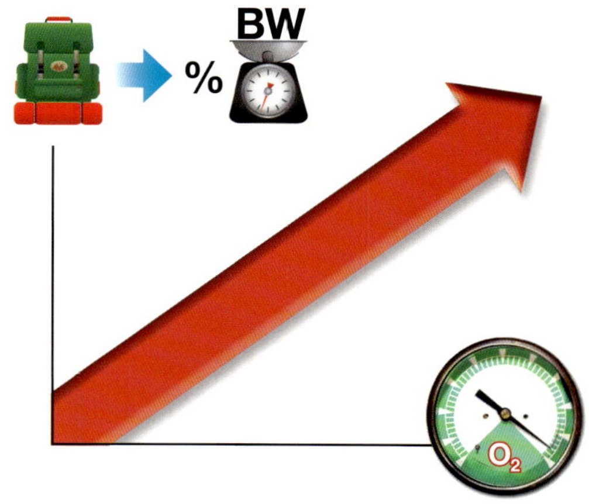

- In a more simple manner, without using complex formulas, we can determine the DER by multiplying maintenance requirements (MER) by a correction factor that depends on the percentage the load weight represents with respect to the dog's body weight and the distance run (see table).

	Distance run (km)														
	15			25			50			100			150		
	Load weight as a % of body weight														
	10	20	30	10	20	30	10	20	30	10	20	30	10	20	30
Weight (kg)	As multiples of maintenance (MER)														
25	1.1	1.2	1.2	1.2	1.3	1.3	1.5	1.5	1.6	1.9	2	2.1	2.4	2.5	2.6
30	1.1	1.2	1.2	1.2	1.3	1.3	1.5	1.5	1.5	1.9	2	2.1	2.3	2.5	2.6
35	1.1	1.2	1.2	1.2	1.2	1.3	1.4	1.5	1.5	1.9	2	2	2.3	2.4	2.5
40	1.1	1.2	1.2	1.2	1.2	1.3	1.4	1.5	1.5	1.9	1.9	2	2.3	2.4	2.5
45	1.1	1.1	1.2	1.2	1.2	1.3	1.4	1.5	1.5	1.8	1.9	2	2.3	2.4	2.5
50	1.1	1.1	1.2	1.2	1.2	1.3	1.4	1.5	1.5	1.8	1.9	2	2.2	2.4	2.5
Average	1.15			1.25			1.5			1.92			2.4		

Pulls 10 kg

Example:

Using the same example as before:

What are this dog's daily energy requirements?

$$DER = MER + ER_{race\ +\ load\ pulling}$$

$DER = 4{,}404.4$ kcal ME/day

$DER = 1.92 \times 2{,}293.4$

$DER = 4{,}403.3$ kcal ME/day

- Other prediction equations would be:

Sledding dogs
Extreme distance and temperature conditions

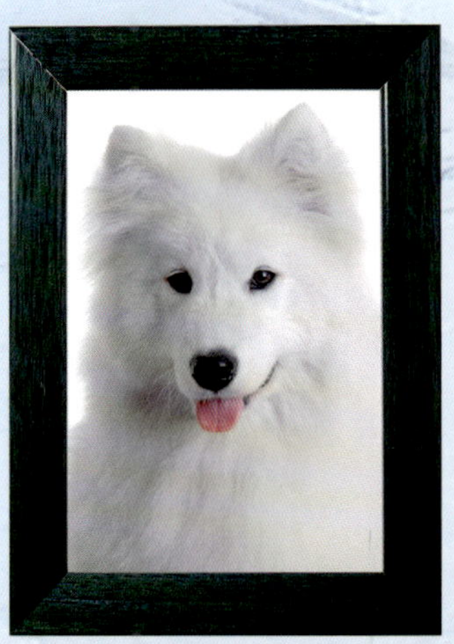

Hunting dogs

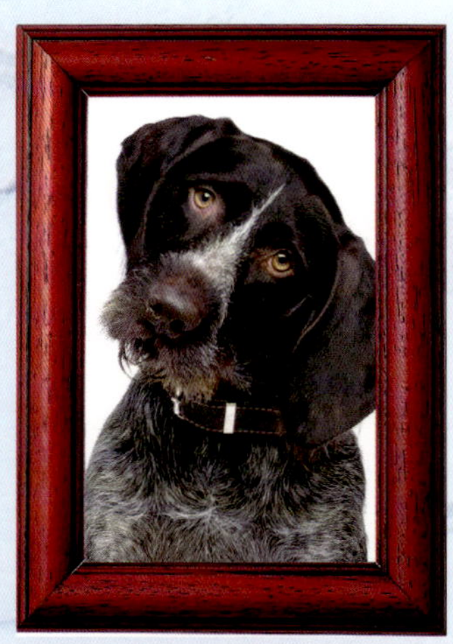

Shepherd dogs

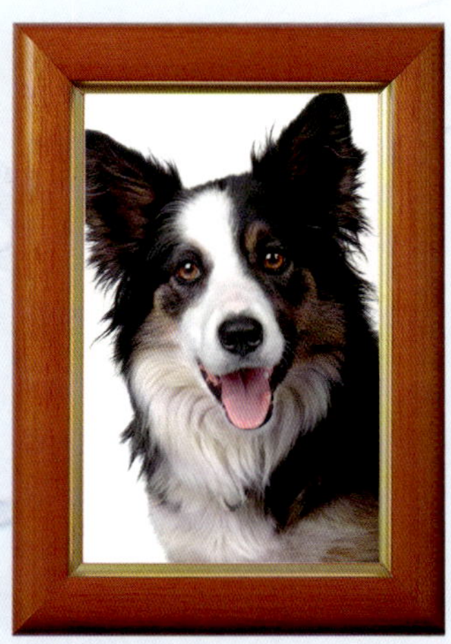

Greyhounds

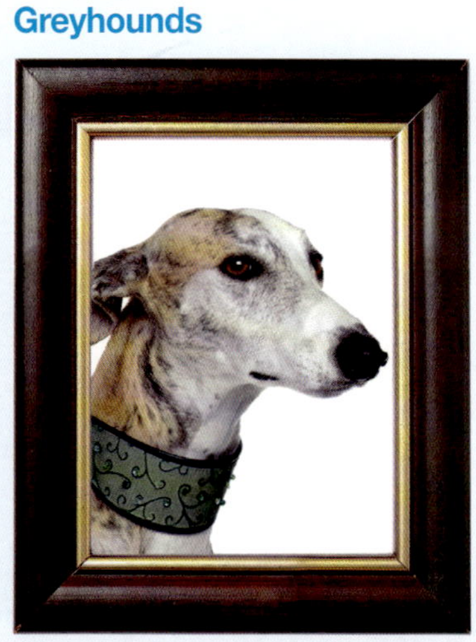

DER (kcal ME/day)	Sledding dogs	Hunting dogs	Shepherd dogs	Greyhounds
DER (kcal ME/day) =	$1{,}050 \times BW(kg)^{0.75}$	$240 \times BW(kg)^{0.75}$	$184 \times BW(kg)^{0.75}$	$140 \times BW(kg)^{0.75}$

Temperature and

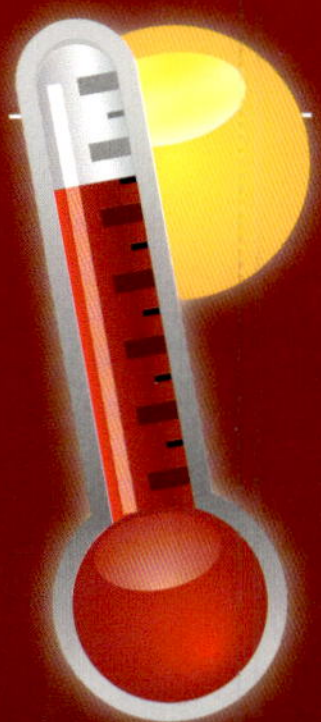

1 High temperatures make it hard for animals to lose heat

- During exercise, almost all of the energy used is proportionally transformed into heat. This heat is thus eliminated by respiration, and to a lesser extent, by dissipation.
- Environmental conditions limit the performance of our athletic pets. High temperatures determine greater water losses and increased work (W) to eliminate the heat produced. In conditions of high humidity, this exchange is reduced.

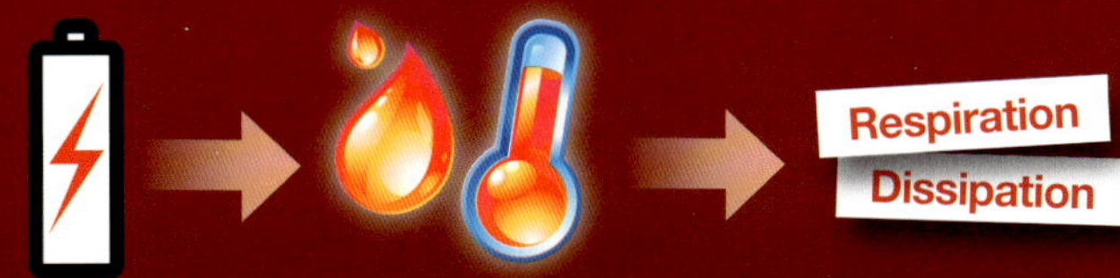

- Adequate hydration is important to maintain the body's normal temperature.

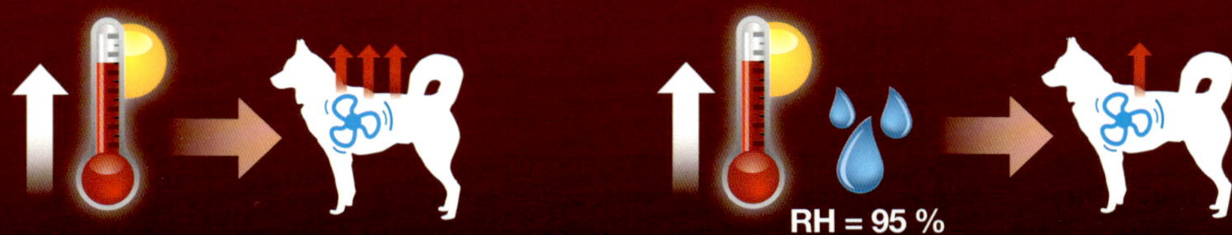

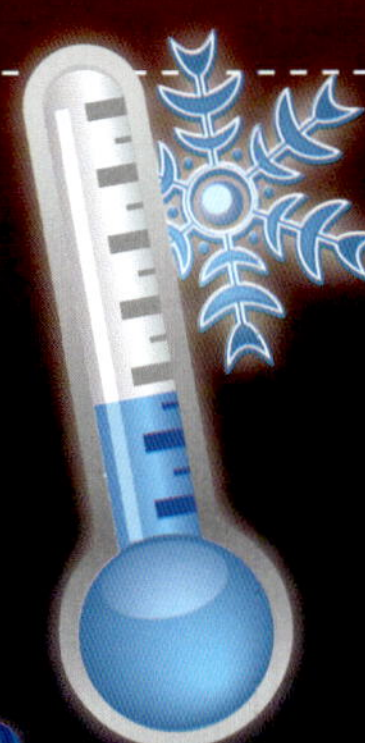

2 How does the cold affect our pets?

Cold temperatures help to maintain body temperature

Conversely, cold temperatures help to eliminate the heat generated during exercise and to maintain the body's temperature.

Cold temperatures require more energy

Dogs that live in cold weather conditions, with temperatures lower than 4 °C, have a 40 % increase in their energy requirements.

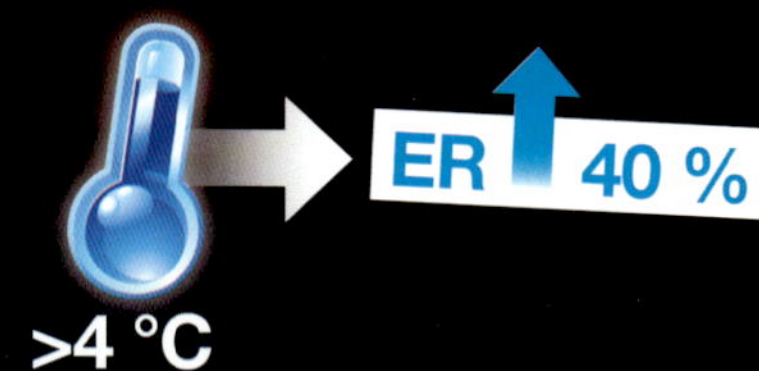

Carbohydrates

- Carbohydrates participate in providing energy by means of glycolysis, which is quadruplicated, as the levels in plasma of glucose are increased by 45 % and those of lactate are reduced by nearly 50 % (there is greater oxidation).

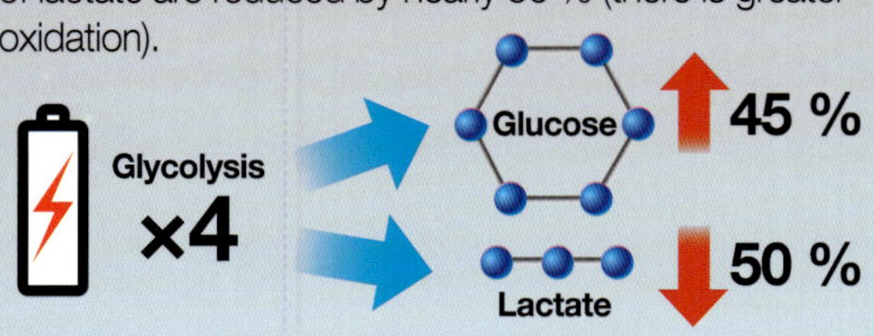

- Contrary to what seems logical, glycemia remains constant because there is synthesis by means of:

FFAs

Glycogenic amino acids
(for example, alanine presents lesser plasma concentrations and greater renal clearance)

Muscular glycogen

Fat

The skeletal muscle is the tissue with the greatest energy demand. However, fats are the primary nutrients that cover this demand; the needs in FFAs under these conditions are increased by 50 %. This has been verified because the levels of ketone bodies in plasma are elevated.

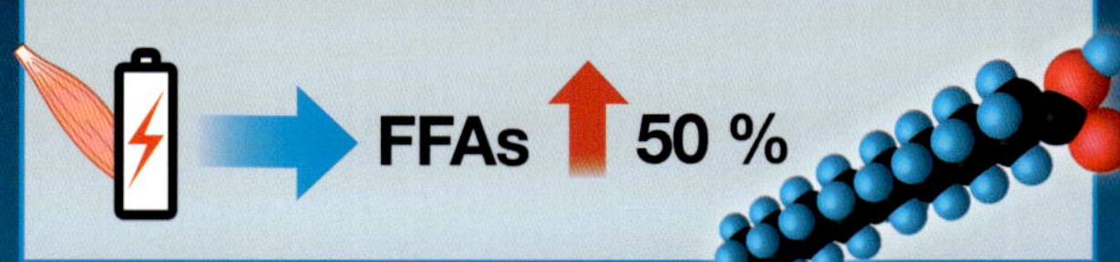

Protein

The exposure to cold temperatures could determine an increase in the amino acid requirements with certain specific objectives:

- Fur growth.
- Allowing for the adaptation of the mechanisms to obtain energy (fat and mitochondria).

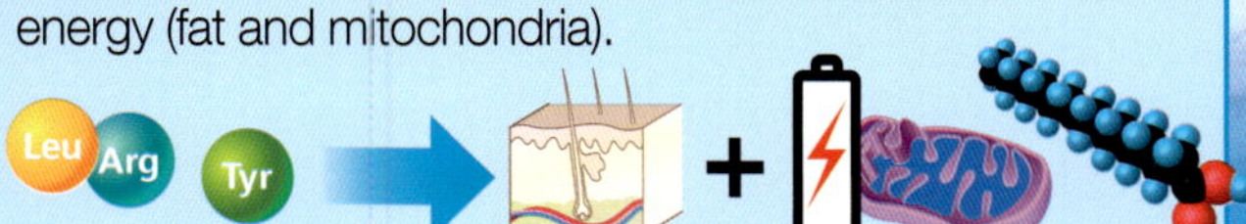

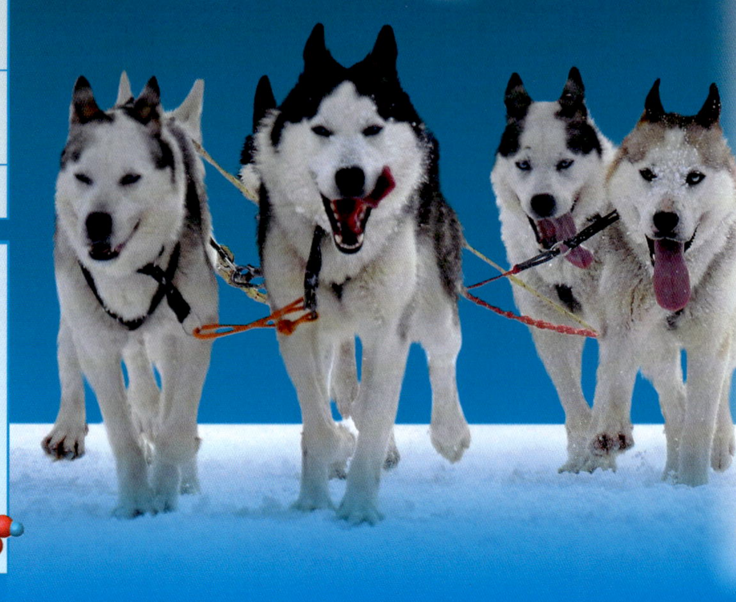

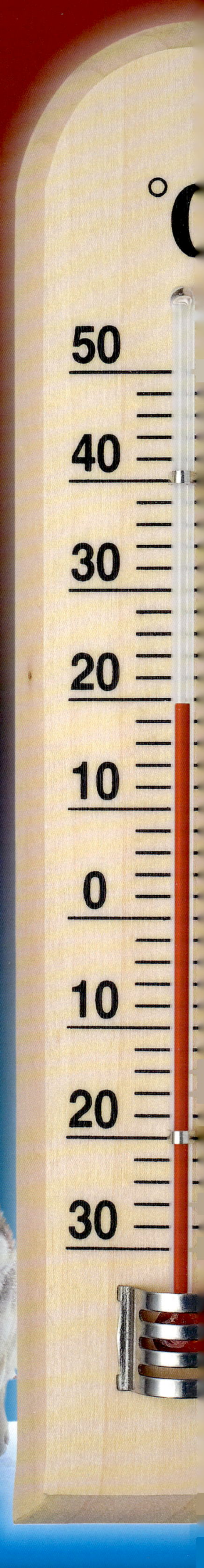

energy requirements in exercise

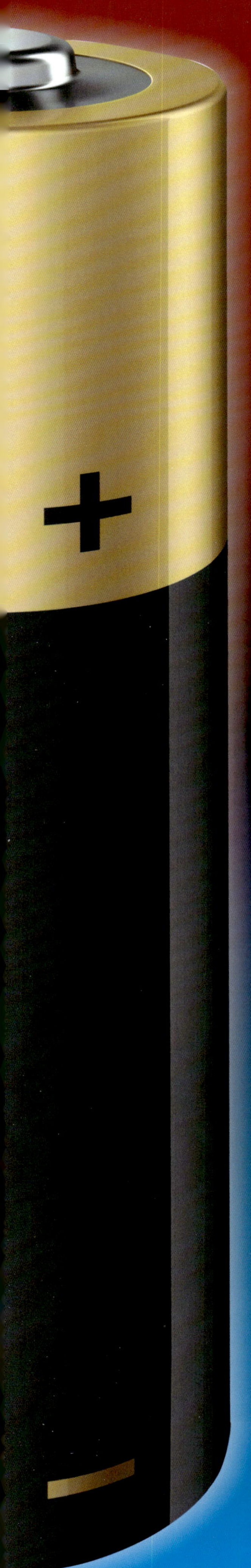

3 The energy used for thermoregulation

✔ As we can see, the recommendations for cold weather conditions are very similar to those for intense work with intermediate resistance.

✔ Taking into account that thermoregulation is related to various factors, we could summarize that the daily energy requirements (DER) are increased outside of the thermo-neutral zone (from 15 to 20 °C, maximum 30 °C, and in the case of nordic dogs, from 10 to 15 °C) according to the following table.

Factors related with thermoregulation

- ✔ Age.
- ✔ Skin thickness.
- ✔ Coverage and type of fur.
- ✔ Type of predominant body fat (brown or white).
- ✔ Acclimation to the environment.

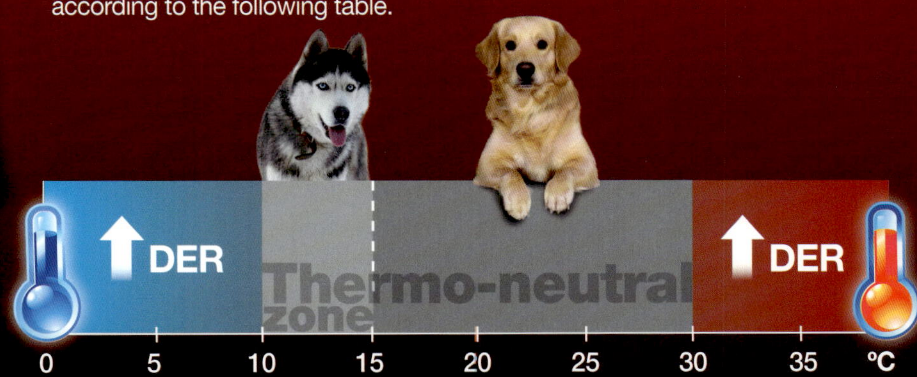

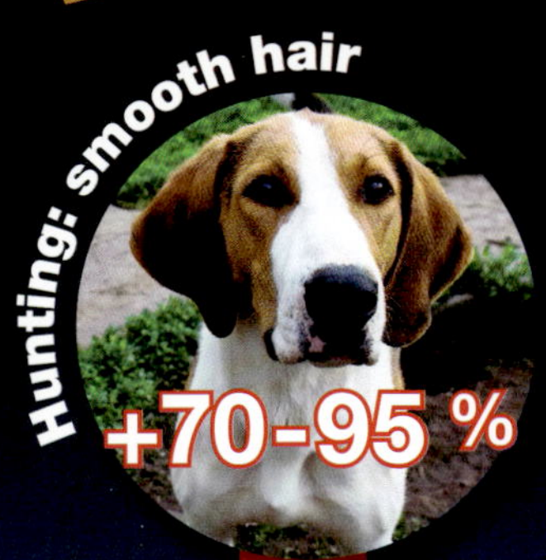

Effect of temperature on the DER

Type of dog		Temperature (limit) Summer (>25 °C)	Temperature (limit) Winter (<7.5 °C)
Hunting	Smooth hair: Pointer, Beagle	+70-95 %	
	Short hair: Labrador	+25 %	
	Long hair: Setter	+59.5 %	
Sledding (-17 °C to 17 °C)			+61.5 %

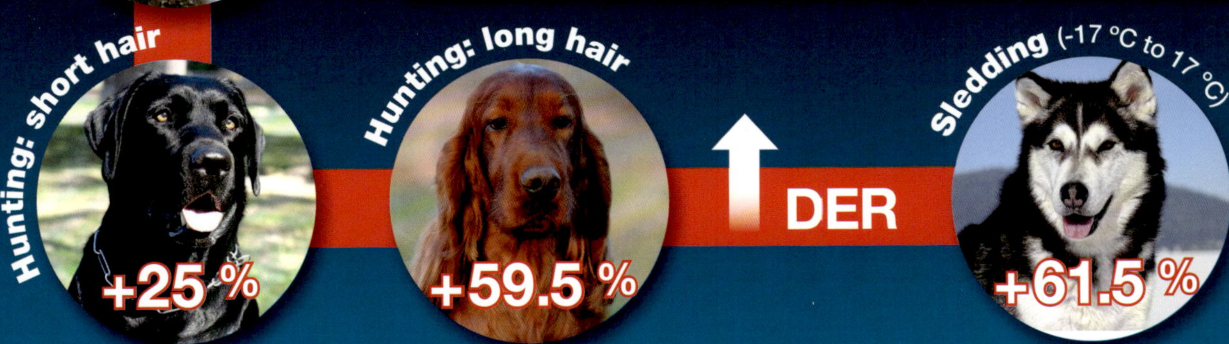

4 Hydrate according to the temperature

In all cases, sporting dogs should be offered water when they have lost 0.5 % of their weight through water loss. As we previously saw, the water requirements are modified with exercise as the energy requirements are increased. As a rule, it is estimated that they need 400 ml of water /1,000 kcal ME in extremely cold temperatures (-45 °C); this value increases 1.5- to 3-fold when the air temperature is greater than 20 °C.

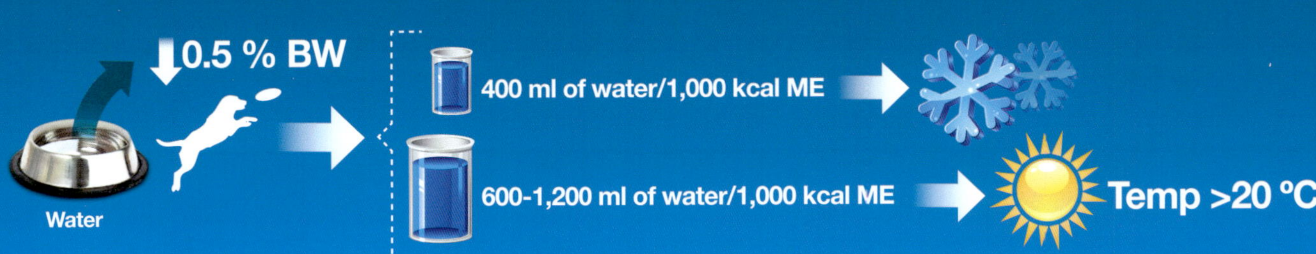

Nutrients

1 Water

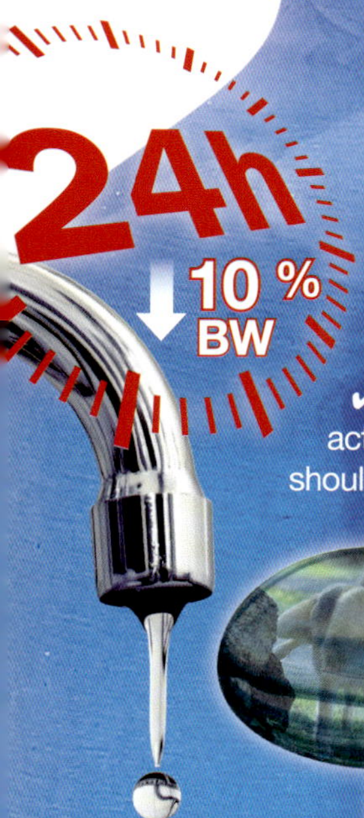

Losses during exercise

✔ Dogs that compete may lose up to 10 % of their body weight in water per day (5 l in one sledding dog), which is 10 times more than normal losses.

✔ Water losses represent a continuous process, while the act of drinking is an intermittent process. For this reason, dogs should always be offered fresh water to compensate for water loss and prevent dehydration.

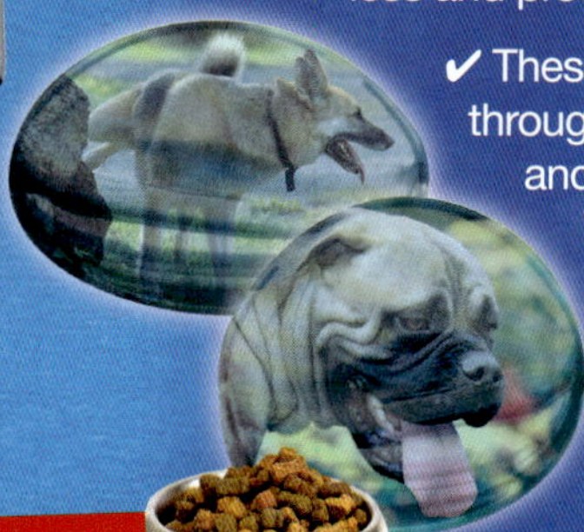

✔ These losses are, primarily, through urination, although respiration and panting also contribute. Water losses through urine are unavoidable due to the high energy content of the food rations (elevated content in solutes, primarily salt and protein).

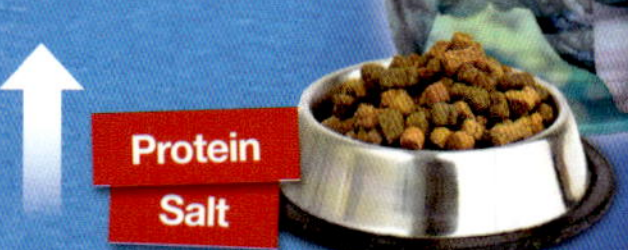

Elimination of sodium to compensate osmolarity

✔ Although dogs do not concentrate their urine, when they are unable to drink water, they experience a physiological elimination of sodium to compensate for the increase in osmolarity. When they are given water, they tend to ingest large volumes in a time shorter than 5 minutes to compensate for and reestablish balance.

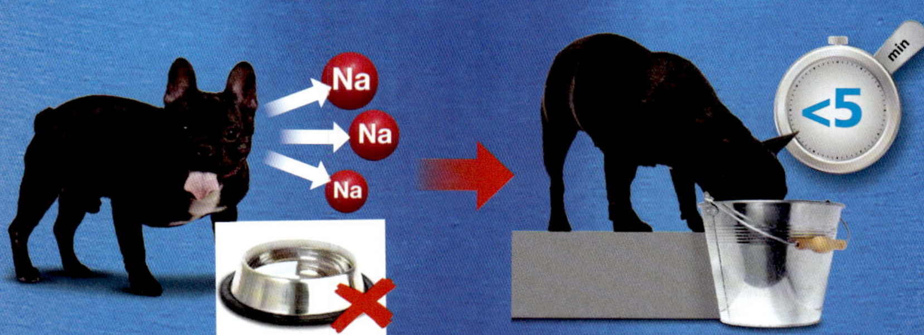

✔ Although dehydration during a race or physical activity increases urinary losses of sodium, there is no need to increase the ingestion of the electrolyte, as its function is reestablished merely by replenishing the water lost.

Consumption of water during a race/physical activity

✔ Generally, dogs consume small amounts of water immediately after each rest break during periods of exercise of one hour at a speed of 10 km/h. This ingestion of water represents a prevision of the requirements derived from the next exercise more so than from the rest period itself.

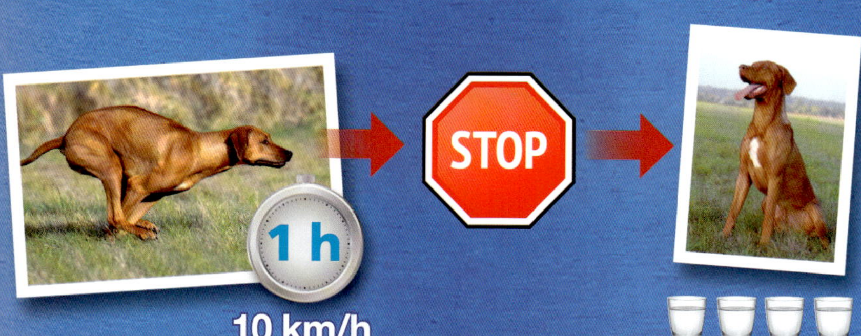

2 Protein and amino acids

Replenishment of protein catabolism

✔ The importance of protein in canine athletes is related to the catabolism-anabolism processes that take place during training periods and the activity itself, more so than to the energy it provides, which is low and inefficient.

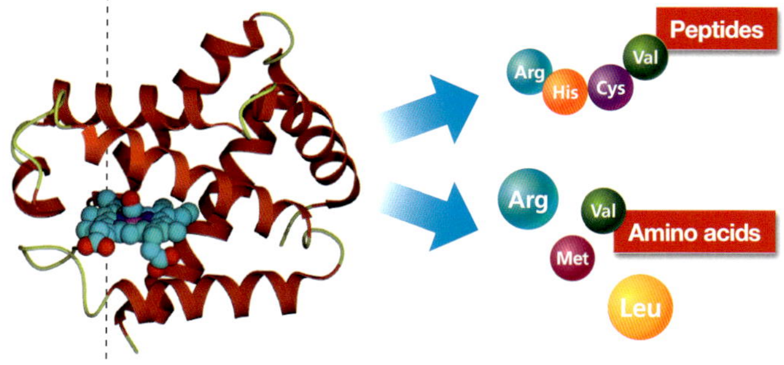

✔ It has been observed that the use of protein is higher in athletes than in sedentary dogs.

Exercise increases the needs in protein, which depend on the following:

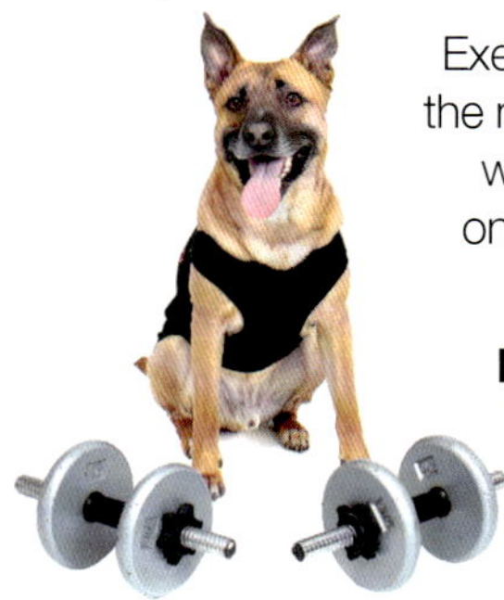

Previous training

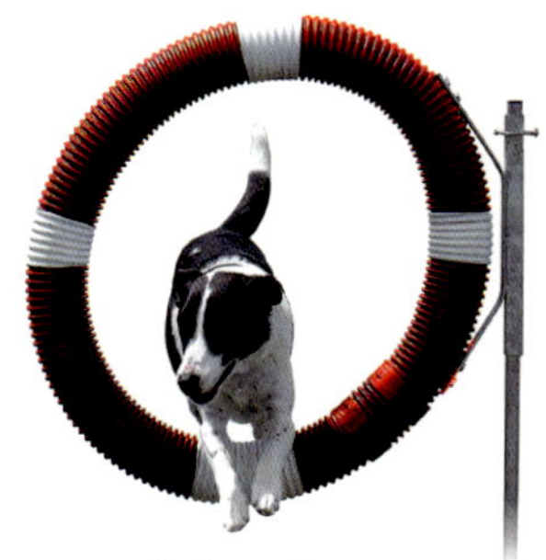

Intensity of the exercise

✔ Protein provides a lower percentage of the energy requirements, but it does so from three essential amino acids: valine, leukin, and isoleukin, which should be provided in adequate proportions in the food rations.

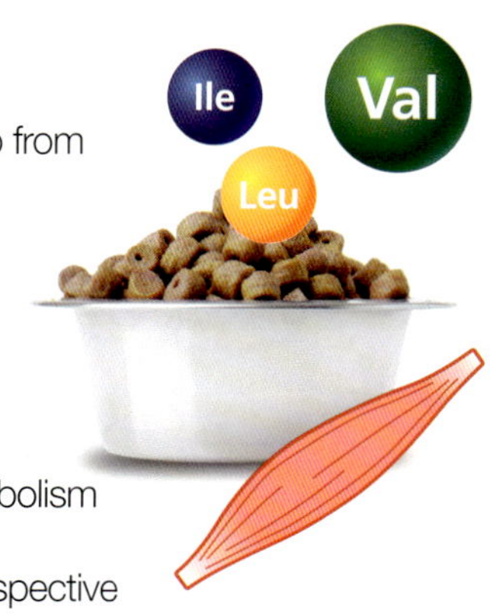

✔ Poor feeding or maximum exercise cause protein catabolism to obtain glucose through gluconeogenesis, with its respective decline in performance, given that structural proteins will be those responsible for taking on this task.

For this reason, incorporating protein in food rations should cover the nitrogen deficiency, and hypertrophy and maintenance of the muscle tissue.

for exercise: water and proteins

Avoiding excess proteins in the diet

✔ Unlike what occurs with ER, the protein requirements in canine athletes increase very little (5 to 15 %), given that energy is obtained from fat and glycogen. Therefore, excess protein in their food rations makes no sense and leads to the risk of greater losses of liquid, through urine, to compensate the increased urea from the catabolism. This situation is not ideal in an athlete due to the thermo-regulating effect of water.

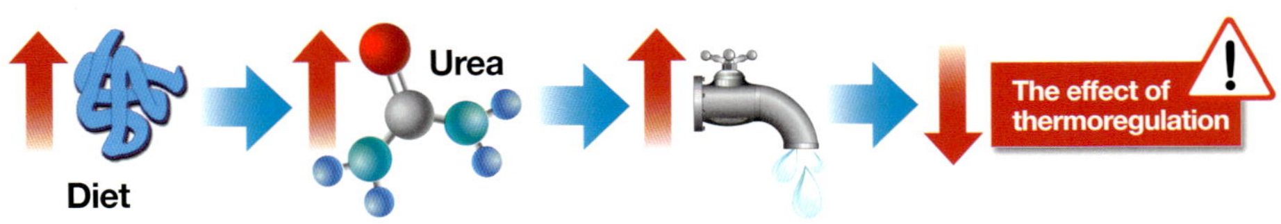

Animal-based protein is a better choice

✔ The origin of the source of protein is also important. Dogs that are fed plant-based protein (grains and soy) develop anemia more frequently due to the fragility of the erythrocytes. The cause is a lack of cholesterol in plasma, with mediation of the lecithin-cholesterol-acyltransferase enzyme.

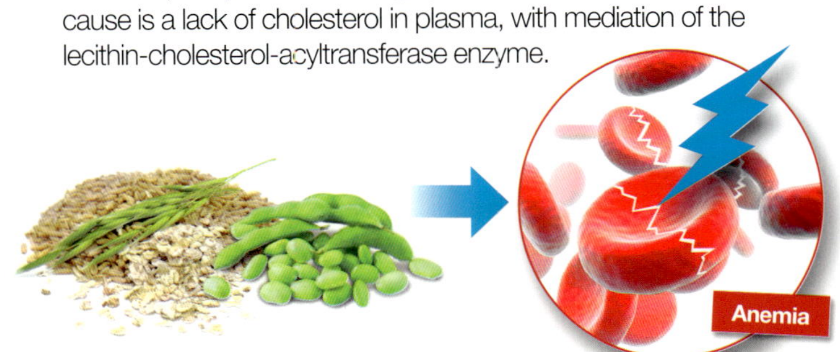

Recommended protein values

✔ The protein requirements have been correlated with fat levels. The best results are achieved when protein represents a minimum of 24 % of the energy (60 g/1,000 kcal ME), although at 40 %, the hematological values are better.

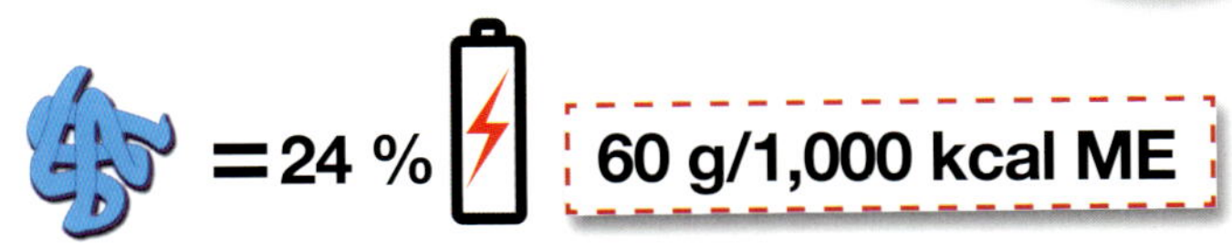

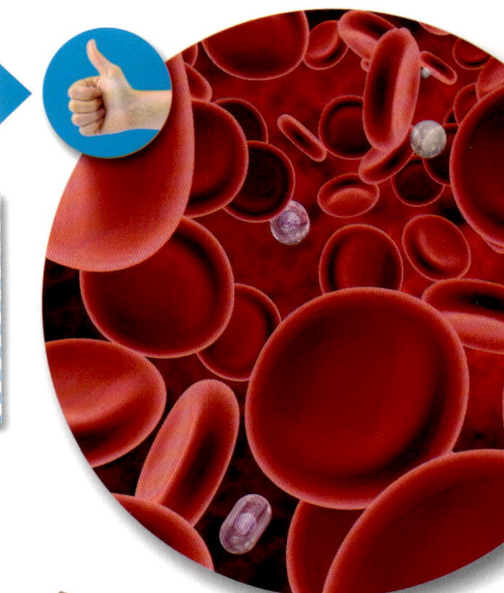

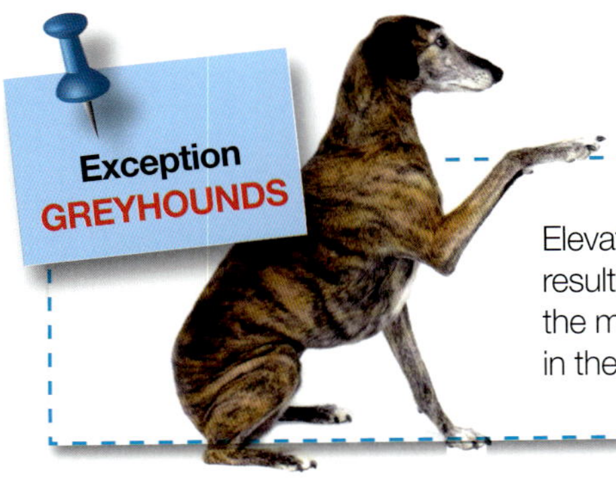

Elevated levels of protein worsen their results expressed as km/h, although the mechanism responsible is a change in the proportion of carbohydrates.

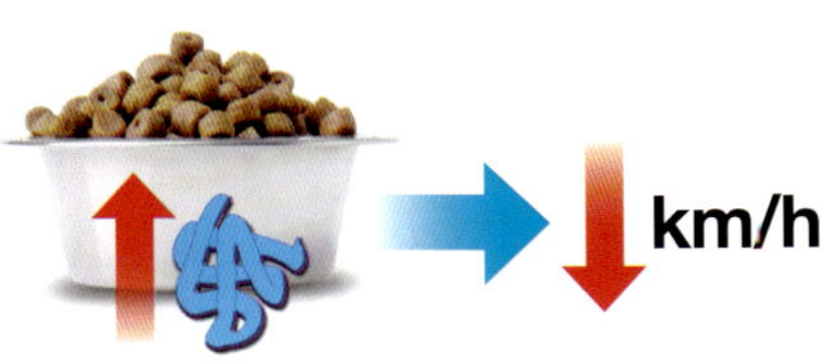

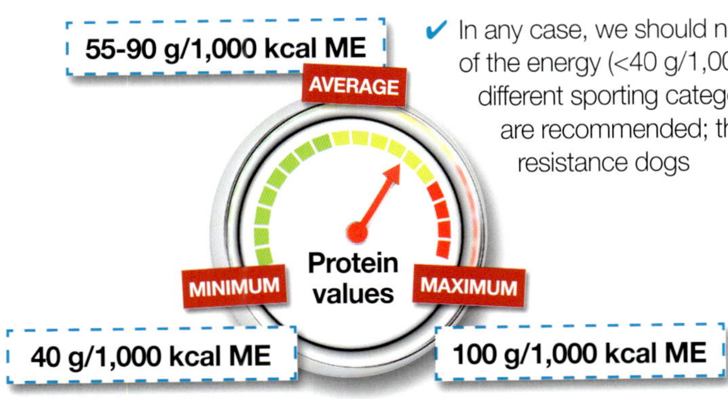

✔ In any case, we should never go under the lower limit of 16 % of the energy (<40 g/1,000 kcal ME). As an average value, for the different sporting categories, between 55- 90 g/1,000 kcal ME are recommended; this value should be increased by 6 % for resistance dogs (for example, sledding dogs). It is estimated that we start with the lowest values and proportionally increase the amount of protein for each 30 additional minutes of exercise.

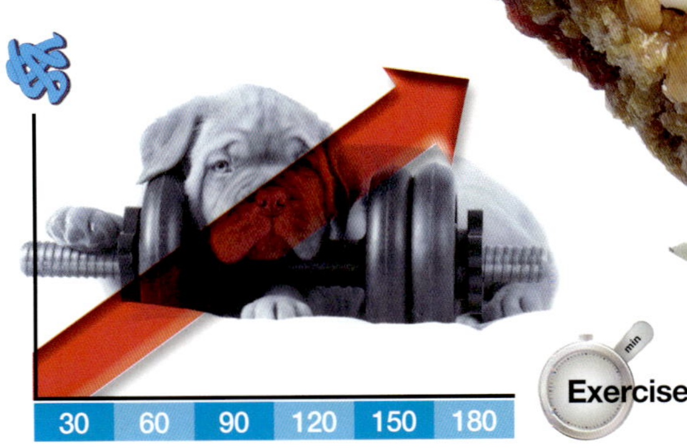

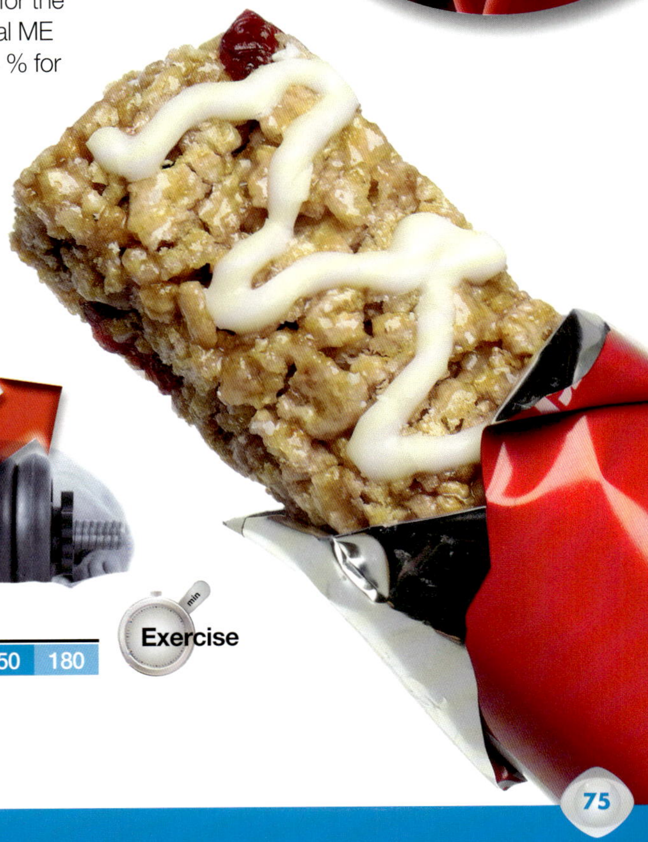

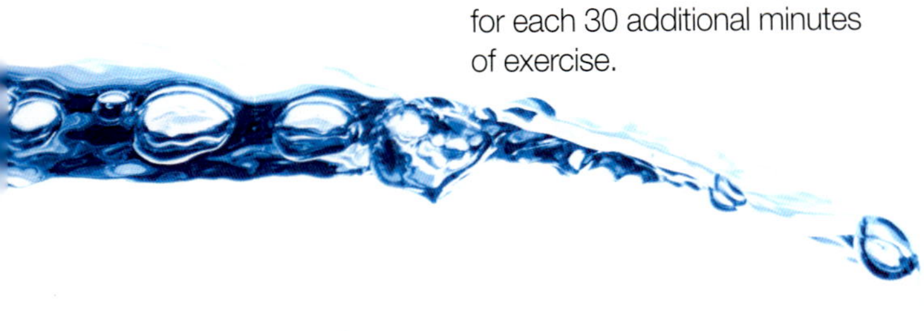

Nutrients for exercise:

1 Fats are fundamental in the food rations of sporting dogs

✔ Approximately 70 to 90 % of their energy comes from metabolizing fats, especially in resistance sporting dogs, primarily due to the following:

- Elevated energy density
- High palatability
- They improve the digestibility of the rest of nutrients

✔ Their presence in food rations is necessary, as the amount of dry material that can be ingested by a dog per day is limited to 3.5 % of its body weight and this is a limiting factor on their performance, which leads to the food rations being highly concentrated.

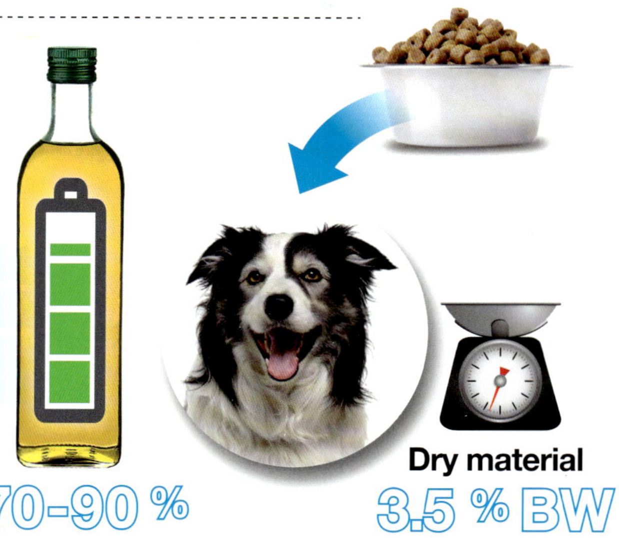

2 Their deficit leads to the obtention of energy from the tissues

✔ If there is a deficit in energy, it will be obtained from different tissues: there will be a loss of structural proteins and body fat. At the same time, the lack of fat coverage modifies the dog's insulating capacity, for which it will have to use part of its maintenance energy for thermoregulation, especially in conditions of extremely cold temperatures.

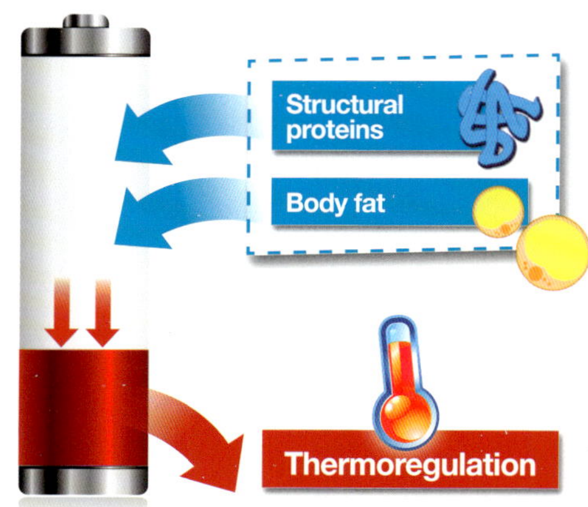

✔ Dogs fed with high proportions of fat have higher levels of FFAs in blood and respond faster when exercising. This is due to the fact that their levels of basal insulin are lower. Insulin levels are directly correlated with the carbohydrates present in the food ration, and this hormone inhibits the release of FFAs from fatty tissues. This fact affects performance and is an important concern in our canine athletes.

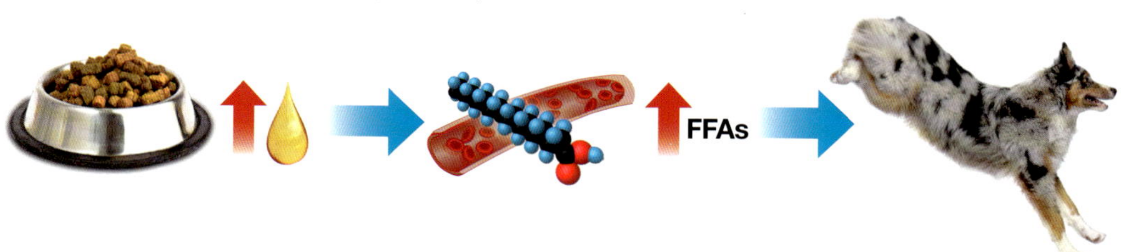

3 Training + fats = greater mitochondrial performance

✔ It has been observed that training and a diet rich in fats (up to 65 % of the energy of the food ration; approximately 80 g/1,000 kcal ME) allows for an increase in the aerobic metabolism, associated with an increase in the size and oxidative capacity of the mitochondria by 20-30 % more. The relationship between the resistance to exercise and feeding, therefore, has been demonstrated.

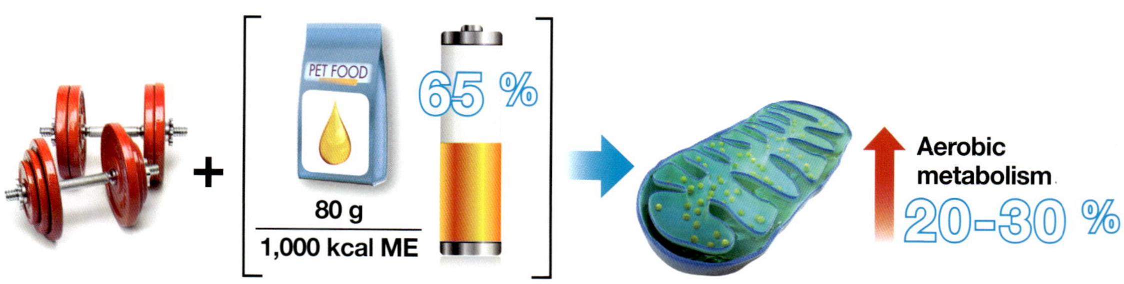

fats and FAs

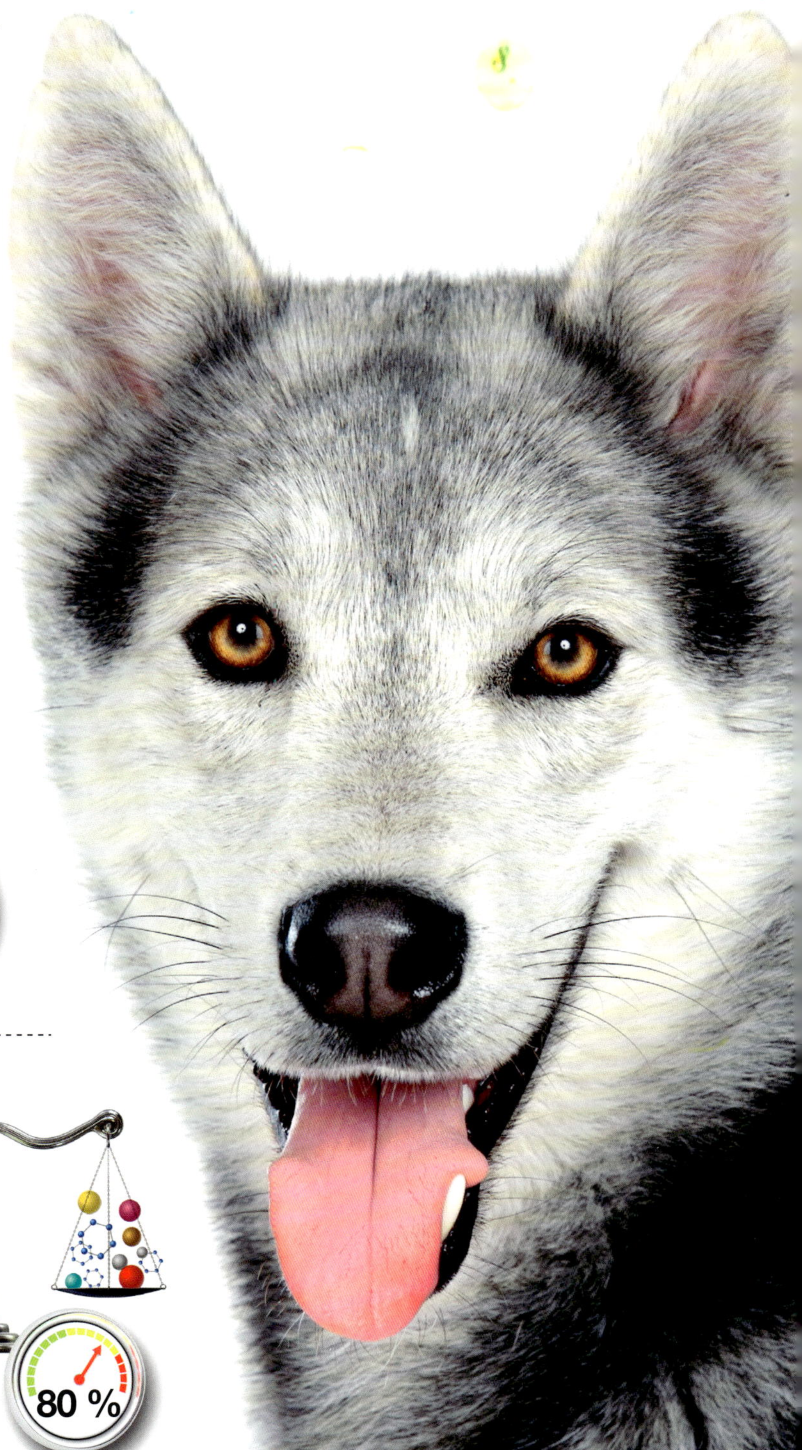

4 The adequate fat profile

- ✔ Regarding the fat profile, it is recommended that the levels of EFAs be 5 g/1,000 kcal ME with a saturated:unsaturated ratio (SFAs:UFAs) of 25:75, taking into account that the richness in FFAs favors oxidative damage.

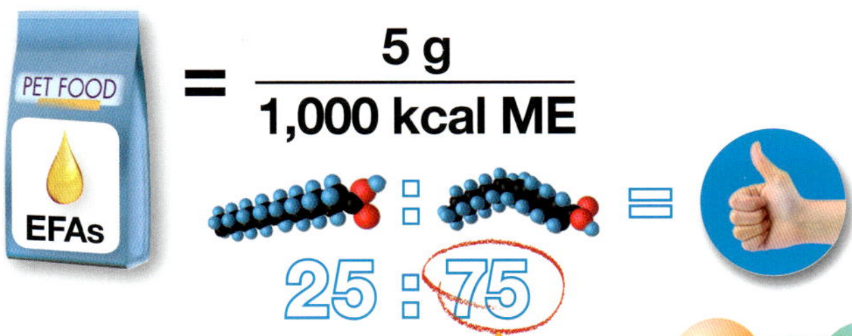

- ✔ To avoid oxidative damage, it is recommended that the ingestion of antioxidant substances be increased (vitamins E and C and selenium).

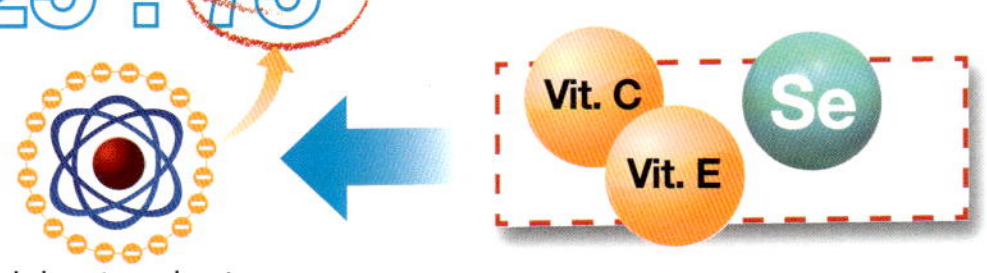

- ✔ In addition, elevated levels of SFAs (> 60 %) affect the sense of smell in our dogs: changes are produced in the ATPase activity of the sodium-potassium pump in the membranes of the brain synapses. This observation is of great interest in hunting and working dogs (dogs that search for drugs, explosives, or people).

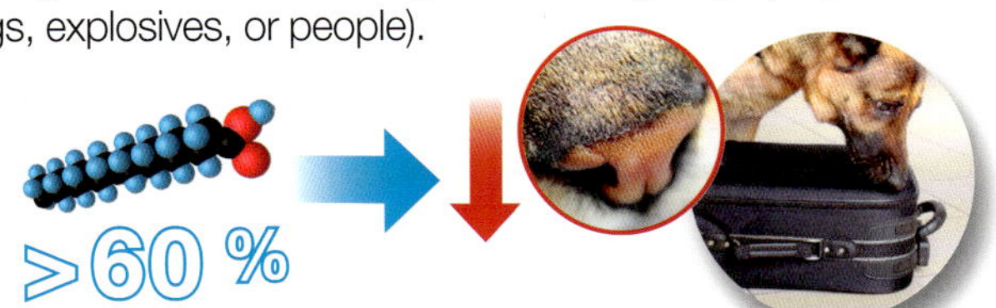

5 Adaptation and tolerance of fats

- ✔ In spite of the benefits, high levels of fat in food rations are not free of disadvantages. The primary one is steatorrhea and anemia.
- ✔ Incorporating increasing levels of fat and ensuring correct balance in the rest of the nutrients, allows for adaptation and a greater tolerance to fat, even at levels over 162 g/1,000 kcal ME (this represents 80 % of the ingested calories), in the dog.

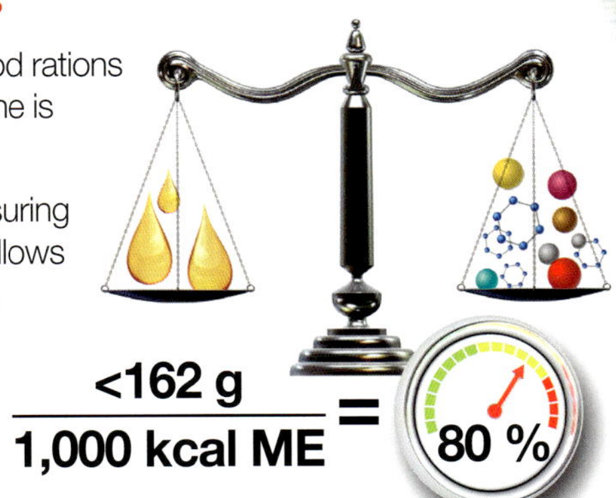

- ✔ Adaptation to these high levels of fat is individual; any change in the quality of the stool or a decrease in ingestion are a reflection of the dog's tolerance limit to fat.
- ✔ Fat requirements, therefore, vary with the activity of the dog:

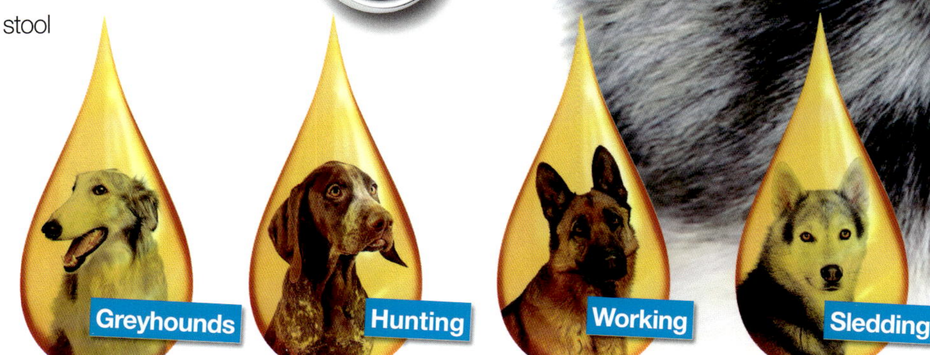

Type of exercise	Intense and brief	Moderate and occasional	Moderate and continuous	Resistance testing
g fat/1,000 kcal	20-25	38-75	60-100	>125-155
% of the ME	20	30-50	45-60	70-80

Nutrients for exercise:

In certain physiological situations or with athletic activity, carbohydrate requirements may increase. Sporting dogs need as much as double the carbohydrates (CH) compared to the same dog on maintenance.

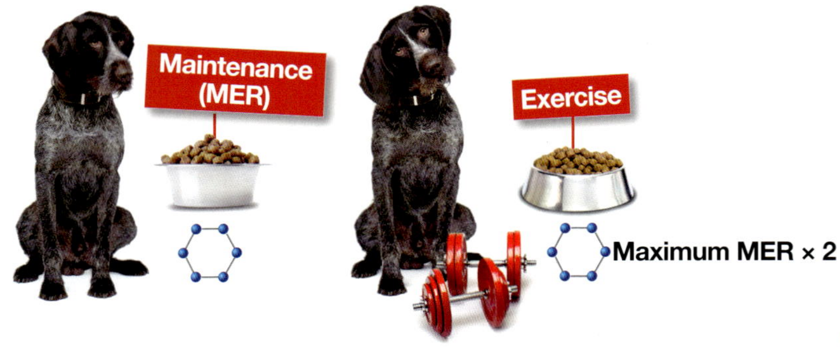

1 Carbohydrates and racing greyhounds

Greyhounds depend on glycogen

Racing dogs (Greyhounds) depend primarily on their glycogen stores for their activity. They use rapid anaerobic pathways to obtain energy. The distance covered vary between 200 and 1,000 meters with average speeds that surpass 60 km/h. Doing this kind of physical activity, they consume almost 80 % of the stored glycogen in about 50 seconds.

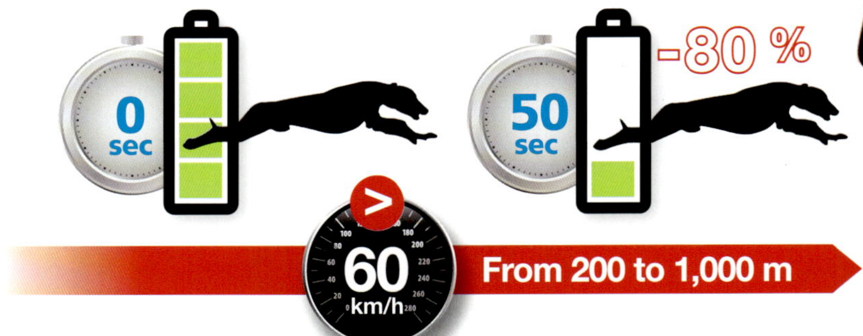

Strategies to increase the muscular glycogen load

- ✔ If we increase the muscular glycogen stores through training and diet, we can obtain sporting benefits, although there are certain doubts about this hypothesis as it all depends on what type of exercise the dog is going to perform.
- ✔ There are at least two feeding strategies, extrapolated from human sports diets, to obtain this muscular glycogen load:

Åstrand Method

Diet low in CH (<28 g/1,000 kcal ME) and depletion of glycogen with intense exercise. Later, for 4 to 7 days, a diet high in CH (250 g/1,000 kcal ME) and low activity. Different studies show that the previous depletion could be counteractive for health and performance.

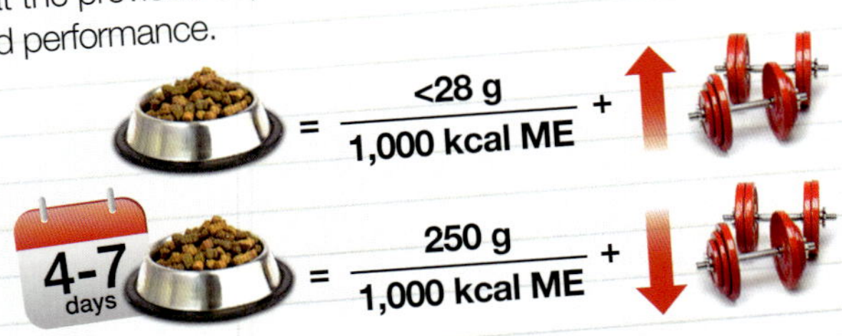

- ✔ Just like in human athletes, racing dogs obtain better results when the levels of CH in their food rations are increased, given that the storage and release of glycogen is higher.

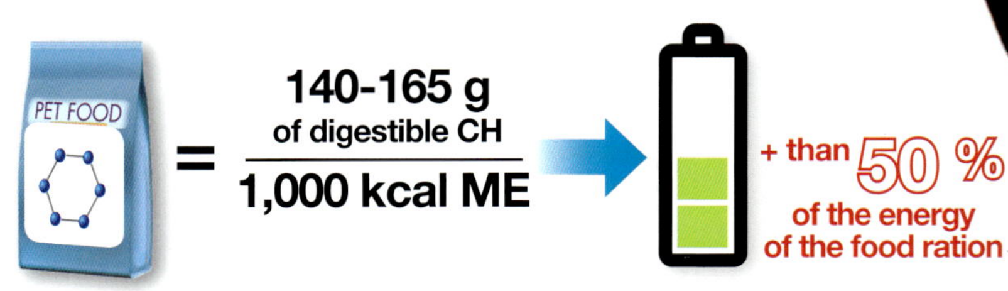

Sherman/Costill method

The diets include high levels of CH (>150 g/1,000 kcal ME), and exclusively CH when the test or competition is close.

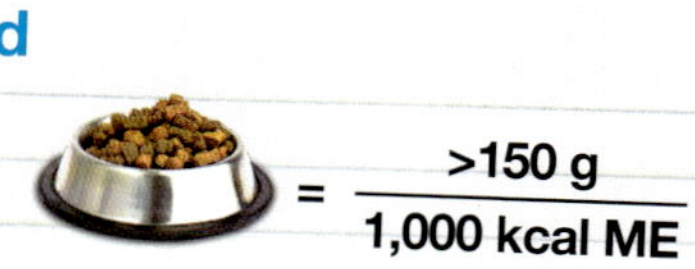

- ✔ Carbohydrates represent, therefore, the base of their diet given that the energy requirements are not that high: 1.1 × MER (from 0.9 to 1.2).

Risks of excessive carbohydrate load

These excessive carbohydrate loads in racing dogs are not free of risks. Lactate generated during anaerobiosis causes rhabdomyolysis, with increased concentrations in plasma of creatine kinase. The muscular tissue swells, edemas are produced and, most importantly, the alternative pathways to obtain energy are inhibited (lipolysis and glycolysis).

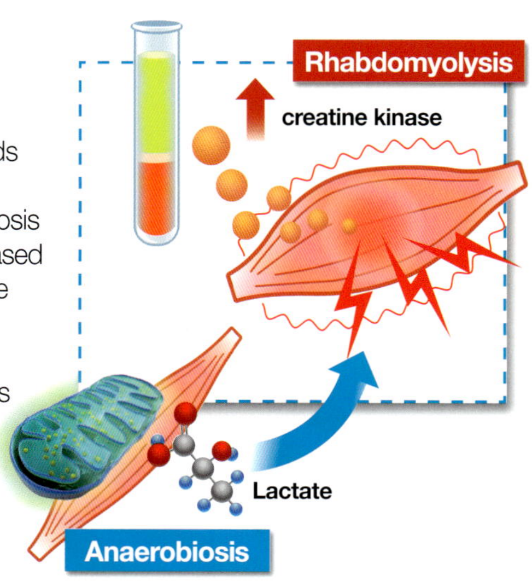

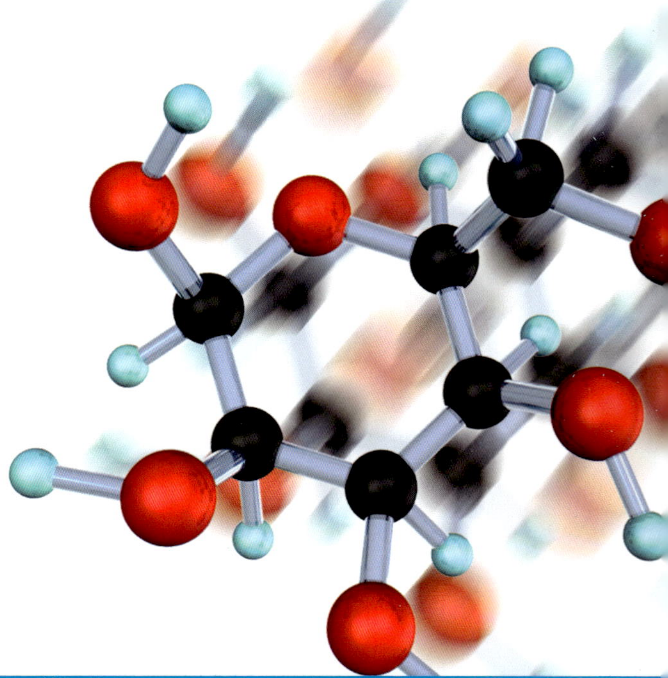

carbohydrates and fiber

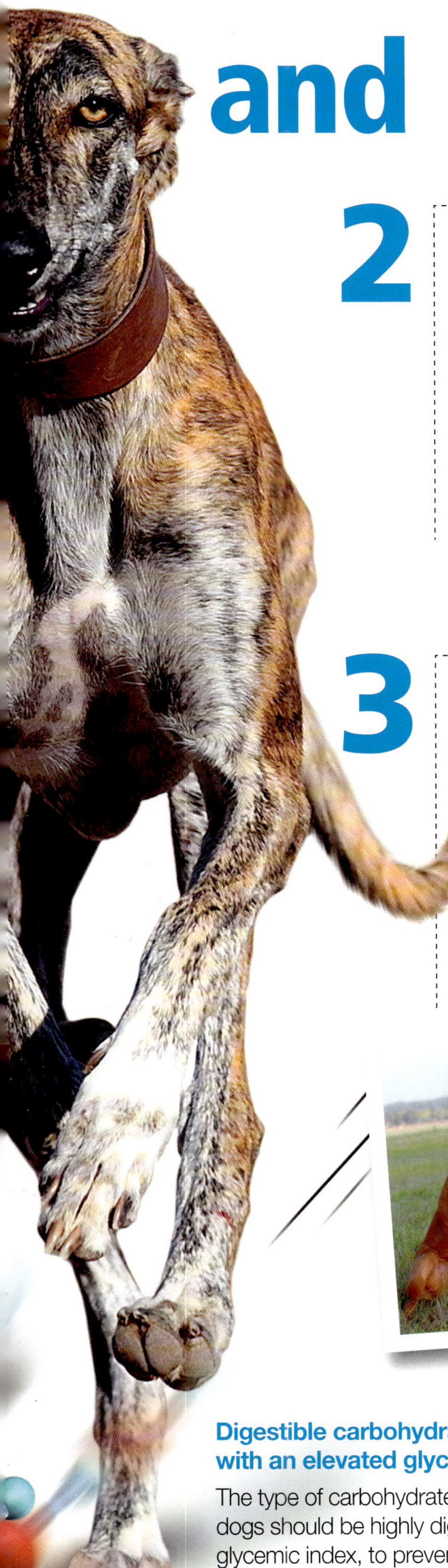

2 Carbohydrates in resistance animals

- ✔ In resistance animals, it seems more appropriate to allow for the storage and release of glycogen to be done at the expense of FAs, and for this reason, the role of carbohydrates in their food rations is not excessively important.
- ✔ A minimum of 40 g/1,000 kcal ME is considered adequate in resistance dogs and a variable concentration of 75-135 g/1,000 kcal ME in those animals that perform moderate exercise.

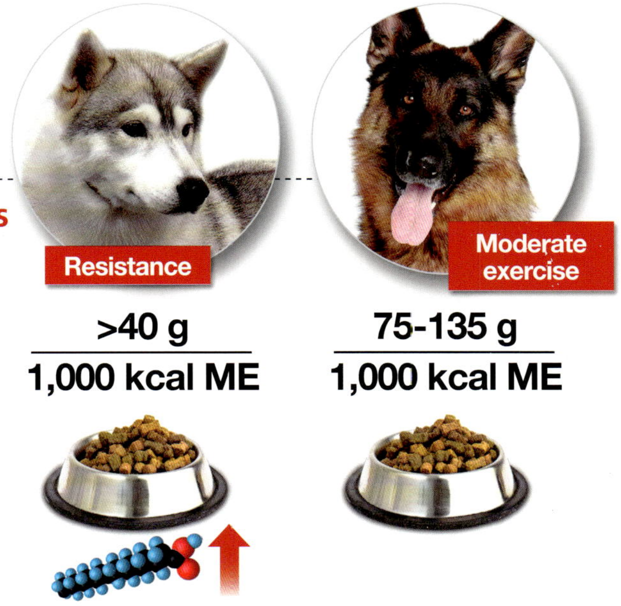

3 Glucose to replenish glycogen

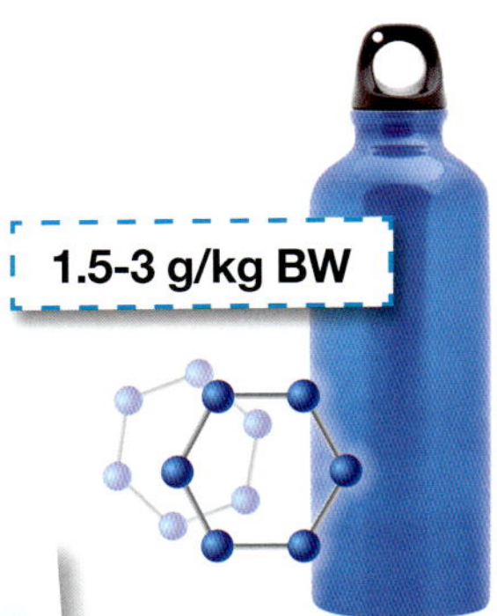

Before, during, and after exercise

Carbohydrates, especially glucose and its polymers, are important in replenishing (resynthesis) glycogen after exercise and in thermoregulation. The use of glucose solutions at variable concentrations (1.5 to 3 g/kg of body weight) before, during, and after exercise allows for the following:

- ✔ Faster replenishment of glycogen.
- ✔ Avoids the loss of athletic performance associated with a decrease in glycemia.
- ✔ Improves thermoregulation.

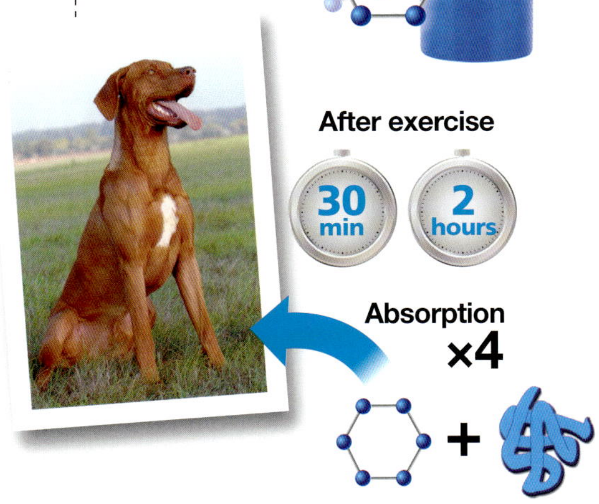

Maximum efficiency 30 minutes after exercise

- ✔ There is a period of time where this process has an efficiency that is up to 4 times higher due to the muscular blood flow being higher: this takes place between 30 minutes and 2 hours after exercising. This practice is of great interest for our resistance athletes because it allows them to rapidly replenish glycogen during short rest periods.
- ✔ There is a hypothesis that suggests that the simultaneous ingestion of protein (due to its effect on insulin release) during this period increases the capacity to store glycogen, but its effectiveness has not been demonstrated. There are different supplements of this type on the market, both as oral solutions as well as "energy bars".

Digestible carbohydrates and with an elevated glycemic index

The type of carbohydrate that we should use in racing dogs should be highly digestible, and with a fast glycemic index, to prevent the non-digestible residue from causing the following:

- ✔ Undesired fermentations (gas).
- ✔ Increased fecal mass (weighing the athlete down).
- ✔ Water loss through the feces.

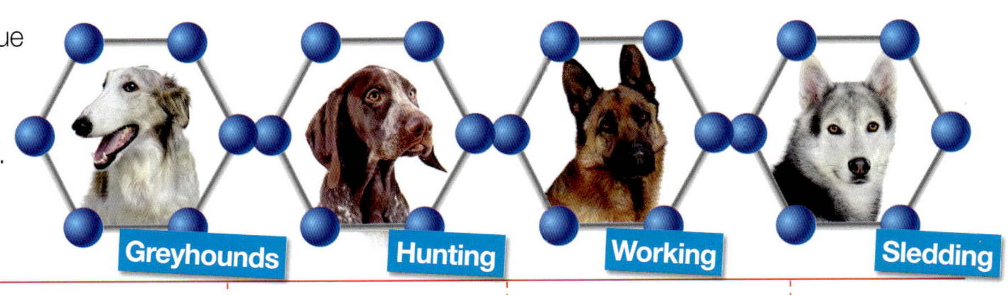

Requirements in CH

Type of exercise	Very intense and brief	Moderate and occasional	Moderate and continuous	Resistance testing
g carbohydrates/1,000 kcal	125-185	85-155	100	45
% of the ME	55-65	30-50	35	15

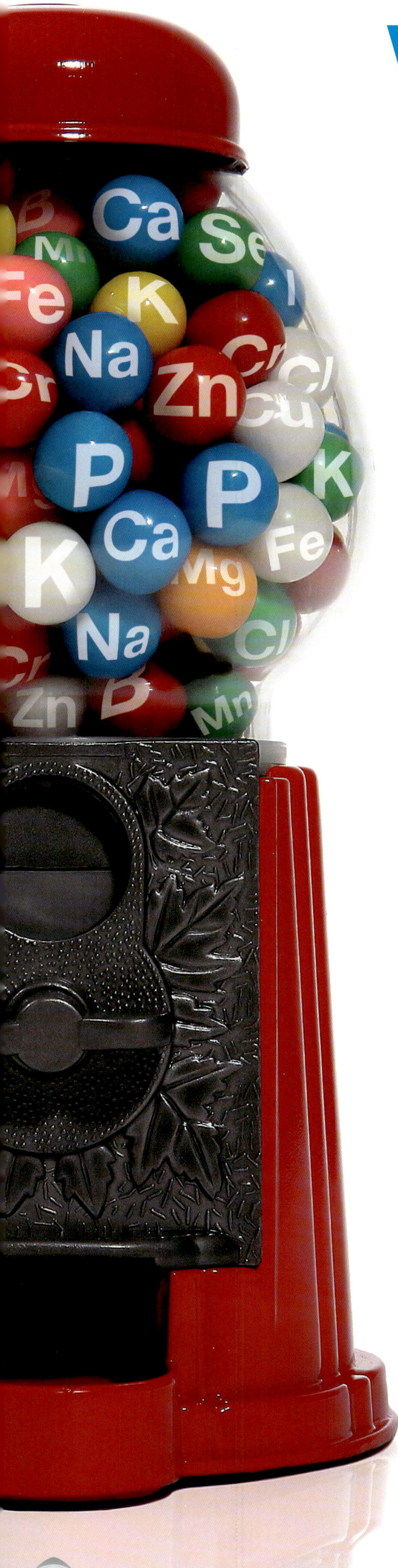

Vitamins and

1 Are more vitamins and minerals needed?

✔ The information available about the importance of these nutrients is scarce, although it seems obvious. It is unknown whether their requirements are modified during exercise.

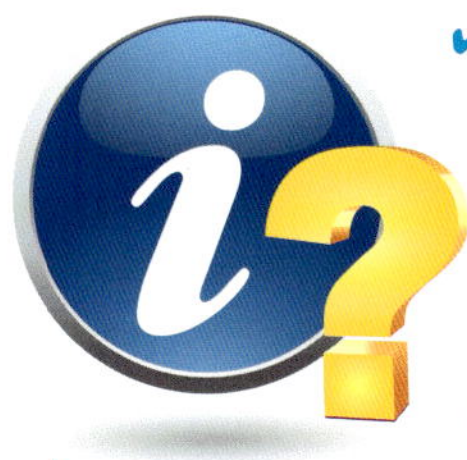

✔ Currently, there is no specific justification to increase the minimal ingestion of vitamins relative to the energy consumed in sporting dogs, given that in the balanced food rations given to these animals their requirements are slightly increased.

2 Possible increase in the requirements of:

Vit. B

Vitamins from the B group, as a consequence of their broad metabolic functions.

Iron, there are suspicions that its requirements are increased with exercise; it is a co-factor of the oxygen transporters, myoglobin and hemoglobin.

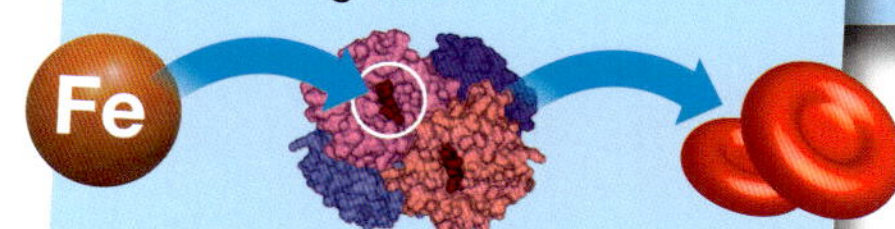

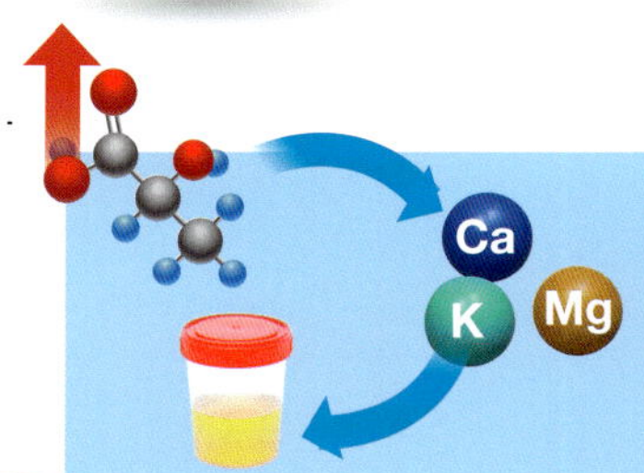

Certain minerals, by certain metabolic processes in conditions of maximum exertion. The metabolic acidosis that is generated (by the increase of lactate) causes a greater elimination of calcium, magnesium and potassium through urine.

3 Vitamin E

Vit. E

✔ Dogs that have increased levels of vitamin E in plasma (reference values × 2) before starting any resistance training, have double the probability of ending the race or training and the probability of having to stop and be eliminated is reduced by half. In this sense, incorporating at least 125 IU/1,000 kcal ME into the food for resistance dogs is recommended, although there is no evidence on its use in the prevention of muscle damage.

✔ The amount of vitamin E in the food rations must be evaluated, due to its antioxidant effect, given that in this type of diets, the levels of fat and UFAs are usually considerably high.

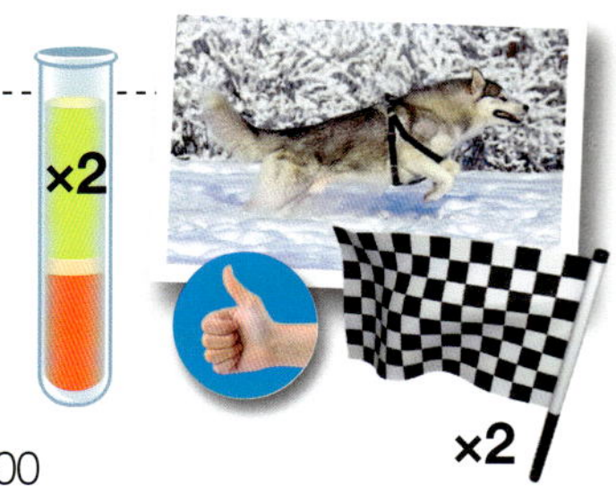

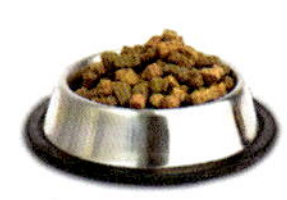 = 125 IU / 1,000 kcal ME

4 Vitamin C

Vitamin C should always be administered with vitamin E and at a concentration of 40-65 mg of vitamin C/1,000 kcal ME to avoid any negative affect on performance. Problems begin when the recommended dose is multiplied by ten.

Vit. C

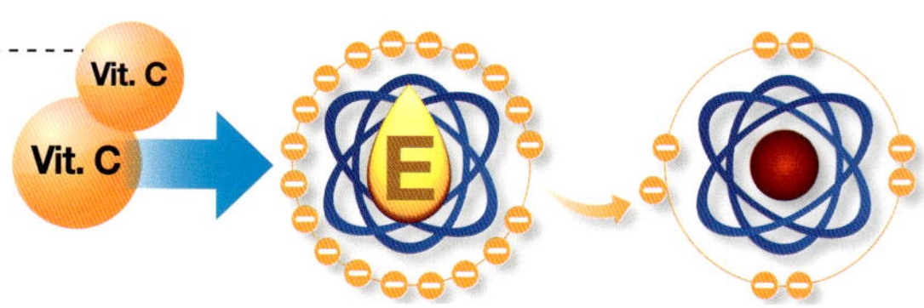

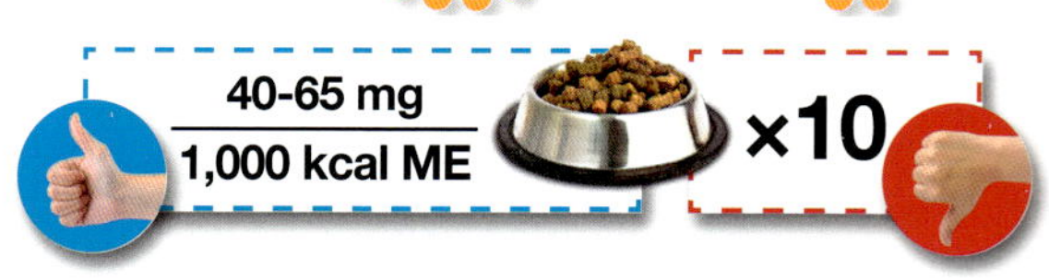

5 Selenium

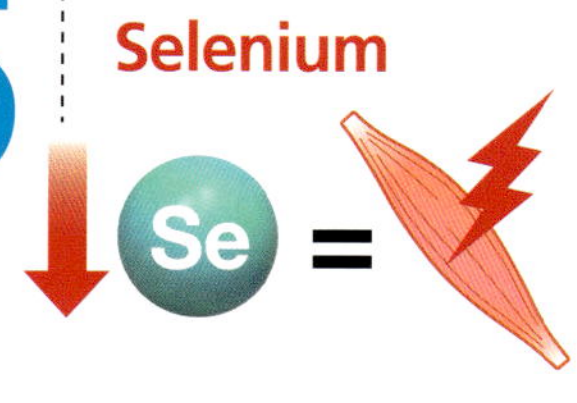

Some studies done on humans have shown that a deficiency in selenium in athletes is related to muscle damage and worsening of functional performance. Based on the benefits that are obtained in patients with cancer (recommendations by the NRC 2006 increased up to 10 times), it seems recommendable to incorporate up to 325 mg/1,000 kcal ME in athletic dogs.

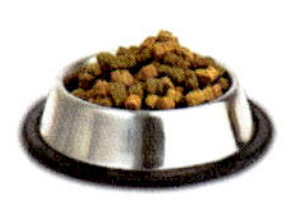 = 325 mg / 1,000 kcal ME

minerals for exercise

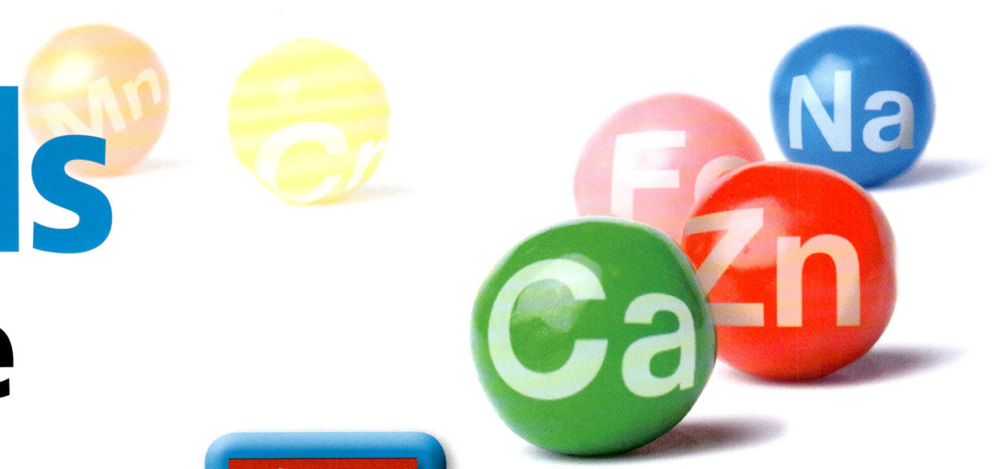

6 Important to combat oxidative damage

Sports or exercise, in their different modalities (aerobic and anaerobic), generate free radicals. These cause oxidative damage and are compensated in a natural manner by the organism. When the physiological limits are surpassed, chronic muscle fatigue appears. To prevent this effect, antioxidant supplements and training are combined.

Training

- ✔ Training has positive effects on the antioxidant enzymatic systems in the muscle, heart, fat, plasma and liver, but it does not avoid or prevent muscle damage.

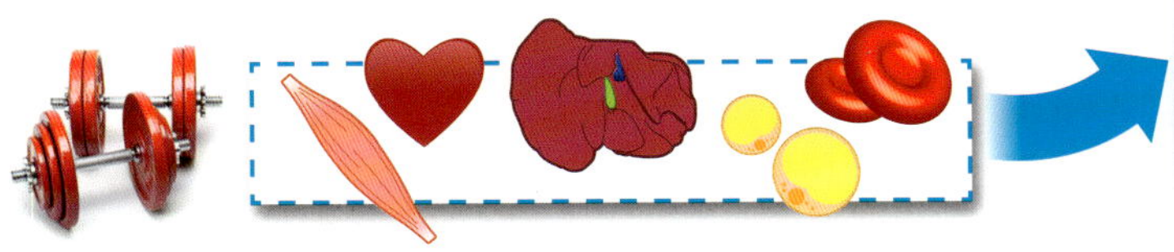

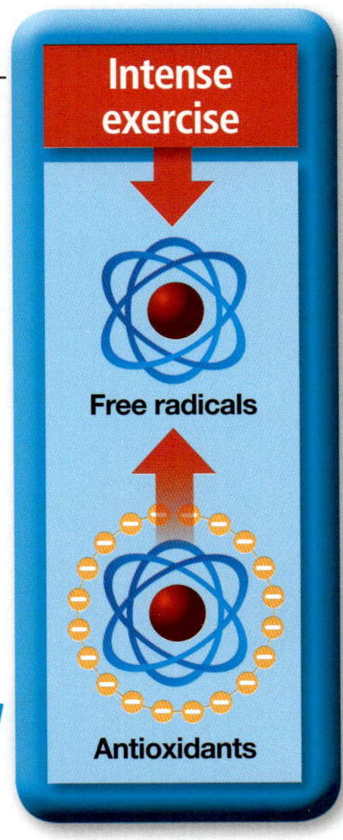

Antioxidants

However, an excess in antioxidants or the use of only one, has negative effects on the performance or causes pro-oxidant effects, respectively. The best option is to use a multiple antioxidant compound with at least vitamins C, E and selenium.

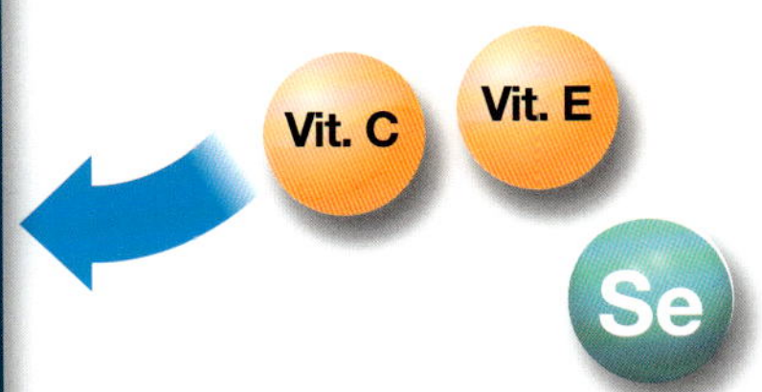

7 Electrolytes

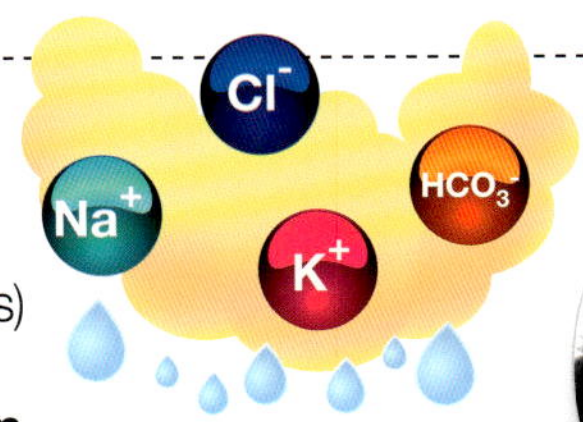

- ✔ Electrolytes such as sodium, potassium, chloride and bicarbonate are lost through saliva (up to 30 % of the losses) and the panting of dogs. In very high temperatures (50 °C) the losses through saliva are very high, especially of **sodium**. In these cases, 1-2 g/1,000 kcal ME of sodium (more than five times the recommendations by the NRC 2006) are recommended, ensuring an ingestion of water of 900 ml/BW (kg)$^{0.75}$.

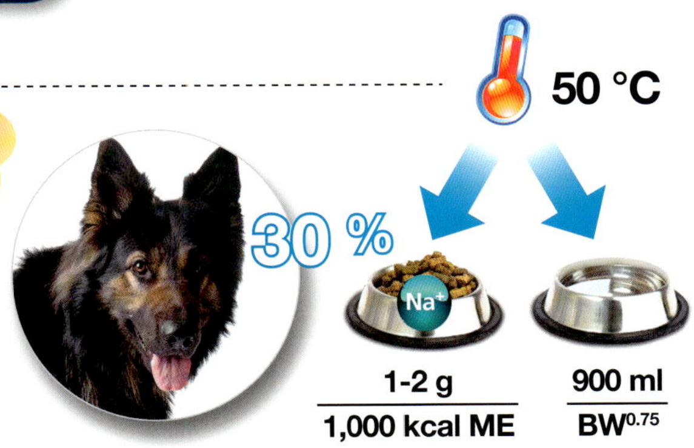

- ✔ The losses of **potassium** through urine are very high after exercise; however, the concentration of sodium is not affected. When evaluating these electrolytes in accordance with the energy used for the exertion, we do find that their urinary excretion is reduced.

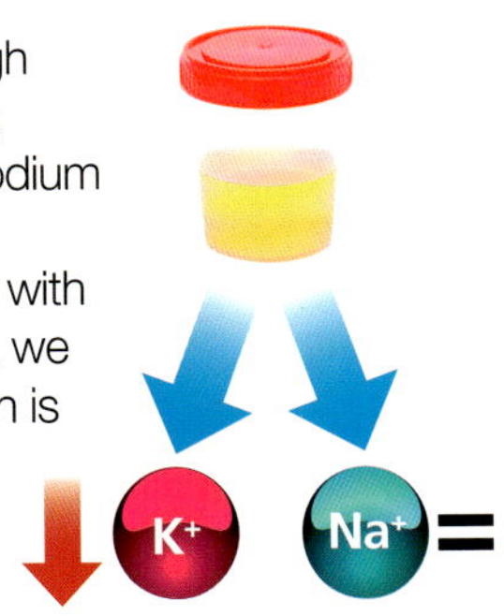

- ✔ There is no consensus on the ideal composition given that hypertonic solutions cause changes to digestive motility, with vomiting and diarrhea, and isotonic solutions cause changes to ingestion due to the activation of the thirst center of the brain (for example, eating snow). In any case, neither is successful in replacing the electrolytes lost after exercise.

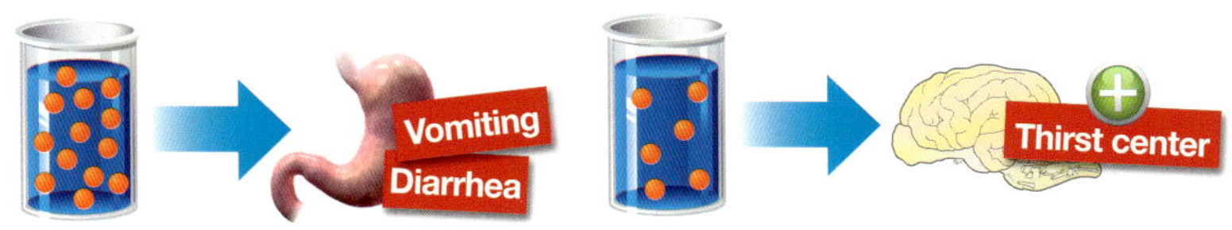

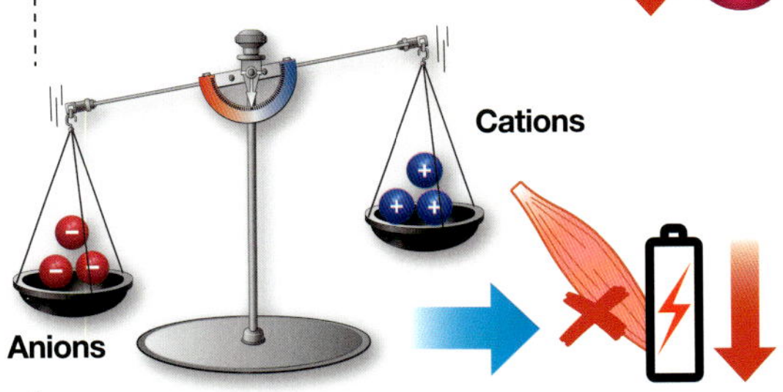

- ✔ An acid-base imbalance harms muscle contraction by affecting the membrane potential, which leaves less energy (strength) available to exercise. Also, these changes in the osmolarity of the plasma impede a correct dissipation of body heat. However, if the animals ingest a complete and balanced food for their activity, the oral administration of replacement solutions to avoid this process does not make any sense.

- ✔ Some studies offer varied information about electrolyte requirements, taking into account the factors involved (type of race/exertion, environmental temperature, load, distance ran, time, etc.); the following table serves as a summary:

Electrolyte	Unit/1,000 kcal ME	Safe upper limit
Sodium/chloride	0.2-1.6 g	8 g
Potassium	0.04-4 g	Not available

- ✔ The use of high doses of trace elements has also been documented in the two primary categories of sporting dogs (Greyhounds and sledding dogs). The recommendations surpass, especially in Greyhounds, by several times, the recommendations from NRC 2006.

	mg trace element/1,000 kcal ME					
Type of dog	Iron	Copper	Zinc	Manganese	Iodine	Selenium
Sledding	15	1.8	14-15	0.8	0.04	Not available
Greyhounds	72-91	1.9-5.7	16-48	4-11	0.3-0.4	0.1

Management

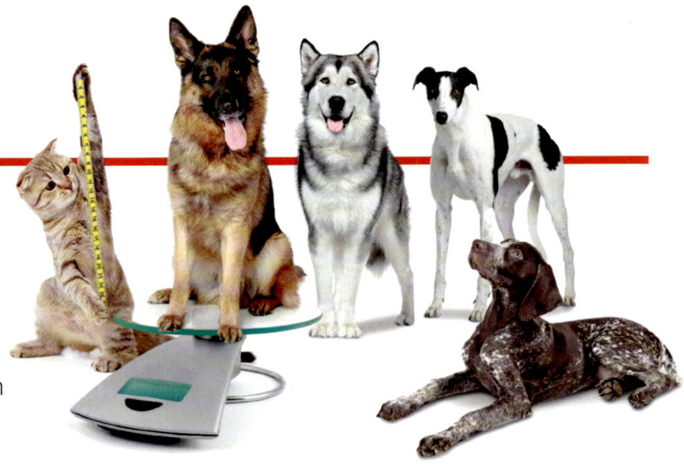

1 Each athlete is an individual case

There are many studies on when is the best time to feed a sporting dog, but it must be taken into account that each athlete is an individual case. The weight, body condition, and degree of hydration will indicate to us whether the regimen is correct or not.

2 A small amount of extra weight as an energy strategy

One strategy is for the resistance dog to start a test or competition slightly overweight (5-10 %, BCS 6/9), knowing that the extra fat will be a source of energy while exercising. The downside is that it represents additional weight for the dog and could possibly affect their performance negatively. On the contrary, Greyhounds have a body condition (BCS) of 3-4/9.

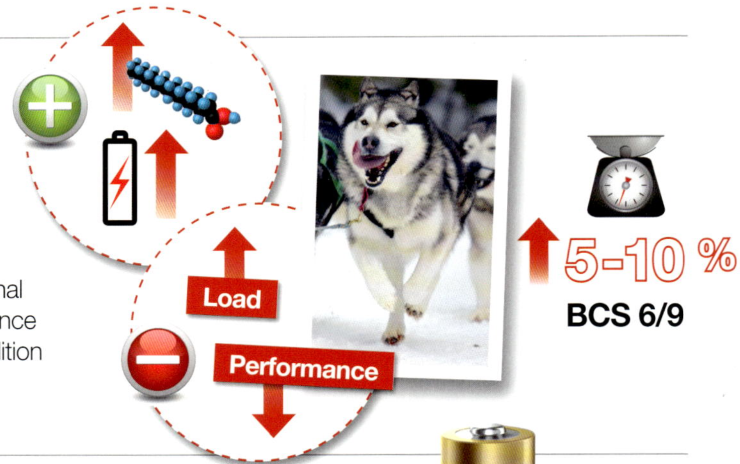

3 The period of adaptation to the diet is fundamental

- ✔ As we have previously seen, the profile of the diets for these dogs is variable. Respecting any changes to the pet's feeding is essential to avoid any digestive problems and allow for the body to adapt to the new food.
- ✔ The greatest limitation is the relationship between the following:

  - High energy requirements, especially in resistance dogs
  - The composition of the diet
  - The physical capacity of the stomach

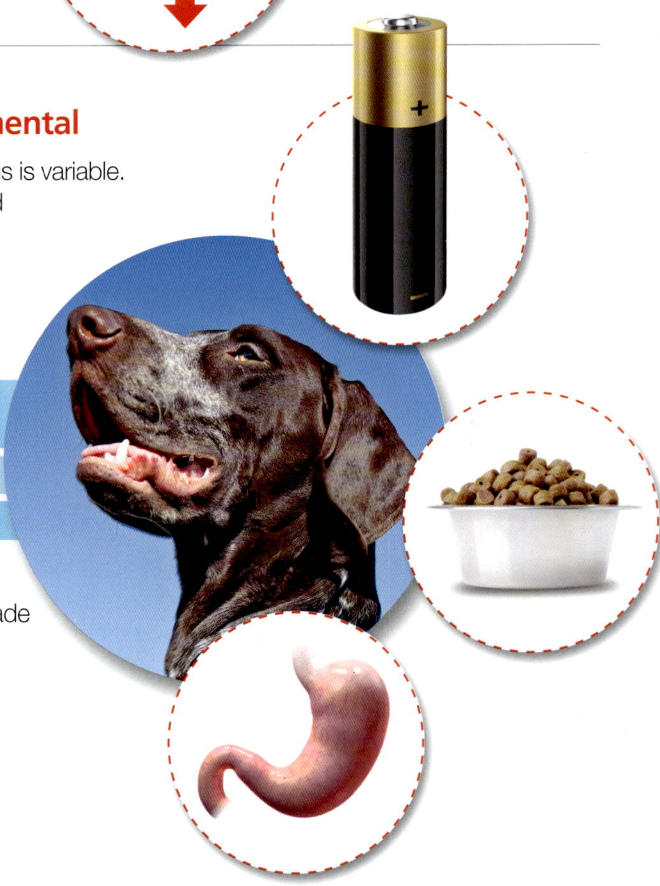

- ✔ In this sense, any modifications to the type of food should be made with a minimum period of 6 weeks before the sporting stage or season starts. Most diets available on the market for this type of athletes have very high energy concentrations, that oscillate between 5 and more than 6 Mcal/kg DM.

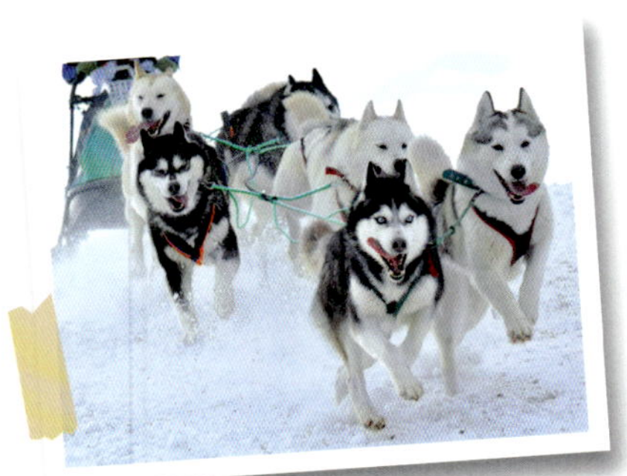

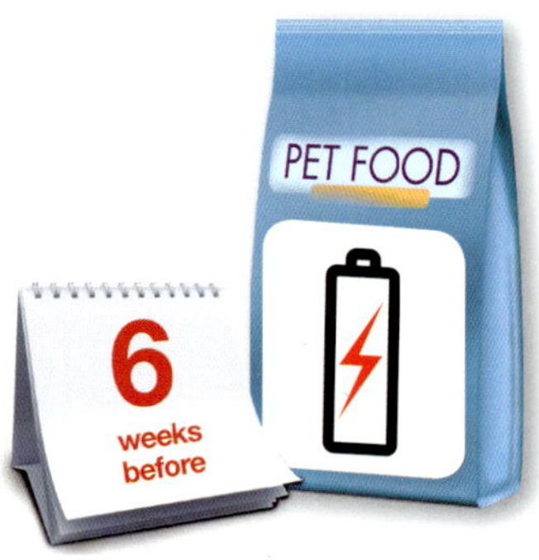

$$\text{Energy} = \frac{5 \text{ and } >6 \text{ Mcal}}{\text{kg DM}}$$

# of feeding in sporting dogs

4 When should food be given?

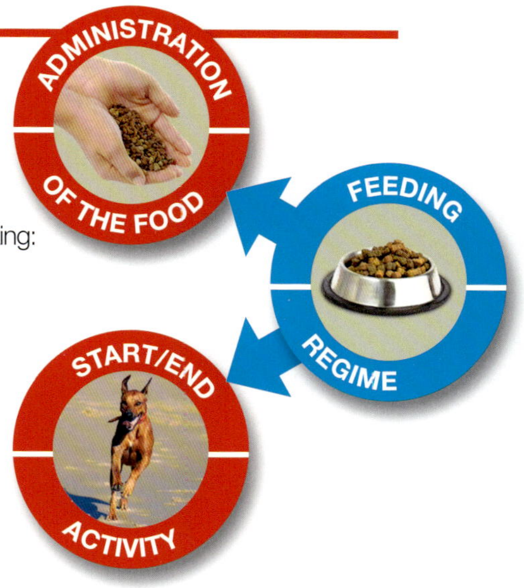

- ✔ The feeding regime is conditioned by the period of time between the administration of the food and the start/end of the activity, given that it affects the use of nutrients. For example, the postprandial temperature increase affects performance while working: the elimination of body heat is worse due to the increase in visceral vasodilation.
- ✔ The levels of insulin depend on the presence of food. We must keep in mind that insulin acts on the use of carbohydrates and the levels of FFAs in plasma, as well as its mobilization from adipose tissue. If we administer the food within 4-6 hours before exercise, rapid use of glucose (depletion of glycogen) will take place, but also poor use of the fats. This will affect the resistance athlete's performance.
- ✔ On the other hand, if we feed and provide water to our dogs 4-6 hours before the competition or test, we will have two advantages:

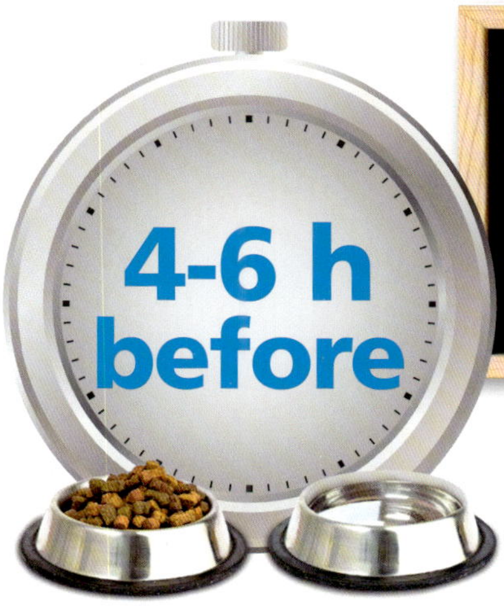

ADVANTAGES

- Sufficient time for them to defecate and urinate, which removes excess weight on the animal.
- We reduce the risk of the occurrence of diarrhea caused by stress.

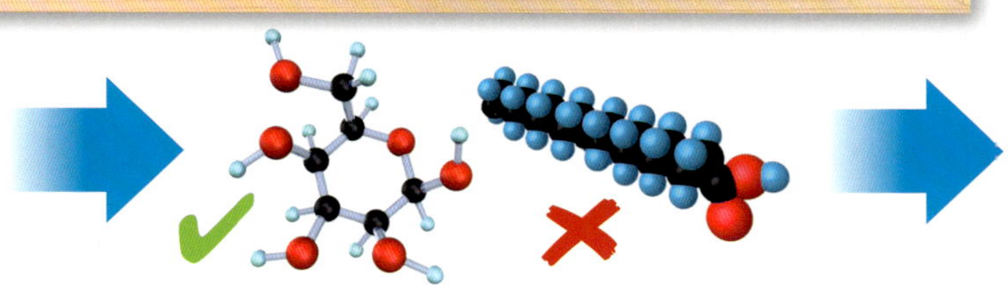

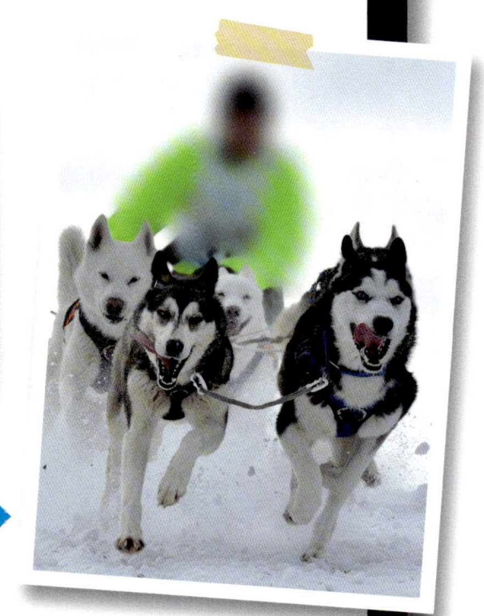

5 Guidelines for correct feeding

- ✔ According to the aforementioned, guidelines for the correct feeding of these dogs are summarized in the following table:

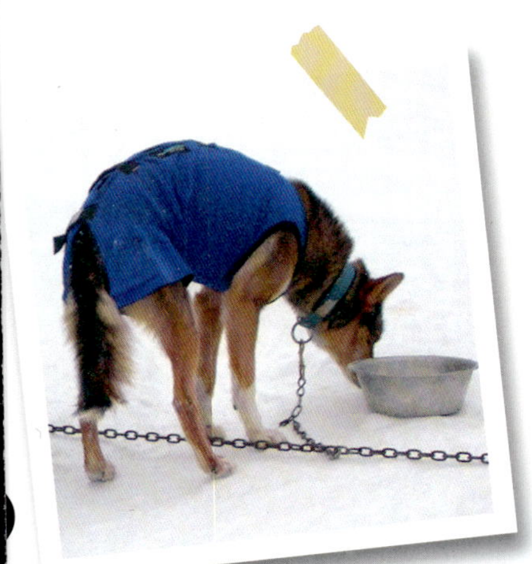

	Management of feeding		
Food type	**Before exercise**	**During exercise**	**After exercise**
Diet for sporting dogs	≤4-6 hours	Variable	≥2 hours
Amount	**1/4-1/3 volume**	**Small volumes**	**2/3 volume**
Water (isotonic)	No	Yes	After 5 minutes and gradual
Oral solution rich in glucose	10 minutes	Yes	30-120 minutes
Amount		**Glucose 1-3 g/kg**	

To be taken into account

There is no fixed rule given that it depends on the type of competition and of the specific performance of each animal. Their temperature and hydration status must be checked continuously: dehydrated dogs cannot regulate their temperature correctly. It is fundamental that these dogs are monitored by their trainers and veterinarian.